Emotions in the Human Voice

Volume 1: Foundations

Emotions in the Human Voice

Volume 1: Foundations

Edited by
Krzysztof Izdebski

Original Cover Art by Daniele Cascone,
Original Chapter Art by Marta Semkowicz

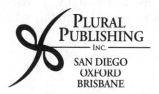

PLURAL
PUBLISHING
INC.

SAN DIEGO
OXFORD
BRISBANE

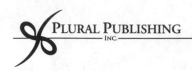

PLURAL PUBLISHING
INC.

5521 Ruffin Road
San Diego, CA 92123

e-mail: info@pluralpublishing.com
Web site: http://www.pluralpublishing.com

49 Bath Street
Abingdon, Oxfordshire OX14 1EA
United Kingdom

Library of Congress Cataloging-in-Publication Data:

Emotions in the human voice / [edited by] Krzystof Izdebski.
    p. ; cm.
  Includes bibliographical references and index.
  ISBN-13: 978-1-59756-073-3 (v. 1 : alk. paper)
  ISBN-10: 1-59756-073-1 (v. 1 : alk. paper)
  ISBN-13: 978-1-59756-118-1 (v. 2 : alk. paper)
  ISBN-10: 1-59756-118-5 (v. 2 : alk. paper)
  [etc.]
  1. Voice–Psychological aspects. 2. Emotions. I. Izdebski, Krzysztof.
  [DNLM: 1. Affect. 2. Verbal Behavior. 3. Auditory Perception. 4. Emotions. 5.
Phonation. 6. Voice Quality. BF 582 E545 2007]
  BF592.V64E44 2007
  153.6–dc22

....   2007043352

CONTENTS

FOREWORD

The human voice—what a masterpiece of creation! We laugh with it, we cry with it, we sing with it, we pray with it, we scream with it, we whisper with it—yet, how little do we know about its effect upon the listener. The voice represents our ultimate means of communication from birth to death, yet how little do we know about its impact on human culture and society. While our voice connects us to our fellow humans and other species, we know but little about the mechanics of this transaction.

Even in antiquity, Greek and Roman philosophers were aware that the voice is the mirror of the soul. But it was not until the 20th century and the age of communication that serious investigations were initiated into the relations between the human voice and emotions. Recent research has revealed that the effect of the mother's voice creates a bond with the fetus in utero during the second trimester of pregnancy (Antonia Pietronelli, 1992). With each year of our physical development, the voice and emotions play a more complex role in our adjustment to an ever-more complex world.

The recent Pacific Voice and Speech Foundation Annual Voice Conference on Voice and Emotion held at the Pixar Animation Studios in California represented the first serious attempt to study the complex relations between voice and emotions on a multidisciplinary level. The success of this meeting sparked a global fire of interest to bring together the vast knowledge from various cultures and various specialties, which has not been readily available to interested individuals.

This search extended to academicians and to clinicians, to scientists and to practitioners, to teachers and to writers. In Europe, contributors hail from Scandinavia and Finland in the north; from Italy and Spain in the south; from the United Kingdom, the Netherlands, Belgium, and France in the west; from Russia in the east; and from Germany, Austria, Poland and Switzerland in Central Europe. In the western hemisphere, chapters arrived from the United States, Canada, and Brazil; in the Far East from Japan, and Singapore, and Viet Nam; in the Pacific region from Australia and the Philippines; and in the Middle East from Israel.

The authors represent an equally diverse group of authorities: psychologists, linguists, speech and voice pathologists, physicians, phoniatricians, acousticians, vocal artists and performers, voice coaches, and experts from the fields of radio, computer science, commerce, television, and motion pictures. Over the past several weeks, I have had the opportunity to review this amazing collection of manuscripts, and I am amazed by the wealth and diversity of the submitted information. While the human voice is always one part of the equation, the emotions vary from joy to pain, from sorrow to happiness; from adults to children; from men to women; from spontaneity to stability; from pleasantness to roughness; from health to disease; from the brain to the organs of phonation; from neurology to psychophysiology; from development to recognition; from actor to anime, and from laughter to love. The information is here and the choice is yours.

All of us share a sincere debt of thanks to the Editor, Dr. Krzysztof Izdebski, an enthusiastic and indefatigable champion of the field of voice, and a dear friend to many of the participating authors. Dr. Izdebski spearheaded the meeting held at the Pixar Studios and has done the lion's share of preparing this book. While all readers will benefit by their study of *Emotions in the Human Voice*, Dr. Izdebski deserves our respect, our admiration, and, above all, our gratitude.

Hans von Leden

PREFACE

When my long-standing friend and colleague, Tom Murry of New York City, asked me in April of 2004, while we were munching on those tiny canapés during a coffee break at a voice course in Paris, France, to put into a *book* the experiences of the XV Annual Pacific Voice Conference entitled *Emotions and Voice* held at the Pixar Animation Studio in Emeryville, California, in March of that year, I was not sure if he was still my long-standing friend, had had an episode of hypoglycemia, or suddenly became my newest tormentor. A year later, as his semi-casual request came to completion, I can truly state that Tom had a vision, which he expressed in that Parisian April milieu with a straight, professorial, but somewhat emotive statement, that simply meant, "KI, you can do it! And I count on you." I am not sure that at the time I heard his voice as a challenge or just a call for a potentially interesting volume collecting conference-related papers. Soon, however, I was to find out.

Upon my return to Northern California, I started to reconstruct the taste of the canapés, Tom's voice, and the events of the XV Annual Pacific Voice Conference. My recollections were positive, so I began to look optimistically for the missing links and started to compile a list of potential contributors, who for whatever reasons were absent from our March 2005 happening but who knew a lot. As soon as I began to put all the materials together and outlined a book, I realized the challenge placed on me by Tom.

This challenge came to me as a big surprise, as I am accustomed to writing, to publishing, to presenting, and to creating year after year new and narrowly focused scientific content that has made the Annual Pacific Voice Conferences (PVCs, an educational activity of the San Francisco based Pacific Voice and Speech Foundation that I chair) a hit. What struck me, when I really sat down to chart out this endeavor, was the vastness of the material on human emotions but how circumscribed the information was relating to *voice and emotions*. Yes, Diane Bless of Madison, Wisconsin, was correct when we first discussed the program of the conference in the fall of 2004 (no, there was no food involved then, just a phone and her ever-friendly voice and loyal support) in saying that the topic of voice and emotions is terrific and right on time.

Luckily, the faculty of the XV PVC responded, and soon I was able to locate and enjoy the enthusiasm of other emotion researchers who for many reasons were unable to be present at the Emeryville happening, and who agreed to contribute to this volume. Specifically, I felt that I am on the right track after connecting with and experiencing the enthusiasm and dedicated intellectual help on this project of Branka Zei Pollermann of Emotion Research Group in Geneva,

Switzerland. Her contribution to the entire concept was pivotal, and I hence dare to nominate Branka for the Honorary Editor.

Looking for further support, I recruited Hans von Leden. Hans is originally from Lower Silesia (a place where I too lived as a child, though long after his departure), and now he is my fellow Californian, though, alas, of southern part, the city of angels, Los Angeles (where I also lived for a while when attending UCLA). Hans, a cross-cultural erudite, and so aware of our peculiar way of living life, simply told me as he always does, using his measured yet so emotive voice, "Krzysztof, I know you can do it; congratulations, good luck and God bless you."

More wonderful encouragement came from Anne-Maria Laukannen of Tampere, Finland. Now I was sure that this challenge would eventually come to fruition, and after chatting with all the other researchers who so generously embraced the project and promised to deliver in the most collegial and unselfish way, I knew that the book would be a reality.

So there was apparently no way for me to retract. With this generous encouragement and upon Tom Murry's continuous insistence, I called S. Singh at Plural Publishing (again, no fancy food around to distract) and presented to him this project as a matter of fact, and after hearing what was cooking, he simply asked, "Krys, do you think anybody will *buy* the book?" He than passed me to a Lauren Duffy of Plural, who proclaimed, "Oh, I love the whole idea, and I am so excited about this book; when can I have it?" It felt safe, as if we found somebody really, really nice to blame if the book fails to sell. (By the way, Lauren has left Plural by now.)

Really, there have been no books or collections on the subject of emotions of the human voice or on emotions in the human voice, and ours was to be first. The book was to be based on the first-ever truly focused international 2-day conference on this topic, namely, the XV Annual Pacific Voice Conference commingled with Pixar Studios' interest in voice and cartoon characters. Was this conference instructional enough to the digital art industry on how to make the voices of the brilliant cartoon characters created by Pixar more emotional, more believable, and more scientifically correct, or are they smart enough on their own? When I contacted Pixar with the idea of a joint meeting on voice and emotions, I was placed in the hands of Randy Nelson, Dean of Pixar University, who embraced the project and went with it blindly, as if a gathering of hundreds of people interested in the emotions of the human voice naturally belonged to the studio. Randy, I do feel guilty for all the flack you may have gotten as a result of this conference, but we had a great time, we learned from your faculty and your environment, and you are a generous host who is greatly missed. And just to let you know, the participants ask for a repeat.

The theme of the conference caught the attention of a Pixar activity tracker, a smart local newspaper writer (you do know that Pixar is a big, big business, and big businesses are carefully watched, and I assume you may know that Pixar was just bought by Disney, and this is also big news), who politely accused the organization of "going emotional." Emotions are cardinal no-nos of any big business. And the "accusation" was right on, as in addition to all the fantastic scientific sessions and presentations by Pixar faculty, we had an unprecedented opportunity to experience on-line, in real life and in virtual reality, not only a special presentation of the Oscar winning Pixar production of *The Incredibles*, but also to enjoy a 6-hour-long parade of professional voice users (artists) demonstrating vocally coded emotions. This group comprised public speakers, voice-over artists, improvisational actors, stage actors, singers from pop, blues, jazz, country, cabaret, opera, and chorus, storytellers, other performers, cartoon character creators, puppeteers, voice coaches, animators, movie sound creators, and others, all of whom showed their vocally coded emotions in a most remarkable way. Thank you guys, thank you indeed. Pity, then, that the content of these incredible artistic renditions, all focused on highlighting the emotional voice, is missing from this volume.

So what is this book all about? First, it is a *thank you note* to all the contributors, as we all are the editors of equal weight. Next, it is a compilation of the most up-to-date knowledge of what constitutes emotive vocalization *vis-á-vis* currently accepted models of emotions. Obviously, some material is missing and some ideas or results are underrepresented, and obviously, there is room to expand and to improve. Nonetheless, these three volumes stand alone and provide a solid reference source on the emotions of the human voice in the most comprehensive way presented so far; it also unifies all of us into a cross-cultural family of people who believe in the power of emotions. Two more volumes are in the works to complete the missing info.

The choice of the title for the book was a challenge as well, and many versions were possible. I tossed the two words, *emotions* and *voice*, around in my head for many weeks, and I finally came up with some combinations that

meant something to me. So, I asked others to evaluate the power of the final choice of the title. Eventually, *The Emotions in the Human Voice* was selected as the title. Nothing fancy, but these words give a straightforward message and fit among the titles of other publications on the subject of human emotions, e.g., Paul Ekman's 1982 publication entitled, *The Emotions in the Human Face* (I trust you agree with this, Paul).

Though the outline of the March 2005 XV Annual Pacific Voice Conference on Emotions and Voice was organized to flow thematically as if it were a theatrical production, I found myself in a conflict when trying to organize the chapters in a clustered and seemingly logical or sequential fashion. After an honest discussion with Lauren Duffy of Plural (again during a break between our mutual responsibilities while attending a meeting, this time on Coronado Island near San Diego in Southern California, and enjoying ice tea this time rather than French cuisine), we decided on arranging the chapters essentially in alphabetical order by the author's last name. The reasoning was based on the idea that this volume represents an anthology of interrelated topics, that as such it can be read in any order, and that only upon consuming the entire volume will a reader be ready to utter an emotive vocalization reflective of his or her personal view of the value of this volume or specific criticism. Of course this did not happen, and the result is as you see it, namely, three volumes subdivided into more or less cog-wheel style subjects, and as I mentioned two more are to come in 2008.

One more thing shall be mentioned that made my efforts in putting this collection together a real pleasure. This was the willingness of Plural to allow me to design the cover and to include nonscientific illustrations. The acceptance by Plural of this idea placed me on a path to search for illustrators and graphic artists who would be willing to produce a cover and the graphic vignettes to illustrate selected chapters.

I admit that I enjoyed the search very, very much. This search took me into the world of art and graphic design that I deeply respect and admire, and it provided me with an emotional break from thinking about the words and the text only. Once I found the artists that I was looking for, it took very little pressure to persuade both of them to contribute on pro-bono bases. Hence, my special thank-you goes to the cover design creator Daniele Coscone of Italy (www.daniele cascone.com) and to the prolific chapter illustrator, Marta Semkowicz of Wroclaw, Poland (www.mase.pl) for agreeing to participate and for producing extraordinary quality if art. Honestly, it took some emotional work on my part to make this deal, but that is completely another story.

So here we are, ready to indulge in the text placed in front of us. As you come to read these superb contributions, please note that we do vocalize often, in fact daily or nightly, often really freely and spontaneously, and that at times we vocalize on command, and that our vocalizations do carry plenty of emotive content, content that can be truly revealing, even if we do not realize it.

Krzysztof Izdebski

ACKNOWLEDGMENTS

The following people listed here (not in alphabetical order) made this book possible, and for that I am profoundly thankful to all them. Because all of you transcend all kinds of boundaries, professions, systems, religions, age, and all else, I simply ask you to accept a humble "thank you" in your native or emotional language and with chosen prosody. If I missed something, or somebody, please yell at me.

Heather Antonissen, Asa Abelin, Jean Abitbol, Albert Bandura, Magda Goldberger, Zdenek Hufnagel, Beata Woytowicz, Mara Behlau, Brasil, Brad Bird, Diane M. Bless, Sylvie Brajtman, Janina Casper, Manuel Pais Clemente, Piero Cosi, Raul M. Cruz, Danielle Coscone, Peter Docter, Maria Dietrich, Carlo Drioli, Steffi Frigo, Anna Paczynska-Izdebski, Grzegorz A W Izdebski, the Singh Family, Piotr Sokolowski Enskoog, Siri Elliason, Karamindan Ghuman, Isabel Guimaraes, Rozalina Gutman, Ioulia Grichkovtsova, Lorrie Griffie, the Seshadri Family, the Asenov Family, Anastasia Vavilova, Venislava Georgieva Georgieva, Hristina Djambazova, Brindis Gudmunsdottir, Lucinda Halstead,

Sabine Hoffmann, Josef Schlomicher-Their, Anna Maria Hortis-Dzierzbicka, the Deutchman Family, Ellen van der Honert, Mirja Ilves, Julian Konrad Matheus Izdebski, Alexandra Michalina Catherina Izdebski, Kazuhiko Kakehi, Arvid Kapas, Gwen Korovin, Jody Kreiman, Marika Kuzma, Anne Maria Laukkanen, Petri Laukka,

Heather Lauren, Inneke Mennen, Marilyn C. Izdebski, Norman Boone and the Boones Family, Marilee Monnot, Luiza Renata Motter, Dominique Morsomme, John W. Mullennix, Thomas Murry, Clifford Nass, Randy Nelson (special thanks for being so PIXAR), Marcos de Sarvat Family, Susana Naidich Family, Kevin Pelphrey, Robert Peterson, Daniela Powsner, Anna Petrini, Jeff Pigeon, Beata Ptaszynski, Raquel M. Ramsey, Ruth Rainero, Lorraine Ramig,

Joe Rauft, Kevin Reher, Brian Rosen, Gary Rydstrom, Lilla-Theresa Sadowski, Annett Schirmer, Marta Semkowicz, Tapio Seppänen, Sumi Shigeno, Julia A. Sidorova, Jennifer Spielman, Andrew Stenton, Claude Steinberg, Kimberly M. Steinhauer, Victoria Stevens, Fantisek Sram, The Juergen Wendler Family, Uyi Thompson Stewart, Rebeca Stockley, Brad Story, Dave Stroud, Veikko Surakka, Marc Swerts, Mihoko Teshigawara, Juhani Toivanen, Miriam van Mersbergen, Ingrid Verduyckt, Jerry Weissman, Willy Wellens, Magda van Opstal.

Britta Yilitalo, Hans von Leden, Herbert H. and Sigrid Dedo, Michael Chcial, Edward Damrose, Jeanelle Mifsud, the Thomas Shipp Family, the PIXAR staff, the Bay Area Italian American Community, the Tonnela Family, Gary Pratt, the Monty Upshaw Family, M.T. Sylvia, Maria Pignato, Timothy Willcutts.

Fred Harris, Kito Gamble, Molly Holm, Michael Grossman, Lydia Hyde, Kathleen

Antonia, Joel Ben Izzy, Lisa Jenai Hernandez, Lucy Beck, Pam Fry, Karen Mellander-Magoon, Franc D'Ambrosio, Sylvie Sandy Cressman, Heather Lauren, Kathy Kennedy, Dorota Rózanska, Faye Carol, Carolyn Bloom, Martin Stirling, Facing New York,

Jacob Johnson, the Schindler Family, the E. David Manace Family, the James E. Kline Family, Trinh Green, Gabriela Heimensen, Kirstem Mott, Rick Sklader, Mieczyslaw Dzierzbicki, Krzysztof and Natalia Izdebscy, Faculty, staff and management of Pixar and Ex'Pressions,

I also want to thank all my voice patients residing all over the world, representing so many different countries, culture, languages and ethnic roots, and all the people I met in my life with feminine or masculine names and voices, who came to see me because their voice was suffering, and all those other fine people I met in my life, that remain emotional about the way they talk.

CONTRIBUTORS

Åsa Abelin, Ph.D.
Senior Lecturer
Department of Linguistics
Goteborg University
Goteborg, Sweden
Chapter 4

Matti Airas, M.Sc. (EE)
Laboratory of Acoustics and Audio
　Signal Processing
Helsinki University of Technology
Helsinki, Finland
Chapter 12

Paavo Alku, Ph.D.
Professor
Laboratory of Acoustics and Audio
　Signal Processing
Helsinki University of Technology
Helsinki, Finland
Chapter 12

Jo-Anne Bachorowski, Ph.D.
Associate Professor
Department of Psychology
Wilson Hall
Vanderbilt University
Nashville, Tennessee
Chapter 6

Pascal Belin, Ph.D.
Department of Psychology
University of Montreal
Institut Universitaire de Geriatrie de
　Montreal
Montreal, Canada

Centre for Cognitive Neuroimaging
Department of Psychology
University of Glasgow
Glasgow, UK
Chapter 10

Bruce L. Brown, Ph.D.
Professor of Psychology
Brigham Young University
Provo, Utah
Chapter 2

Daniele Cascone
Illustrator
http://www.danielecascone.com
Cover illustration

Genevieve Caelen-Haumont, Ph.D.
Director of Research CNRS
International Research Center MICA
Hanoi, Vietnam
Chapter 15

Shirley Fecteau, Ph.D.
Center for Non-Invasive Brain Stimulation
Department of Behavioral Neurology
Beth Israel Deconness Medical Center
Harvard Medical Center
Boston, Massachusetts
Chapter 10

**Krzysztof Izdebski, FK, MA, Ph.D.,
CCC-SLP, FASHA**
Chairman: Pacific Voice and Speech
　Foundation
San Francisco, California

Clinical Associate Professor,
Voice and Swallowing Center,
Department of Otolaryngology, Head
    and Neck Surgery
Stanford University, School of Medicine
Stanford, California
Chapters 1, 3, and 14

Kati Järvinen
Department of Speech Communication
    and Voice Research
University of Tampere
Tampere, Finland
Chapter 14

Arvid Kappas, Ph.D.
Professor
Jacobs University Bremen
Campus Ring 1
28759 Bremen, Germany
Chapter 8

Monja Knoll
Center for the Study of Emotions
University of Portsmouth
Portsmouth, UK
Chapter 13

Petri Laukka, Ph.D.
Department of Psychology
Uppsala University
Uppsala, Sweden
Chapter 11

Anne-Maria Laukkanen, Ph.D.
Professor of Speech Technique and
    Vocology
Department of Speech Communication
    and Voice Research
University of Tampere
Tampere, Finland
Chapters 12 and 14

Deryle Lonsdale, Ph.D.
Associate Professor

Department of Linguistics and English
    Language
Brigham Young University
Provo, Utah
Chapter 2

Michael Owren, Ph.D.
Associate Professor
Department of Psychology
Georgia State University
Atlanta, Georgia
Chapter 6

Jaak Panksepp, Ph.D.
Bailey Endowed Chair of Animal Well-
    Being Science
Department of VCAPP
College of Veterinary Medicine
    Washington State University
Pullman, Washington
Chapter 13

Natalia Poliakova, M.Ps.
École de Psychologie
Université Laval
Quebec, Canada
Chapter 8

Branka Zei Pollermann, Ph.D.
Psychologist
Department of Psychiatry
Geneva University
Director
Vox Institute
Geneva, Switzerland
Chapters 3 and 15

Annett Schirmer, Ph.D.
Assistant Professor
Department of Psychology
Faculty of Arts and Social Sciences
National University of Singapore
Singapore
Chapter 5

Marta Semkowicz
Illustrator
http://www.mase.pl
Original artwork on pages xxii, 42, 74, 100, 136, 152, 178, 214

Tapio Seppänen, Ph.D.
Professor
Department of Electrical and
    Information Engineering
University of Oulu
Oulu, Finland
Chapter 7

Elizabeth Simpson
Neuroscience and Behavior Student
Department of Psychology
University of Georgia
Athens, Georgia
Chapter 5

Matthew Spackman, Ph.D.
Associate Professor of Psychology
Department of Psychology
Brigham Young University
Provo, Utah
Chapter 2

Brad H. Story, Ph.D.
Assistant Professor
Speech Acoustics Laboratory
Department of Speech and Hearing
    Sciences
University of Arizona
Tucson, Arizona
Chapter 9

Juhani Toivanen, Ph.D.
Academy Researcher
Department of Electrical and
    Information Engineering
University of Oulu
Oulu, Finland
Chapter 7

Eero Väyrynen, M.Sc. (EE)
Researcher
Department of Electrical and
    Information Engineering
University of Oulu
Oulu, Finland
Chapter 7

Hans von Leden, M.D.
Professor of Biocommunications
    (Emeritus)
University of Southern California
Los Angeles, California
Foreword

Teija Waaramaa, M.A., Ph.D.
Researcher
Department of Speech
    Communications and Voice Research
University of Tampere
Tampere, Finland
Chapter 12

Jörg Zinken, Ph.D.
Department of Psychology
University of Portsmouth
Portsmouth, UK
Chapter 13

INTRODUCTION

This is one of the shortest introductions the reader of any scientific volume will ever experience. The reason for this brevity is obvious; namely, as the editor of these volumes, I am extremely proud to have been charged with the task of creating this book, yet I clearly recognize that it is not my book, and that it was created by all of us, all of us who are concerned with the topic of emotions expressed, conveyed, produced, perceived, or generated in the context of the human voice.

The concept that the voice is a carrier of emotions is not a new one. In fact voice, emotions, sexuality, guilt, etc., have been discussed in the Talmud, in the Bible, in Hinduism, in Buddhism, in the Koran, and in many other writings on philosophy or on religious doctrines. Many of the contemporary scholars credited with the development of modern thought and scientific truth about life, or about the evolution of life and of the psychological correlates of life (e.g., Darwin, Freud, Fromm, Jung, etc.), have addressed voice and emotions. So, is there anything we can say about this topic that has not been said before?

These volumes provide the *answer*. We are clearly aware that emotional information is and can be conveyed by a variety of means of human communication. Communication involves content, prosody, gesture, facial expressions, paralinguistic aspects, and cultural know-how. We now know that cross-modality inputs affect the production and perception of another modality. We also know that not all aspects are universal, and that it is OK to be restricted by cultural constraints. With respect to voice and emotions, these modalities are, however, still unclear.

Voice is today a fully acknowledged tool of labor, as so much of our interactions are conducted in the absence or the presence of another person, namely, on the phone or over Internet voice transmission, with the voice signals alone carrying all the clues of our well-being or about our emotional state. Hence, it is not a perplexing question, why we are then ready to make assumptions, judgments, choices, firing and hiring, judicial opinions, criminal recommendations, or purchase choices and other crucial decisions about life based on the emotions we experience regardless of this vocal information?

This work addresses some topics of vocally coded emotions and certainly neglects many pertinent questions. This book is not a final word in the quest of understanding what constitutes vocally conveyed emotions, but in my opinion, it is a darn good approximation of the current (2006/7) state of the art on this subject. Two more volumes addressing pragmatic applications of vocal emotions, more on neural controls and on various aspects of commercial applications, media, man-machine interactions and song, stage and TV are in the works, and are planned to be out at the end of 2008.

Nonetheless, much will still remain to be discovered and learned. One thing that will become obvious when these volumes are consumed by the reader is the fact that, during the act of acoustically conducted communication, emotional information may be coded and expressed both by the content and by modulation of speech. And although it is almost given that the left brain is in charge of language, emotions are shown to be lateralized to the right part of the brain, and much is to be learned about cross-brain integration.

Moreover, similarities in acoustic profiles, intonation, and emotion flow now permit us to assess the extent of how hemispheric lateralization of speech prosody depends on functional instead of acoustical properties. This brings at least one fundamental question into focus; namely, are there acoustical properties of emotions, and if there are, what are they and how do they differ or influence the functional concepts of emotions? The other fundamental question is that of the discovery of what constitutes an emotion in itself. To trivialize this entire concept, I dare to paraphrase Chomsky and Halle who in the epilogue to their then most fundamental work on English phonology (*The Sound Pattern of English*, 1968) proclaimed that the work they had just published suffers from "fundamental scientific inadequacy." Is this volume destined to suffer a similar course? So as not to make this an excuse, I will also dare to quote a Latin doctrine, "*Per risum multum debes cognoscere stultum*," rightly or wrongly stating that the perception of voice cues in the laughter of the emotionally disturbed can point to the source of the type of emotional disturbance that produced such a sound. So then, to cover up my own ignorance, I dare to say, "*Nulla aetas ad discendum sera*" or "It is never too late to learn." With this hope I turn the rest to the reader, and I plea for forgiveness of our ignorance of the scope of the subject we so do love.

Krzysztof Izdebski

To my two special children,
Alexandra Michalina Catherina
and
Julian Konrad Matheus,
whose voices over
their combined 29 years of life
have never failed
to express their emotions,
emotions and voices
I had so many chances
to misinterpret.
Oakland, San Francisco,
and all the many places all over the world,
I found myself working on these volumes

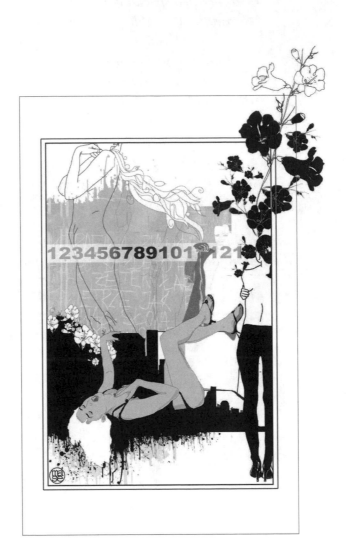

CHAPTER 1

Erotic and Orgasmic Vocalization: Myth, Reality, or Both?

Krzysztof Izdebski

Abstract

Vocalization provides a nonverbal pathway for emotive states. The process of mating and sexual advances or of sexual pursuit and execution lends itself perfectly to emotive forms of vocalization, referred to here as *seductive or erotic vocalization*. Although erotic/seductive vocalization is a fact of life, scholarly studies about this form of human behavior are essentially nonexistent, though ample data can be found on the mating process and the associated mating sounds produced by other species.

Here, a preliminary look at this neglected aspect of human vocal behavior is presented in the form of an ad hoc model of what I broadly dare to term *erotic vocalization* (ER). In later writings, I will attempt to explore through this model vocalizations associated with the various stages of human sexual behavior, but in this instance I only focus on the vocalization associated with an orgasm, even more specifically, vocalizations associated with the female orgasm. The overall proposed model hypothesizes that each stage of sexual/seductive interaction exhibits a specific vocal/verbal phase in addition to nonverbal behavior, that each phase is subject to a specific emotional load that will be reflected by the diversity of vocalization types, and that these patterns are not typical or random; though universal like all emotions, they are person, culture, and gender dependent.

At this stage, more questions are posed than are answered, as only scant and marginal scientific literature exists on any aspect of human erotic vocalization, with the specific studies pertaining to orgasm and vocalization being either anecdotal or simply nonexistent. Therefore, at this introductory stage, this chapter covers the acoustic and perceptual analysis of the sounds associated with the female orgasm. The analysis presented here is based on acoustic signals containing EV derived from movie renditions, from postings on the Internet, and from real-life situations provided by consenting adults.

These preliminary findings and the literature review suggest that what, when, and how we choose or do not choose to vocalize during the various stages of sexual behavior is person specific and the production of these sounds and their reception affect our interpersonal relationships and the quality of the sensual experiences during all stages of interaction, including the love-making stage. The acoustic results and the observations from the available literature suggest the existence of a distance between the commercially portrayed erotic vocalizations and those evoked in real-life situations, and that commercial renditions of EV, especially the pornographic ones, not only depart from reality, but may contribute to a formation of a collective "erotic fata morgana,"; these misleading renditions may form unrealistic expectations that can be potentially disruptive to the expectations about sexual life and how EV ought to be. This distance between reality and commercial renditions may be especially vivid when considering the concept of love and love-making versus the sexual events that can be described by the verbalization of a four-letter word. One must assume that pornography, despite its derogatory or often destructive portrayal of the idea of love and sexuality, is however here to stay. So the way to cope with this distortion is not to fight it, but rather to correct it.

Introduction

There are many movie renditions of erotic love containing some sort of EV, outside the pornography industry. One, however, that seems to take precedence for the purpose of this chapter is *When Harry Met Sally* (1989). In this movie, Harry, played by Billy Crystal, brags to his baseball swinging male pal that he makes women "meow" in bed. The bewildered fellow repeats, "You make women meow?"[1] Later in the movie, when munching in a diner with Sally (played by Meg Ryan), Harry claims that he can recognize a fake orgasm, and when Sally asks him "How do you know?" he replies, "Because I know." "Oh . . . "

"You do not think that I can tell the difference?" asks Harry. "*No!*" comes out loud and clear from Sally.

The scene that follows is considered to have assured the commercial success of the movie. The scene in point features a female orgasm (yes, of course, a fake one acted out on the spot by Ms. Ryan) in an apparent act designed to challenge Harry's claim of possessing knowledge of being able to tell what is real and what is not. The sounds of Sally's fake orgasm are heard by all the guests in the diner, who continue to munch casually on their deli-style culinary creations, as if listening to Muzak. They actually have their ears perked up, and at the final moment dare to gaze in Sally's direction in utter astonishment. The sounds of Sally, her face, her gestures, and the bewildered look of Harry and of the onlookers (or rather on-hearers) are apparently what this movie is most remembered for. Let's face it, Harry, a *male*, is not alone in proclaiming his expertise, as a mature (and hence by definition, one can suppose, a somewhat more experienced) female diner guest, who was certainly impressed by the quality of the vocalization that was just broadcast from a nearby table, tells a bewildered server, "I will have what she is having." Good for her, or should we say, we will see (Fecteau, Armony, Joanette, & Belin, 2005)?

The quest for experiencing love, or an orgasm as a sign of erotic expression of the act of love-making between two adults, and better yet, an orgasm decorated by a vocal ornamentation, seems to be a universal wish of either gender, as this sound apparently signals that the partners are satisfied. This quest is not a modern one, as love with all its attributes has been discussed from antiquity onwards, including some serious treatises by some of the brightest minds in our intellectual past (Fisher, 2004).

Yet the scholarly specifics on the subject of romantic love (Aron, Fisher, Mashek, Strong, & Brown, 2005; Bartels & Zeki, 2000, 2004; Fisner, Aron, & Brown, 2005; Fisher, Aron, Mashek, Li, & Brown, 2002) or love-making are only beginning to surface, and are still ex-

---

[1] This almost derogatory attitude of Harry and his labeling the erotic female voice as "meowing" may actually reflect an unfortunate reality, as his statement relates somewhat to the observations reported by Provine (2003) in his book on laughter. On page 78, Provine describes the results of a psycho-perceptual experiment in which his students had to describe in semantic terms the sounds of human and nonhuman (primate) laughter they just heard. While humans laugh predominantly with or with combinations of voicing, primates according to Provine laugh in a frictionlike manner (i.e., without distinct F_0 presence), and their laughter is judged as a breathy sequence of sounds. While the students recognized the sounds of human laughter as laughter and they did it with a very high degree of accuracy, the breathy laughter of the primates was judged not as laughter, or even as a sound of an animal, but was considered to represent (albeit by a small group of participants) as a sound associated with masturbation or with having sex. So how about that meowing?

tremely rare (Hostege et al., 2003), and those that address the vocal emotions associated with sounds of sex are a real rarity (Fecteau et al., 2005, Fecteau, Belin, Joanette & Armony, 2007).

The literature available about vocalization and love essentially amounts to casual discussions of the various charkas; in my book, and despite the respect I hold for the notion of ethnological wisdom, the style and the description of the aspects of these charkas do not conform to the scientific rigor of investigations we are accustomed to.

So, just to digress for a moment, let me address some modern concepts of what we now assume to know or to comprehend scientifically about the concept of *romantic love*, especially from the brain point of view (Aron et al., 2005; Bartels & Zeki, 2000, 2004; Fisher et al., 2005). The Rutgers and Stony Brook Group of researchers asked just these types of questions and provided some answers based on functional magnetic resonance imaging (fMRI) responses of people who were intensely in love. The results of this study based on a cohort of 17 subjects showed that the intense feeling of being in love activates the brain in the right ventral tegmental area and in the right caudate nucleus and that such activation is dependent on the intensity of passion present. These same subjects' responses to facial attractiveness were found to activate the left ventral tegmentum. These brain regions are the dopamine-rich areas, and such areas have been considered the areas associated with reward and motivation. This finding thus suggests *that love is a motivation* and therefore love is dopamine rewarded, and because love is a motivation, it differs from emotion; hence, it also differs from pure sex drive.

This all indicates that sex and making love with or without love are distinctly different brain controlled entities. And, I dare to say, we know the real thing feels better. The researchers further stated the obvious fact that romantic love changes with time, and that it resembles euphoria in the early stage. They also stated the less obvious fact that romantic love shares biobehavioral similarities with the concept of mammalian attraction, hence giving space to mate selection, and that the corticostriate system is an anatomical substrate for the complex factors that contribute to the process of romantic love and of mate choice. Hence, in general their work suggests that romantic love uses both subcortical reward and motivation systems to choose a specific individual, while the limbic cortical regions attend to the individual emotional factors and the reward functions in the human brain show localization heterogeneity (Aron et al., 2005; Holstege et al., 2003). These concepts of attractiveness are supported elsewhere (Bartels & Zeki, 2000, 2004) by the London researchers who also showed using fMRI that when romantic love is experienced, there is really no space for negative emotive states, and that human attachment employs a push-pull mechanism (Sherer, 1988). Because of this mechanism, we overcome social distance and negative emotions by deactivating negative networks and bond in love through the reward circuitry. And this according to Bartels and Zaki (2000, 2004) explains the power of love to motivate and to exhilarate. I'll bet you that the opposite occurs in a divorce situation, namely that all the negative networks are reactivated to the fullest, and I do not wish you to prove or experience this hypothesis at any cost.

As it was just shown, being in love has nothing to do with actual love-making, and both concepts were already subject of discussion in the early writings, but I am of course looking for the vocal connections, no matter how remote.

So, apparently the Sumerian tablets include the phrase "the voice of your name . . . "and poems written during Egypt's New Kingdom (1539–1075 BC) but most likely composed much earlier depict love and romance using metaphors, repetitions, and other poetic techniques, [i.e., "To hear your voice is pomegranate wine to me" (Walker, 2004)] in the context of ancient writing on love. Moreover, in the Torah, God tells Abraham, "All that Sarah has said to you, hearken to her voice" (Genesis 21:12), supposedly meaning that there shall be no inequality between a man and a woman in all matters including the matters of love. In the Bible (Genesis 4:1, NASB, 1995) we can read "Now the man had relations with his wife Eve . . . "), and Islam also tells of sexual lust. Lust, in the current concept, has also been studied by fMRI, and was shown to be a sign of general and not specific mating, as it lights up different parts of the brain (Fisher et al., 2002). As the old Chinese proverb says, "Love is of all passions the strongest, for it attacks simultaneously the head, the heart and the senses." For example, Al-Suyuti, a 12th century commentator of Koran interpretations, wrote with passion about the sensations of love-making and about the eternal reward of sleeping with sev-enty *houris* (virgins/angels), all with "appetizing vaginas" (Warraq, 2002).[2]

Reading Ibn Warraq further (2002), we learn that the modern philosopher Nietzsche was not very fond of Christianity, as he felt that among other issues, Christianity was in conflict with the beauty of human sexuality, and that Christianity was dead wrong in being so. Apparently, the ancient Jews (from whom the Christian doctrine derives) felt that sex is like food and that overusing sex may be harmful. Moreover, according to the writings of Ibn Warraq (2002), St. Augustine, a Catholic doctrinarian, apparently was at one time also pro-sex, until he changed his mind; Kant, in his discussion of love (yes, *love*, and not love–making; see previous discussion) distinguished between *amor complacentiae* and *amor benevolentiae* and spoke of pleasure [Green, 1992; perhaps even in terms of "pure pleasure" (B. Zei-Pollermann, personal communication, 1992)], referring to the first concept, while he spoke of the sense of duty with respect to the second one. It also appears to me that even the conservative yet modern Catholic doctrine keeper, Pope John Paul II, also felt that as long as love-making leads to procreation and is executed with respectful passion, pleasure and its expressions in the process of experiencing love, even while making it, are not a sin or an ungodly event but a reward (Jan Pawel II, 1995).

Modern scientific explanations of the concept of romantic love or being in

---

[2]This rendition comes from an article by Ibn Warraq (2002) who in my opinion produced a convincing argument on religion and sex with regard to the three major western religious doctrines, (To learn more, the reader is referred to Ibn Warraq, "Virgins? What Virgins?" *Guardian Unlimited*, Saturday, January 12, 2002, http://www.guardian.co.uk/saturday_review/ story/0,3605,631332,00.html) No wonder that some moderns try to use this "appetizing" reward as an incentive for ungodly acts of terrorism and suicide, which are by the way forbidden by the Koran (see above.).

love including the neural basis for this emotion or lust and motivation do exist (Aron et al., 2005; Bartels & Zeki, 2000, 2004; Fisher, 2004; Fisher et al., 2005; Fisher & Thomson Jr, 2007) as discussed before. There are some studies on the brain effects of actual love-making (Holstege et al., 2003), but again no relationship to vocalization was found, despite assumptions that voicing enhances the experience. The experience in itself has been also shown to have caused a peculiar onset of temporary amnesia, apparently due to blood pressure changes (Gallagher, Murphy, & Carroll, 2005), which prompted another paper on the same subject paper entitled in a quite witty way, "Make Love to Forget" (Bucuk et al., 2004). This is not a bad idea, though not exactly matching the opinion of Lord Chesterfield (1694–1773) who declared, "Sex: the pleasure is momentary, the position ridiculous, and the expense damnable" (Brainy Quotes, 2007).

But to return to the core of this chapter, the voice, and in fact the erotic voice, a general question can be asked: Why is there so little in a scholarly way about this specific topic? Another question posed can be simply, "Who cares?" Another question that can and really should be asked is, What constitutes Harry's apparent ability to recognize facts from fiction? What acoustic or emotional detector(s) did Harry possess to claim such expertise? Was his apparent expertise a reality, or was it merely a myth or wishful thinking? Perhaps it is the amygdala, the thalamus, and the hypothalamus, or is it the cortex and the cerebellum, or all of the above, that tell us what we "hear" when in bed, and if we hear it at all, even when the sound is present.

If the answer is yes (to Harry's possessing specific receptors), we shall then ask if indeed there are true and typical vocal characteristics associated with an orgasm, and if it is so, can these acoustic/perceptual clues alone be enough to separate truth from fiction?

The ability to separate these two types of vocal expressions on the basis of the sound alone may be perhaps not a trivial point at all, as emotions are recognized more accurately when the face and voice are combined, while most of the erotic sounds discussed here are typically produced in semidarkness or at least with a dim lighting, a concept advanced elsewhere (Hughes, Dispenza, & Gallup, 2004). Hence, the acoustic characteristics of the sound may constitute a crucial input for the brain and may be enough to distinguish between the negative and the positive vocally mediated emotions, that is, the emotions of fear and/or of pleasure (Fecteau, Armory, Joanette, & Belin, 2005, Fecteau, Belin, Joanette & Armony, 2007).

If the answer is no, we can then ask, Why not? Well, we can continue to ask and to ask and to ask, almost ad nauseam, because there is no literature to provide quick, or as a matter of fact, hardly any answers. Even the mighty and non-peerreviewed Internet fails.

We can also ask what these sounds mean, what these sounds are for, and how the true sounds may differ from the fake ones. We can also wonder if the erotic sounds sold to us by the entertainment industry represent reality or are distant from reality or do they simply promote a "collective confusion," a concept I discussed with Dr. Victoria Stevens, a contributor to this volume who has been working on the subject of unrealistic wishful thinking for a while (Stevens, personal communication, 2006). So, are we simply duped by the film/entertainment industry into believing in and longing after a pattern of erotic vocalization that is not real, or not a part of the healthy sensual and respectful sexual life, instead of recognizing that if it sounds good it, it must be true? Or is the collective erotic fata morgana taking over?

We can for example also ask what role voice plays in our intimate emotional life, if such erotic vocalization really exists, if it can be defined objectively, and if so, if it differs in the diverse cultural and gender settings. We can ask further if heterosexual vocalization is different from erotic homosexual vocalization, since the so-called homosexual voice may differ from the expected male vocal norms in specific settings (Eckert & McConnell-Ginet, 2003; Gaudio, 1994; Jacobs, 1996; Kulick, 2000; Levon, 2004; Linville, 1998; Munson, Jefferson, & McDonald, 2006; Podesva, 2003; Podesva, Roberts, & Campbell-Kibler, 2002; Rogers, Smyth, & Jacobs, 2000; Smyth, Jacobs, & Rogers, 2003), and since the "acoustic cues associated with perceived sexual orientation generally agreed with acoustic findings as a function of actual sexual orientation" (Linville, 1998), suggesting, though cautiously, that speech of at least some openly gay men or women may demonstrate characteristics that are discernible as descriptive of sexual orientation to the listeners (Munson et al., 2006; Rogers et al., 2000; Smyth et al., 2003).

Acoustic cues associated with perceived sexual orientation generally agreed with acoustic findings as a function of actual sexual orientation, and while results need to be interpreted cautiously, recent findings also suggest that members of the openly gay or transgender community may demonstrate certain speech features that are discernible to listeners (Munson et al., 2006).

We can also ask if the homosexual nation responds to same-sex erotic vocalization in a manner similar to how heterosexuals respond. This hypothesis is not out of line, as there is mounting evidence that gay men respond differently than straight man do to human pheromones such as AND and EST (Savic, Berglund, & Lindstrom, 2005). AND is detected in male sweat, and EST in female urine. This study showed on the basis of positron emission tomography that homosexual men showed hypothalamic activation to AND, and that was in congruence to the heterosexual women, but no differentiation was found when gay men were presented common odors. This is of significance, as animal models clearly show that the choice of sexual partner is highly dependent on sex specific pheromone signals processed in the male and female mating centers located in the anterior portion of the hypothalamus (Stowers, Holy, Meister, Dulac, & Koentges, 2002).

We can also ask how voice parameters reflect emotions associated with all aspects of sexuality, whether across-genders or within-gender preference. Why? Because empirical evidence suggests that voice quality changes as a function of initial meeting, flirting, seduction, first kiss, first act of making love, first arguments, etc. And why would we suspect otherwise, as these acts are emotionally loaded, and we know that that calls for a codependence there. We can ask and ask, and pose an essentially unlimited string of questions, because there are hardly any answers in the scientific literature to any of the aspects of vocalization and sexual behavior.

It is the beginning of 21st century, and we are debating and starting to accept in some U.S. courts the concept of domestic partners and that of the legitimacy of a gay marriage; we are now again excited about incorporating "intelligent design" in teaching (Blavatsky, 1999; Dembski, 1999); we are inundated by various forms of sex in daily life and in the majority of commercials; we have advanced to a screen version of Alfred Kinsey's scientific quest to study human sexuality; and we were told almost a decade ago by the president of the United States, Mr. Bill Clinton, that oral sex is not sex, yet there is a real void in the knowledge of the role of vocalization (nonverbal communication so vital to sexuality) in human sexual interactions.

Though essentially a pre-Columbian research area of human behavior, the subject of erotic vocalization evokes eager interest, and at the same time surprise, with whomever I happen to discuss my attempt to write this chapter. Interestingly, my declaration of a willingness to pursue this topic was quite often associated by a curious "What ?!" during my year-and-a-half-long pursuit of this subject and the various conversations on this subject with all sorts of lay and educated people from all over the globe. Some even told me that from now on I will not be recognized for my work on phonatory movement disorders that freed thousands of patients from unsuccessful psychotherapy treatment (Dedo & Izdebski, 1983; Izdebski, 1992) or for organizing the Annual Pacific Voice Conferences (http://www.pvsf.org), but that I will be referred to as "Dr. Orgasmic." Well, why not? Better than some other names I have been called in the past.

I really encountered only a few of my fellow humans of both genders who had the guts to discuss vocalization and sex with me, and who did not giggle or initially display some sort of embarrassment that eventfully subsided. One, however, after displaying initial enthusiasm and willingness conduct common research, later declined fearing academic authorities disapproval. Yet to my utter surprise, nobody dared to deny the role that erotic vocalization plays in their lives. Some, after a pause, even provided information from their own experiences, one of which I incorporated into this text.[3]

But, unlike Harry, most of my male discussants were honestly ambivalent with regard to their expertise of separating the facts from fiction, and those women who volunteered to describe their experiences gave accounts that fell far from the commercial movie renditions of how we sound when we are in love and making love, and not making sex.

Literature

Yes, it is much easier to learn in our modern society about explicit or hidden mating behaviors and their vocal correlates of chimpanzees, apes, lizards, finches, or other species than of the human species, and yes we know more about why a family of flies are gay than why humans are gay (Nikitopoulous, Arnhem, van Hooff, & Sterck, 2004; Villella, Ferri, Krystal, & Hall, 2005). Apparently is OK to be gay if you are a fruit fly; (Villella et al., 2003). It is better for the industry; but is bad if you are a fruitcake, or want to get married to the same sex partner (Murray, 2006)— was there a pun intended?

Yet voice, verbal and nonverbal behavior, courtship, and eroticism are integrally expressed and interwoven in human

---

[3]One potential collaborator stated that anything regarding seduction in voice would be dangerous to her curriculum vitae. How about freedom of speech or academic freedom?

behavior (Abitbol, 2006; Anolli & Ciceri, 2002; de Weerth & Kalma, 1995) and some cultures, specifically the ones that teach Tantra or Taoism, place a significant value on the role of vocalizations in sex. In researching this topic, I came across a posting on the Internet that struck me as funny, if not profound. I actually contacted this person and she verified that it was her own idea and not plagiarism. The posting said, "The Scriptures tell us to love, Kamasutra teaches us how to" (J. Strzelak, personal communication, 2006, October 20). Semantically, these may be confusing concepts, but this witty play on words evoked a giggle in me, and I wanted to share this experience.

So, what explains the apparent silence on this subject in our modern world? While some more or less anecdotal paragraphs embedded in various texts on human sexual behaviors or in consumer literature exist, these often simply amount to a description of erotic speech that accompanies sex acts. This type of speech expression is generally referred to as "dirty talking." Talking, dirty or not, during the orgasmic stage of love-making may not be advisable according to some, as talking can be distracting (Hutcherson, 2005), and the same apparently goes for watching the TV while making love. But the impact of music on love-making is unclear, and playing music is at times advised, not only as a means of erotic enhancement, but also as a means of masking the sounds of love-making from for example children or neighbors. So, there goes the attraction for the modern apartment lifestyle, or the open window policy.

Some cursory information on seductive vocalization comes from Abitbol (2006), who casually though passionately addressed seduction and seductive voice throughout his recent publication, but his rendition lacks scientific explanations of what it is that constitutes seductive vocalization. A more rigorous account can be found in the chapter by Anoli (see Chapter 13 in Volume 3 of this publication).

We know both empirically and scientifically that emotional loading will alter the characteristic of the basic vocal signal; hence, seductive speech, a form of communication expressive of a specific emotional state, is by definition an enabling operator expected to affect vocal characteristics. Moreover, erotic vocalization, since it is an expression of "the ultimate pleasure" may be expected to display characteristics of pleasantness and attractiveness, a concept discussed elsewhere with respect to voice (Lonsdale, Brown, & Spackman, 2007). This concept of vocal attractiveness may result from a set of the innate stimuli colored by environmental situations, that in turn may further influence the voice quality.

To comprehend how the voice contributes to, if not decides on, how we may be influenced by its quality in the process of selecting a casual sexual mate, or even a lifelong partner, was a subject of a remarkable study by a group of East Coast researchers (Hughes, Dispenza, & Gallup, 2004; Hughes & Gallup, 2003). (For more on this topic see Chapter 13 in Volume 2 of this publication.)

These researchers were interested to discover what constitutes vocal attractiveness in a sexual context, and through their research they were able to demonstrate a close link between body shapes, sexual behavior, and vocal signals. They concluded that the information contained in voice can us tell much about the sexual choices we make, including how we determine choosing a mate. Their data implied that sexual behavior, promiscuity, and frequency of sexual encounters can be predicted by our vocal patterns. Sounds scary?

Furthermore, the work of Anolli and Ciceri (2002; also see Chapter 13 by Anolli in Volume II) on male seductiveness clearly suggests that voice is "the real beef" in the process of seductive communication. And please keep in mind that the work of Hughes et al. (2004) pointed out that the erotic voice is here to stay, because voice and voice quality inform partners about mutual emotional states, specifically when the lights are off.

Data

So, how does the voice sound in a specific erotic milieu, and more specifically here, what are the characteristics of the voice during a female orgasm if vocalization is indeed present? Or, in other words, is Hollywood, Sally, or Harry on target, or are we simply being brainwashed and presented with an unrealistic acoustic (and visual) rendition of erotic vocalization and given an acoustic wish list scripted in a different type of sci-fi?

While typically the love-making process lasts on the average 15 minutes, the duration of the typical female orgasm is said to be short, in fact very short, and that of a male is even shorter. The female orgasm lasts more or less eight (yes *eight*) seconds, and it may or may not be accompanied for its eternity by vocalization (although the mean measured orgasm

duration in a laboratory setting in at least one study was measured to last 19.9 seconds as expressed by vaginal blood flow; Levin & Wagner, 1985).[4]

So how much sound and information can be associated with the 8- to 20-second time frame, and what message can be sent out in that time, that apparently makes the partners want each other more eagerly over and over again, and what information is contained in the voice that assures the partners that everything is just great; and do we really hear the message?

Well, before I attempt to describe these acoustical and perceptual characteristics, I first wish you to consider some basic physiologic factors that should be kept in mind when analyzing and discussing erotic vocalization.

The Physiology of Female Orgasmic Response

Female orgasm represents a physiologic release of vasocongestion relieved by the vaginal muscles and myotonia through contractions of pelvic floor muscles that surround the lower third of the vagina; the contractions include the rectal musculature. Each contraction occurs at about 1-second intervals and there are typically between 5 and or 13 such contractions, making the duration of an orgasm somewhere between 5 and 13 seconds, averaging at 8 seconds [see previously referenced blood flow study (Levin & Wagner, 1985)]. Orgasmic pleasure, which may depend significantly on

---

[4]No, I do not think the name "After Eight" given to a chocolate-mint candy has anything to do with this magic number, but who knows? Also the Chinese prefer eight as a magic number (apparently referring to flying stars) and apply this number to feng shui, medicine, architecture, and arts. Hence, orgasmic vocalization must be ipso-facto more or less short and to the point, or something like a sound bite during an expensive political campaign, or during a sporting event aired on national TV. And therefore I dare to deem it to be convincing out of intrinsic constraints.

psychological factors (Bridges, Critelli, & Loos, 1985; Mah & Binik, 2005), has been shown to relate to the intervals and the intensity of the contractions, and hence the accompanying vocalization, if present, must follow these time constraints. Individual variations are the *norm*, but a certain pattern can be expected. It appears hence that all the sounds or words that may occur afterwards are more or less the afterthoughts.

Based on the work of Masters and Johnson (1966), the orgasm is also associated with bodily responses outside the immediate genital area, and vocalization is considered to be one of these so-called extragenital orgasmic responses; in fact, recently a two-dimensional model of orgasm that incorporates context has been proposed (Mah & Binik, 2002).

The other response comprises a sexual flush present in 75% of women, and the respiratory and heart rates change, with the respiration rate increasing to as high as 30 to 40 breaths per minute, the pulse rate reaching between 110 and 180 beats per minute, and blood pressure ranging between 30 and 80 mm/Hg systolic and 20 and 40 mm/Hg diastolic (which is below the average values for some women; Murray, Brahler, Baer, & Maretta, 2003).

Since the work of Kinsey et al. (1998), some new ideas about orgasm have surfaced. For example, orgasm is no longer considered a purely physiological response but as a combined systems response, indicating that the stimulus, although usually a physical one, may include imagery as well (Gallagher, 1986).

And the research of others now seems to define an orgasm, in addition to representing peak intensity of excitation resultant from stimulation from visceral and somatic sensory receptors, as a part of a response to cognitive processes, therefore not restricting the orgasm solely to the genital system (Komisaruk & Whipple, 1991).

Masters and Johnson (1966) delineated two major differences between men and women, namely that only men could ejaculate, and that only women could have a series of orgasms in a short period—an idea challenged later (Whipple, Hartman, & Fithian, 1994; Whipple, Ogden, & Komisaruk, 1992). In their study of the orgasmic response involving a cohort of 751 subjects, Hartman and Fithian (1972) showed that male and female orgasmic patterns are undifferentiated within the orgasmic parameters measured, and that response patterns were individualized; everyone showed an individual orgasmic pattern, with the widest variation between people occurring in the cardiovascular functions. Vocalization was not discussed.

Again with respect to orgasmic length, gender differences are found, showing that a male orgasm lasts on average 10 to 13 seconds, while muscle contractions (measured physiologically in a laboratory setting) that determine female orgasm duration last between 7 and 51 seconds, although the same women reported subjectively a perception of their orgasms lasting between 7 and 107 seconds (Bohlen, 1983). This laboratory vs. subjective duration has been also discussed elsewhere (Rellini, McCall, Randall, & Meston, 2005).

While it is agreed in general that the orgasm is short, the speed with which women can experience an orgasm can be reached at times very quickly (e.g., 15 seconds at the fastest end) or more slowly (an average of 20 minutes at the other end), and the role of foreplay in orgasm duration and intensity is unclear (Miller & Byers, 2004).

And yes, it is a challenge for many partners to recognize if their lover is having an orgasm. Moreover, both groups (males and females) admit faking an orgasm.

And yes, it is also recognized that women who report a variety of orgasmic experiences (at least three types are spoken about) may have sequential or multiple orgasms, and it appears that women make subjective distinctions between orgasms resulting from stimulation of different body zones (i.e., vagina, clitoris, or Graefenberg spot; Singer & Singer, 1978; Masters & Johnson, 1966) or from self-induced imagery (Whipple et al., 1992). Whether these responses are associated with differences in vocalization remains to be seen.

Anger possesses specific vocal characteristics and is usually considered an unpleasant experience and an unpleasant emotion. So why mention anger in a chapter on love? Interestingly, anger can evoke a very negative emotional response that can inhibit orgasm, while in some individuals it can provide the stimulation that produces arousal. This controversy has been used to explain why some couples fight and then have sex, because fighting acts as an erotic stimulus, and if therapy is used to end the fighting, the partnership may end unless other methods of erotic stimuli are developed to replace the fighting. Communication problems are recognized as playing a significant role in many sexual dysfunctions (Kelly, Strassberg, & Turner, 2006), and men may behave in a degrading manner towards partners after being exposed to sexually explicit films (Mulac, Jansma, & Linz, 2002).

Because erotic stimulation is a part of lovemaking, it can be asked how much the voice in itself can act as the stimulator of erotic behavior; the work of Hughes and Gallup (see Chapter 15 in Volume 2) strongly suggests that voice can guide us to choose a mate. Thus, so as not to contradict myself, I dare to say that some voice and speech usage in the process of lovemaking can be useful, especially when it speaks to one's emotive centers. It is conceivable to think of the voice as an erotic stimulus, in the same way as chills can be caused by listening to certain music (Panksepp & Bernatzky, 2002), or as a turn-on, as it goes in some songs ("Sexy noises turn me on and on/Talk to me and you can't go wrong/I love the sound of your voice when you make love to me . . . "; Salt N Pepa, 2002).

The Literature Again

Yes, some of what will be reviewed next can be easily challenged on scientific grounds, but often that is all there is. Some of it however appears solid. It has been claimed that the 8-second female (and for that matter, shorter for the male) orgasm can be prolonged, as some leading sex experts suggest. When possible, and when learned, the female orgasm can be elongated to about or beyond 60 seconds, and the ability to stretch this experience is possible, claim some, when the experience is accompanied by deep breathing and by focused vocalization (Chia & Abrams, 2005; Dessilets, 2003).

Such deep breathing happens apparently when relaxation takes over, and this state is only possible because of the openness and the softness of the woman's heart, which controls her relaxation (Chia & Abrams, 2005). The softness and openness happen because the two chakras, the throat chakra and the sex chakra, are intricately linked and significantly affect each other; activating the voice chakra will help to activate the sex chakra. When this activation takes place, both partners will be encouraged to breathe and to make sounds coming from the depths of their bodies. Interestingly, a hormonal connection between the vagina and breast in the female has been documented, as the oxytocin, the hormone that triggers the female breast milk reflex, may be released at orgasm even in non-lactating women (Trinkl, 1999).

This work incorporates previous knowledge of the role oxytocin plays in the mammalian reproductive life, as this hormone facilitates among other things bonding, acceptance, and pari-formation in various mammals. In humans, oxytocin was shown to stimulate milk ejection during lactation and uterine contraction during birth, and the hormone is released during orgasm both in men and women. Moreover, there is evidence (albeit controversial) that the female glottic mucosa during menses shows a composition similar to that of the vaginal mucosa (Abitbol, 2006). Others however challenge any expression of sex hormone receptors in the human vocal cord (Schneider et al., 2006).

In fact, some of this reasoning appears to be circular, specifically with regard to the possible relationships between vocalization and orgasms, as these arguments incorporate (in a sense, work) within the traditional Taoism and Tantric philosophies that equate throat with vagina and believe that the two chakras, the throat chakra and the sex chakra, are intricately linked and hence significantly affect each other. Activating the voice chakra will help activate the sex chakra. As far as I can determine, there is no scientific evidence for this reasoning. To illustrate this point I will paraphrase from Dessilets (2003) who writes, that the activation of

the voice (the throat) also lends to opening this gate and that she is not referring to the Hollywood style of screaming and moaning, but rather the sounds that are produced when surrendering to pleasure.

In their groundbreaking work on sexual behavior (and also a rare one in which orgasmic vocalization is mentioned), Brauer, Brauer, and Brauer (2001) ask the partners not to forget to vocalize their pleasure during an orgasm with as loud a sound as possible. They transliterate this ideal sound as an "aaaaaHHHaaaaa" sound, and they tell the reader that the voice has to come from the depths of the abdomen. They agree with Saida Dessilets that this erotic sound can give an orgasm an extra boost. They also believe that vocalization (nonverbal communication) during lovemaking plays a role in arousal, while talking (speech, verbal communication) is destructive at the point of an orgasm. Quite a contrary point can be made regarding the portrayal of sounds found in *When Harry Met Sally*, as so many *yeses* were uttered at an elevated dB level. Assuming that erotic *yes* is speech, the content of speech, not limited to the *yes,* but often containing quite a vulgar array of words and verbal screams, profanities, or other obscene "dirty talk monologues," is frequently presented in porno-flicks during lovemaking (or rather sex-making) scenes. Of course, I do not only deplore this degradation of human intimacy, but I am in agreement with the value of vocalization and not of speech, as based on my own "studies"; also it has been shown that lack of communication is of significance in sexual dysfunction (Kelly et al., 2006; see Appendix A).

Brauer et al. (2001) also encourage couples to moan and groan. In fact, they profess the sound's profound value in lovemaking to the point that they actually teach lovers how to vocalize during the act of lovemaking. These sex experts also propose that couples should take time to learn and to practice (and when not in bed) how to vocalize to an orgasmic success, meaning how to achieve a long and rich orgasmic experience. They propose making an "aaaaaHHHHaaaaa" sound with the mouth open, as this will help to increase the G-spots sensation. Hyperventilation and groaning during intercourse have been recently shown to alter brain metabolism as a result of hypocapnia, with groaning and hyperventilation during sex being interpreted as a psychophysiological mechanism that deepens states of sexual trance.

Silence during lovemaking acts as learned control (perhaps because of fear of being heard or because of built-in embarrassment), and silence is thought to limit pleasure. Hence, other experts on sexuality also agree that sexual vocalization is useful and brings plenty of fringe benefits to the lovers, as it frees feelings, and the sounds of moaning, groaning, or sighing facilitate deep exhalation, and hence enhance the orgasm. In addition, vocalization seems to help to diffuse the arousal throughout the body and to serve as a feedback to the partner that things are going well. So it seems that screaming is not the way to go (Dessilets, 2003). This is not a surprise, as screaming is often perceived by the brain as not a pleasant experience (Fecteau et al., 2005; Passie, Hartmann, Schneider, & Emrich, 2003).

Support that sex vocalization is good for you comes from the most recent work by Fecteau et al. (2005; 2007) who used functional magnetic resonance imaging (fMRI) to investigate brain activity of healthy controls exposed to positive and negative emotional vocalizations. To investigate which part of the brain participates, these researchers presented the subjects with various vocal signals that, among others, included sexual vocalizations (no speech was contained in these sexual vocalization signals), as well as laughs, cries, fearful screams, and non-emotional vocalizations (e.g., coughs). They used an event-related design to avoid mood induction, and very short stimuli (mean sound duration was 1.6 sec). After completing the scanner portion of the experiment, participants rated these vocalizations on emotional valence. Laughs and sex vocalization were described as expressing positive emotions, while cries and fearful screams portrayed negative emotions, and the non-emotional signals were described as neutral. When comparing the fMRI activations related to the positive signals such as laughs and sexual vocalizations to that of neutral vocalizations, Fecteau et al. (Fecteau, Belin, Joanette & Armony, 2007) found greater activity in the bilateral amygdala, the right superior temporal gyrus, and the right primary auditory cortex/middle superior temporal sulcus (see Figure 1-1, illustrating the amygdala activations associated with each category of vocalizations). Hence, pleasure appears to be a bilateral phenomenon but with the right brain possibly mediating the acoustics of the pleasure. So this innovative study may be in fact the modern evidence for the traditional wisdom that using the left brain during sex, or expressing words or being verbal during orgasm, is not what it is all about. (It would be of great interest to repeat this experiment using both real and fake sounds and those extracted from so-called dirty talk. Awaiting the anticipated results invites a bet that Hollywood erotic sounds, i.e., those containing yelling or speech, would evoke an emotionally

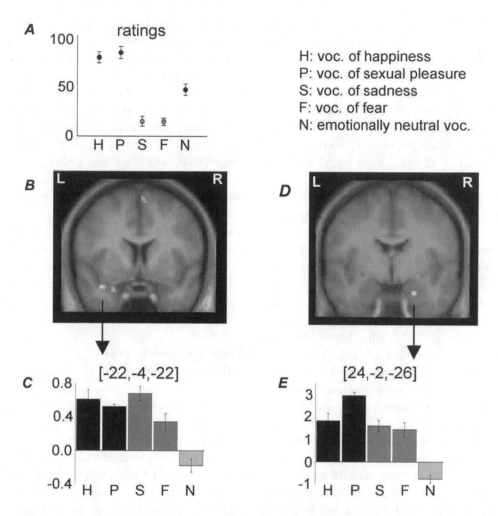

Figure 1–1. fMRI illustrating the amygdala activations associated with each category of vocalizations). Hence, pleasure appears to be a bilateral phenomenon but with the right brain possibly mediating the acoustics of the pleasure. Reprinted with permission, Fecteau, 2007.

valid response as well, but that the left brain may be the one that would light up more in these cases.) Now, going back to the reality of the results of Fecteau et al. (2006), their work provided evidence of bilateral amygdala involvement in the acoustic processing of valence, the role recognized for the visual stimuli, and bilateral activation being valid for both the negative and pleasant emotive acoustic signals, solidifying the role of this organ in emotion (Gosselin et al., 2005), with evidence that the right amygdala may be more "interested" in responding to happiness and less to fear.

Of interest here may be an observation made by Fecteau et al. (2005) with respect to age and gender differences in judgments of the authenticity embedded in the emotional nonlinguistic vocalizations, the sort of stuff expressed by the not–so–young female guest in the diner in

When Harry Met Sally. As we recall, this lady wanted to have what Sally just had. Well, the work of Fecteau et al. (2005) tells us that older women rated sex vocalization signals as less authentic than the judgments of the younger women, whereas authenticity judgments for men were not age dependent. So is sound of import to the sex partner? There is no obvious answer, but one study seems to be quite puzzling (though maybe just for me). The study I am referring to investigated arousal of healthy young and sexually functioning women who were watching erotic movies with and without sound while their physiological signs of arousal were monitored. And the results demonstrated that the presence or absence of audio input did not increase subjective arousal. On the average it took 2 minutes to reach maximal arousal in these subjects (Laan, Everaerd, van Bellen, & Hanewald, 1994). But when fMRI was used to compare the neural correlates of sexual arousal in 20 male and 20 female subjects via measurements of their brain activity while these subjects watched erotic film excerpts, the level of arousal was found greater in the males. Viewing these erotic segments as opposed to neutral videos was associated, for both groups of subjects, with bilateral blood oxygen level dependent (BOLD) signal increases in the anterior cingulate, medial prefrontal, orbitofrontal, insular, and occipitotemporal cortices, as well as in the amygdala and the ventral striatum. But note that only the males, not the females, showed thalamic and hypothalamus responses to these sexual stimuli. These findings reveal the existence of similarities and dissimilarities in the way the brain of both genders responds to erotic stimuli. They further suggest that the greater sexual arousal generally experienced by men, when viewing erotica, may be related to the functional gender difference found here with respect to the hypothalamus (Karama et al., 2002). If it is really so or not may be hard to prove, or may be actually irrelevant, as the recent evidence on who actually made the erotic movie, that is man or woman, seems to make a big difference to the female or male audiences, with subjective experience of sexual arousal being more pronounced in women to the woman made movies, and with more feeling of guilt, shame or aversion to the male made movies (Laan, Everaerd, van Bellen, & Hanewold, 1994).

More Questions and Still Few Answers

Are vocal patterns portrayed in the media as representative, consciously or subconsciously shaping our notion of how erotic vocalization really sounds, either real or fake? As I tried not to forget the silence on this topic, I dare to ask more, and do it knowingly, as I am unable to answer. Nonetheless, I want to address the fundamental nature of the erotic vocalization, and I want to know not only what constitutes erotic seductive vocalization, but how this vocalization differs within the various stages of erotic behavior and between the various sex preference groups, i.e., straight partners, heterosexuals, gay-lesbians, bisexuals, and transgender individuals. Is there a period of acceleration of these vocal patterns, and are these patterns age dependent? Inferring from hormonal maturity affecting body changes and age-related voice changes, we should expect that sensual/sexual/erotic voice can be further subject to fluctuation based on hormonal voice links associated with gender. But because so much is not clear and not discussed, other questions arrive, including the questions, "Is there an erotic voice at all?" "Is the voice individualized, or are there patterns?" "Is the erotic voice universal, or is it culture specific?" "Is the erotic vocalization common or exclusive to the recognized sexual orientation groups, or does the voice of seductiveness cross the subgroups?" In other words, is the voice of a man seducing a female attractive to a gay man or that of a seducing heterosexual woman attractive to a lesbian? So much about the responses of adult humans to pheromones is unclear (Wysocki & Preti, 2004).

If we take for granted the surfacing scientific evidence that gay men respond with arousal to male hormones, in the same or similar way that straight women respond to male pheromones (Savic, Berglund, & Lindstrom, 2005), can we ask if a seductive male voice can be "dangerous" not only to a woman but to a gay man as well? Or, can a seductive, erotic, or orgasmic vocalization of a straight woman "hook" a lesbian? When letting the mind wander, there seems to be no end to questions, and as there are no answers, this discourse can continue in silence and in the absence of written works.

No wonder then that the mature female diner (in real life the mother of the director of the movie) playing a customer who just listened to the sounds of a faked orgasm produced by Sally, among the pancakes, hamburgers, and BLT sandwiches and a captive audience, not to mention all the film crew, was nevertheless so convinced about the reality of the sounds she just heard that she said with much obvious pleasure to the server, "I will have what she is having,"

apparently not referring to the choices of the diner's menu.

A Model

So what constitutes sexual, seductive, or erotic vocalization? The model I propose here for the purpose of this chapter should be treated at best as an *ad hoc* working trial that aims at incorporating all the recognized stages of sexual behavior possibly reflected by emotive vocalization, namely, introduction (flirt), pursuit (discourse negotiations), foreplay (foreplay), execution (act of lovemaking), outcome (orgasm), and conclusion. Therefore, for this purpose, I define sexual vocalization as voice alone, or as vocalization contained in speech produced during the stages of seductive sexual behavior.

Data Analysis

The wider data corpus on which this model is being built comprises "real" and "commercial" sources. The data analyzed for the purpose of this portion of the model are limited to vocalization associated with orgasm, and come from three sources: (a) personal recollections of erotic sounds reported by various people describing various vocal sounds produced by their partners at climax, (b) analysis of sounds of orgasm taken from Internet postings (e.g., http://www.sounds.com), and (c) from commercial sources (i.e., from various movies).

The available data were gender divided, and at this point the data do not include the sounds produced by the various sex preference subgroups, and the analysis is limited to the sounds associated with the female orgasm, either during intercourse or during masturbation. When possible the erotic vocalization data were contrasted to the habitual voice of the same speaker.

Acoustic analyses were performed using standardized acoustic CSL signal processing paradigms (Kay-Pentax) software systems.

Parameters measured were:

■ All signals were analyzed with regard to time, rate, frequency, F_0/dB contour pattern, associated ventilatory components, and other events such as presence of words, grunts, special effects (i.e., banging, noise), or the like.

■ Time measures comprised: (a) total time of the entire acoustic event (OV), called here *orgasmic vocalization delta time* (OVDT) measured in seconds and (b) duration of each segment containing a phonatory cluster or each segment duration (OVSD) including the duration of the respiratory components, all expressed in milliseconds.

■ Rate (OVR) refers to the rate of repetition of segments (OVSD) within total OVDT. The rate is expressed in Hz.

■ Frequency refers to voice fundamental (F_0) measured also in Hz and reflects the averages and ranges of voice F_0 for the entire OVDT and for the segment with most F_0 variation.

■ Contour pattern.

■ Associated respiratory components: description and duration of perceived respiratory components.

■ Words: description of words present.

■ Special effects: i.e., banging, sounds of vibrators, or the like.

In total, 18 samples of OV were analyzed. Thirteen represented downloaded samples and two were obtained from consenting adults, referred to henceforth as ROS. Of the commercial orgasmic voice samples (COVS) one was from *When Harry Met Sally* (HMS), one was from a hard-core porno (HCP), and one from a soft-core porno movie (SCP). Figure 1–2 shows a spectrograph of this type of vocalization with the portion labeled (a) representing a segment from HMS and (b) representing a ROS sample. A glance at this spectrograph demonstrates clearly a disparity between these two representations with respect to all acoustic aspects, all measures, and all representations.

Findings

Findings for these two groups are summarized and contrasted in Table 1–1 and are described below. In general, the ROS group showed distinct differences in all characteristics measured, as discussed next.

■ OVDT Duration: The duration range for OVDT was 2 to 19 seconds. The average OVDT duration was 9 seconds. The HMS OVDT was approximately 67 seconds, or on the average six times longer than the noncommercial rendition.

■ OVSD Duration: The duration range of OVSD ranged from 380 msec to over 1 second. The average duration was about 700 msec. The HMS duration did not differ substantially for the noncommercial OVSD.

■ OVR never exceeded 1.5 Hz, while the commercial rate was up to twice that rate.

■ OV fundamental (F_0) range for the entire OVDT and for individual segments showed at the most one octave to one and a half octave shifts in the ROV cases and wider ranges for the commercial data.

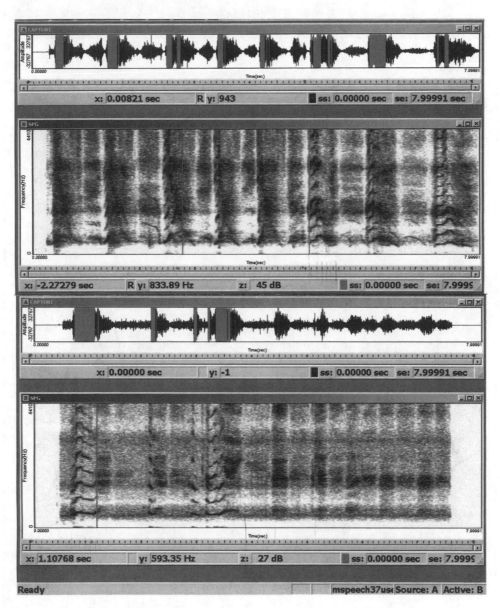

Figure 1–2. Narrowband spectrographs of a segment of ROV **(a)** and a segment of COV **(b)**. Note the differences in all discernible acoustic characteristics. This figure was published in Amygdala responses to nonlinguistic emotional vocalizations. Fecteau, S., Belin, P., Joanette, Y. & Armony, J. L., (2007) *Neuroimage, 36,* 480–487. Reprinted with permision.

Contour patterns for the ROV were more stable or even monotonous looking vocalizations, and showed less F_0 variation (swings), and the overall contours were less unstable than those found in HMS or other commercial OV samples. Hence, a general impression of the ROV patterns was that an OV cluster most often began with a vocalized sound, and less frequently with a sound of air

Table 1–1. Autonomic Effects on Various Organs of the Body

Organ	Effect of Sympathetic Stimulation	Effect of Parasympathetic Stimulation
Eye		
• Pupil	Dilated	Constricted
• Ciliary muscle	Slight relaxation (far vision)	Constricted (near vision)
Glands	Vasoconstriction and slight secretion	Copious secretion (containing many enzymes for enzyme-secreting glands)
Sweat glands	Copious sweating (cholinergic)	Sweating on palms of hands
Heart		
• Muscle	Increased rate Increased force of contraction	Slowed rate Decreased force of contraction (especially of atria)
• Coronary arteries	Dilated (beta$_2$); constricted (alpha)	Dilated
Lungs		
• Bronchi	Dilated	Constricted
Gut		
• Lumen	Decreased peristalsis and tone	Increased peristalsis and tone
• Sphincter	Increased tone (usually)	Relaxed (usually)
Liver	Glucose released	Slight glycogen synthesis
Kidney	Decreased output and renin secretion	None
Bladder		
• Detrusor	Relaxed (slight)	Contracted
• Trigone	Contracted	Relaxed
Penis	Ejaculation	Erection
Systemic arterioles		
• Abdominal viscera	Constricted	None
• Muscle	Constricted (adrenergic alpha) Dilated (adrenergic beta$_2$) Dilated (cholinergic)	None
• Skin	Constricted	None
Blood		
• Coagulation	Increased	None
• Glucose	Increased	None
• Lipids	Increased	None
Basal metabolism	Increased up to 100%	None
Adrenal medullary secretion	Increased	None
Mental activity	Increased	None

Note: From "Disorders of the Autonomic Nervous System: Targeted Pharmacologic and Nonpharmacologic Interventions," by L. D. Foreman. Available from http://www.medscape.com/viewarticle/416459
Data from "Clinical Tutorial #30," by W. Miles. In L. Foreman (Ed.), *NASPE 22nd Annual Scientific Sessions* (p.), 2001.

escaping, and that the cluster specifically toward the final moment terminated with air release (exhalation), while the commercial OV air clusters occurred more or less at random, and not predominantly toward the end of the cluster. Due to sample insecurity, pattern distinctions between self-generated OV (during masturbation) and those from intercourse could not be properly evaluated, but examples that were clearly derived from masturbation samples seemed not to differ in pattern for the intercourse OV. Both however differed from HMS.

The typical F_0 was at about 400–500 Hz levels for the noncommercial OVs. The HMS sound exceeded the F_0 for speech taken from a speech sample by more than two octaves. Though loudness was not measured, the ROV loudness was judged to be not as loud as the commercial renditions.

Contour patterns of F_0 were more often flat or falling in ROV and more rising-falling in non-ROV. Typically, there was a short period of a fast F_0 rise followed by a slowly falling F_0 contour. No strident difference was noted between the intercourse and masturbation samples.

The respiratory (respiratory/ventilatory) component was found to be longer in the ROV samples than it was in the commercial samples. The intensity or force of respiratory component (breathing) appeared stronger in non-ROV samples, and the rate appeared faster in these cases. Both types however showed reduction of rate, and more air expulsion was noted towards termination of the OV event, regardless of the total OVDT duration. Some mixture of vocalization was present in some samples.

Other elements such as speech (*yes, yes, yes, oh God! you are here, fuck,* etc.)

were extremely rare in the ROV samples and were more common in the commercial samples. The same goes for screaming, banging, and the sounds I termed here, special effects, while the presence of other environmental sounds (music and vibrators) was also rare in ROV samples examined. It is important to be cautious when interpreting these data as "average" or "typical," because it is assumed theoretically that emotions are purely individual and that vocal expressions will be expressed on case-by-case basis.

Perceptual Descriptions

Perceptual accounts describing OV provided by adults who were willing to provide these descriptions corroborated most findings obtained on the basis of Internet accessed samples, rightly or wrongly considered to represent real vocal events. The use of these perceptual accounts and entering these observations as a form of antecedent analysis may be questioned as scientifically dubious, but by doing so, in fact, I dared to rule out two OV segments from the Internet accessed data as non-ROV segments, based on their patterns. One of these segments was indeed a fragment (*oh yes, yes, yes* . . .) from the HMS sample analyzed here. The other representation was embedded as an example of orgasmic sound on one of the sites, and this sample differed perceptually and acoustically from the majority of other samples. Reported masturbation sounds were limited to a respiratory component and calm vocalization. Mechanical vs. manual masturbation samples were too few to render any pattern distinction.

Summary

There are several inherent problems with this account: (a) unclear origins of the majority of sounds downloaded from the Internet assumed to represent ROV, (b) lack of contrasting the data with a general model of erotic vocalization, (c) relying on a small sample of verified ROV sounds, (d) incorporating recollection into the process of scientific inquiry, (e) small sample size, (f) even smaller sample of what I termed here commercial OV, (g) lack of matching modal voicing and experimental voicing for the same sample of OV, to mention just few and very obvious drawbacks. Setting these inherent weaknesses aside, the data presented here appear to represent the first organized attempt to address this specific aspect of human vocalization. Findings are in a way surprising and seem to substantiate ancient teachings that vocalization of emotions, including those associated with lovemaking and specifically with orgasm, are brief and gentle, follow respiratory and muscular contraction rates, in a way are very intimate and do not reach the commercially presented vocal crescendos and screams, and are not really associated with or contaminated by dirty talking or in general with any talking at all.

It is mostly the voice and air (exhalatory air) that convey information and signal arrival of an orgasm, perhaps satisfaction, approval, and love. And therefore the amygdala and the hypothalamus appear to be involved perhaps more on the right than the left side as these sounds carry pleasant information.

The almost flat and unornamented F_0 pattern seems to connote peace and its prolongation signals pleasure, while the fluctuations may be attached to individual means of stressing joy, but in a gentle and not vocally violent way, as manifested by pitch elevation; pitch elevation is mostly part of joy. Although the amplitude of these vocal signals was not analyzed here, a generalized view of the signal amplitude seems to show a drop-off at the termination of each segment and with termination of the entire OV sequence. The amplitude variations are not wide.

The rate of OV was found to be rather slow and hence seems to be regulated by the respiratory rather than by the laryngeal component, which seems to have an optimal rate of 5 Hz. In this way, ROV seems to be mediated through the coordination of the sympathetic nervous system, vocalization, and ventilation and not via speech motor cortex, the cerebellum, or the left brain. The sound appears to be the by-product of the respiratory flow, onto which the voice is placed, like throwing a leaf and not a stone onto a stream of water, and making it all flow together without a splash.

In conclusion, the results seem to support the teaching of Tantra and Tao that talking may be distractive, while breathy, relaxed, and focused vocalization and air flow associated with breathing and some laryngeal (glottic) narrowing are more rewarding and reflect more the emotional state of an orgasm than screaming and yelling, "Oh God, yes, yes, yes baby yessss." So being breathy (as in respiration) brings us closer to the sound of the laughter of apes, which in at least one experimental study was interpreted as a sound of lovemaking. It thus shows that the species differ but only by a little.

I don't want to trivialize this subject, but I wish to admit that this chapter was intended to be a "teaser" (no pun intended) rather than a pure scientific inquiry written in a scientific style, and that soon we will be able to get down to a more rigorous and scientific study of the seductive voice in its multitude of manifestations, and of the ROV, the voice we adults want to hear if just once in a while. So finally, how about Harry's "I do know" statement? Let me guess if you now can tell with more assurance if Hollywood knows best. After all, as one female proclaimed wisely (though for the purists the concept of these two loves are at odds), "The Scriptures tell us to love, and Kamasutra tells us how to" (Stralek, 2006) I dare to add silently, "Let's go."

Acknowledgments. I am grateful for the critical and constructive remarks given this chapter by the following scholars: Dr. Branka Zei-Pollermann (Switzerland), Dr. Anne-Maria Laukannen (Finland), Dr. Raul M. Cruz (USA), Dr. Mara Behlau (Brazil), Dr. Shirly Fecteau (Canada and USA).

Postscripts

In discussing this chapter with Dr. Branka Zei-Pollermann of the Geneva Emotion Group, and a contributor to this volume, the following was suggested.

Q: What is the semiological status of sexual vocalization?

A: Is it a spontaneous indicator of an emotional state?
If it is, then it is not surprising that every person will sound different. This is entirely determined by the so-called push force (see Scherer, 1988).

B: Is it produced to intentionally communicate the feelings of the moment?
If it is, then the sound should have a somewhat conventionalized character to transmit the intended meaning (Schroeder, n.d.).

After reading this chapter Branka also suggested that with respect to male orgasmic behavior, she wished to see a physiologically clear link between vocalization and erection in relation to vagal tone and the ups and downs of sympathetic or parasympathetic domination (see Table 1–1) and the corresponding consequences for voice production. For more on this, the reader is referred to the model proposed by Scherer (1988).

Branka also wants to see a distinction between the erection or pre-erection period dominated by the parasympathetic system and the accompaniment of the lax, low, and soft voice, and the ejaculation period dominated by the sympathetic system with the resulting consequences of vocalization in a tense voice, with higher pitch and louder volume, all influenced by the breathing pattern (Foreman, n.d.).

In preparing for this chapter I have searched (and I continue to do so on daily basis as I never seem to be able to finish writing this chapter) endlessly all possible sources. I can willingly admit that I may have failed in my efforts to unveil the obvious, but my inquiry took me into all possible directions. I searched world literature, all kinds of Web sites and links, I conducted physical searches of multiple volumes in the libraries, bookstores, etc, and I found only faint traces of the information I was looking for. I felt a little bit like the secret service investigators portrayed in the 1967 controversial British TV fantasy-drama series starring Patrick McGoohan entitled "The Prisoner," interpreted by some of the fans as a comment on the relationship between the individual and society, or as a study of the nature of mankind. In this for-TV serial the hero was tormented by the authorities, by being endlessly asked for one and only one thing, namely for the *information*. I really encourage the reader to go to http://www.youarenumber6.com to hear this dialog, "What do you want?" The emotional quality of these voices remains superbly executed, and both scary and chilling.

In March 2006 alone, I went through the indexes of 78 different books on sexuality that I found at one of the most prestigious academic bookstores in the nation, Cody's Bookstore on the famous Telegraph Avenue in Berkeley, California, just few steps from the gate where the free speech movement started. Ironically, this monument will be closed forever on July 10, 2006). These efforts located only three (yes, *three*) publications that had a few lines on voice/vocalization and sex, and I am referencing these here. This rare find translates essentially to more or less 100 lines of text on the subject of vocalization among the 15,000 pages or 1,200,000 lines or so of the global text on the subject of human sex on Cody's bookshelves.

I also had live librarians help me to find sources. They used some complicated tricks only librarians are privileged to, trying all possible recognized call words (voice, vocalization, sex, sexual behavior, interaction, intercourse, orgasms, etc., and in all possible combinations) for all available peer-referred journals and without restrictions to any language or the year of publication. All essentially in vain. I also contacted by phone and by e-mail

some leading sex education experts, university based sex advice lines, sex culture organizations or spiritual sensual gurus in the world, and my quest was answered only either with silence, with no sounds or no replies, Results: no specific information was provided. And one such recognized expert on human sexual behavior replied, "Regretfully, we have no information on the subjects of your inquiry" in an e-mail response to my inquiry (Izdebski, personal communication, 2006). Moreover, direct data search of the most prestigious institutes dedicated to studying human sexual behavior was equally disappointing and yielded minimal or no references to the subject of voice and eroticism.

References

Abitbol, J. (2006). *Odyssey of the voice*. San Diego, CA: Plural.

Abitbol, J., Abitol, R., & Abitbol, B. (1999). Sex hormone and the female voice. *Journal of Voice, 15*(3), 424–446.

Anolli, L., & Ciceri, R. (2002). Analysis of the vocal profiles of male seduction: From exhibition to self-disclosure. *Journal of General Psychology, 129*, 149–169.

Aron. A., Fisher, H., Mashek, D. J., Strong, G., Li, H., & Brown, L. L. (2005). Reward, motivation, and emotion systems associated with early-stage intense romantic love. *Journal of Neurophysiology, 94*(1), 327–337.

Bartels, A., & Zeki, S. (2000). The neural basis of romantic love. *Neuroreport, 11*(17), 3829–3834.

Bartels, A., & Zeki, S. (2004). The neural correlates of maternal and romantic love. *Neuroimage, 21*(3), 1155–1166.

Blavatsky, H. (1999). *The secret doctrine: The synthesis of science, religion, and philos-*

ophy. Pasadena, CA: Theosophical University Press.

Bohlen, J. G. (1983). State of the science of sexual physiology research. In C. M. Davis (Ed.), *Challenge in sexual science*. Philadelphia: Christopher Booker.

Bordwell, D. (2006). *The way Hollywood tells It*. Berkeley: University of California Press.

Brainy Quotes. (2007). Lord Chesterfield. http://www.brainyquote.com/quotes/authors/l/lord_chesterfield

Brauer, A. P., Brauer, D., & Brauer, D. J. (2001). *Eso: How you and your lover can give each other hours of extended sexual orgasm*. New York: Warner Books.

Brian, A., Murray, C., Brahler, J., Baer, J., & Marotta, J. (2003). Correlations between activity and blood pressure in African American women and girls. [Electronic version]. *Journal of Exercise Physiology*, *6*(3), 38-44.

Bridges, C. F., Critelli, J. W., & Loos, V. E. (1985). Hypnotic susceptibility, inhibitory control, and orgasmic consistency. *Archives of Sexual Behavior*, *14*(4), 373-376.

Bucuk, M., Muzur, A., Willheim, K., Jurjevic, A., Tomic, Z., & Tuskan-Mohar, L. (2004). Make love to forget: Two cases of transient global amnesia triggered by sexual intercourse. *College Anthropology*, *28*(2), 899-905.

Chia, M., & Abrams, R. C. (2005). *The multiorgasmic woman*. New York: Rodale Books.

Dedo, H. H., & Izdebski, K. (1983). Intermediate results of 306 RLN sections for spastic dysphonia. *Laryngoscope*, *93*, 9-16.

Dembski, W. A. (1999). *Intelligent design: The bridge between science and theology*. Downers Grove, IL: InterVarsity Press.

Dessilets, S. (2003). *Female ejaculation. The ancient art of ambrosia*. Available from: http://www.universal-tao.com

de Weerth, C., & Kalma, A. (1995). Gender differences in awareness of courtship initiation tactics. *Sex Roles*, *32*(11-12), 717-734.

Eckert, P., & McConnell-Ginet, S. (2003). *Language and gender*. Cambridge, UK: Cambridge University Press.

Fecteau, S., Armony, J. L., Joanette, Y., & Belin, B. (2005). Judgment of emotional nonlinguistic vocalizations: Age-related differences. *Applied Neuropsychology*, *12*, 40-48.

Fecteau, S., Belin, P., Joanette, Y., & Armony, J. L. (2007). Amygdala responses to nonlinguistic emotional vocalizations. *Neuroimage*, *36*, 480-487.

Filmsite.org. (n.d.). Sex in cinema: The greatest and most influential erotic/sexual films and scenes. Available from http://filmsite.org

Fisher, H. (2004). *Why we love: The nature and chemistry of romantic love*. New York: Henry Holt.

Fisher, H., Aron, A., & Brown, L. L. (2005). Romantic love: An fMRI study of a neural mechanism for mate choice. *Journal of Comparative Neurology*, *493*(1), 58-62.

Fisher, H. E., Aron, A., Mashek, D., Li, H., & Brown, L. L. (2002). Defining the brain systems of lust, romantic attraction, and attachment. *Archives of Sexual Behavior*, *31*(5), 413-419.

Fisher, H. E., & Thomson, Jr., J. A. (2007). Lust, romance, attachment: Do the side-effects of serotonin-enhancing antidepressants jeopardize romantic love, marriage and fertility? In S. M. Platek, J. P. Keenan, & T. K. Shakellford (Eds.), *Evolutionary cognitive neuroscience* (pp. 245-283). Cambridge, MA: MIT Press.

Foreman, L. D. (n.d.). Disorders of the autonomic nervous system: Targeted pharmacologic and nonpharmacologic interventions. Available from http://www.medscape.com/viewarticle/416459

Gajewski, M. (2006). Na swieta wreszcie w domu. *PANI, Styczen*, *184*(1), 33.

Gallager, W. (1986). The etiology of orgasm. *Discover*, 51-59.

Gallagher, J., Murphy, M. S., & Carroll, J. (2005). Transient global amnesia after sexual intercourse. *Irish Journal of Medical Science*, *174*(3), 86-87.

Gaudio, R. (1994). Sounding gay: Pitch properties of gay and straight men. *American Speech*, *69*(1), 30–57.

Gorky Park. (n.d.). Available from http://www.greatestfilms.org

Gosselin, N., Peretz, I., Noulhiane, M., Hasboun, D, Beckett, C., Baulac, M., et al. (2005). Impaired recognition of scary music following unilateral temporal lobe excision. *Brain*, *128*(Pt. 3), 628–640.

Green, R. M. (1992). *Kierkegaard and Kant: The hidden debt*. New York: State University of New York Press.

Hartman, W. E., & Fithian, M. A. (1972). *The treatment of sexual dysfunction: A bio-psycho-social approach*. Long Beach, CA: Center for Marital and Sexual Studies.

Holstege, G., Georgiadis, J. R., Paans, A. M., Meiners, L. C., van der Graaf, F. H., & Reinders, A. A. (2003). Brain activation during human male ejaculation. *Journal of Neuroscience*, *23*(27), 9185–9193.

Hughes, S. M., Dispenza, F., & Gallup, G. G., Jr. (2004). Ratings of voice attractiveness predict sexual behavior and body configuration. *Evolution and Human Behavior*, *25*, 295–304.

Hughes, S. M., & Gallup, G. G., Jr. (2003). Sex differences in morphological predictors of sexual behavior: Shoulder to hip and waist to hip ratios. *Evolution and Human Behavior*, *24*, 173–178.

Hutcherson, H. (2005). *Pleasure: A woman's guide to getting the sex you want, need, and deserve*. New York: G. P. Putnam's Sons.

IMDb. (n.d.). *Biography for Dennis Potter.* Available from http://www.imdb.com/name/nm0693259/bio

Izdebski, K. (2006). Personal conversation.

Izdebski, K. (1992). Symptomatology of adductor spasmodic dysphonia: A physiologic model. *Journal of Voice*, *6*, 306–319.

Izdebski, Z., & Ostrowska, A. (2004). *Seks po polsku*. MUZA SA, Warszawa

Jacobs, G. (1996). Lesbian and gay male language use: A critical review. *American Speech*, *71*(1), 49–71.

Jan Pawel, II. (John Paul II, The Pope). (1995). *Encyklika evangelium vitae*. Kraków, Poland and Libreria Editrice Vaticana, Vatican.

Karama, S., Lecours, A. R., Leroux, J.-M., Bourgouin, P., Beaudoin, G., Joubert, S., et al. (2002). Areas of brain activation in males and females during viewing of erotic film excerpts. *Human Brain Mapping*, *16*(1), 1–13.

Kelly, M. P., Strassberg, D. S., & Turner, C. M. (2006). Behavioral assessment of couples' communication in female orgasmic disorder. *Journal of Sexual Marital Therapy*, *32*(2), 81–95.

Kinsey, A. C., Pomeroy, W. B., Martin, C. E., Gebhard, P. H., & Bancroft, J. (1998). *Sexual behavior and the human male*. Bloomington: Indiana University Press.

Komisaruk, B. R., & Whipple, B. (1991). Physiological perceptual correlates of orgasm produced by genital and non-genital stimulation. In P. Kothari (Ed.), *Proceedings of the First International Conference on Orgasm*. Bombay, India: VRP.

Kulick, D. (2000). Gay and lesbian language. *Annual Review of Anthropology*, *29*, 243–285.

Laan, E., Everaerd, W., van Bellen, G., & Hanewald, G. (1994). Women's sexual and emotional responses to male- and female-produced erotica. *Archives of Sexual Behavior*, *23*(2), 153–169.

Levin, R. J., & Wagner, G. (1985). Orgasm in women in the laboratory—Quantitative studies on duration, intensity, latency, and vaginal blood flow. *Archives of Sexual Behavior*, *14*(5), 439–449.

Levon, E. (2004). *Examining a gay prosody: Issues in theory, methodology and identity.* Paper presented at Lavender Languages and Linguistics XI, American University, Washington, DC.

Linville, S. E. (1998). Acoustic correlates of perceived versus actual sexual orientation in men's speech. *Folia Phoniatrica et Logopaedica*, *50*, 35–48.

Lonsdale, D., Brown, B. L., & Spackman, M. P. (2007). Emotion and vocal attractiveness. In K. Izdebski (Ed.), *Voice and emotion* (Vol. 1, chap. 2). San Diego, CA: Plural.

Mah, K., & Binik, Y. M. (2002). Do all orgasms feel alike? Evaluating a two-dimensional model of the orgasm experience across gender and sexual context. *Journal of Sexual Research*, *39*(2), 104–113.

Mah, K., & Binik, Y. M. (2005). Are orgasms in the mind or the body? Psychosocial versus physiological correlates of orgasmic pleasure and satisfaction. *Sexual Marital Therapy*, *31*(3), 187–200.

Masters, W. H., & Johnson, V. E. (1966). *Human sexual response*. Boston: Little, Brown.

Miller, S. A., & Byers, E. S. (2004). Actual and desired duration of foreplay and intercourse: Discordance and misperceptions within heterosexual couples. *Journal of Sexual Research*, *41*(3), 301–309.

Mulac, A., Jansma, L. A., & Linz, D. G. (2002). Men's behavior toward women after viewing sexually-explicit films: Degradation makes a difference. *Communication Monographs*, *69*(4), 311–328.

Munson, B., Jefferson, S. V., & McDonald, E. C. (2006). The influence of perceived sexual orientation on fricative identification. *Journal of the Acoustical Society of America*, *119*(4), 2427–2437.

Murray, B. A., Brahler, C. J., Baer, J., & Marotta, J. (2003, August). Correlations between activity and blood pressure in African women and girls. *Journal of Exercise Physiologyonline*, *6*(3).

Murray, S. (2006, June 8). Gay marriage amendment fails in Senate. *Washington Post*, p. A01.

Nikitopoulos, E., Arnhem, P., van Hooff, J. A. R. A. M., & Sterck, E. H. (2004). Influence of female copulation calls on male sexual behavior in captive Macaca fascicularis. *International Journal of Primatology*, *25*(3), 659–677.

Panksepp, J., & Bernatzky, G. (2002). Emotional sounds and the brain: The neuroaffective foundations of musical appreciation. *Behavioural Processes*, *60*, 133.

Passie, T., Hartmann, U., Schneider, U., & Emrich, H. M. (2003). On the function of groaning and hyperventilation during sexual intercourse: Intensification of sexual experience by altering brain metabolism through hypocapnia. *Medical Hypotheses*, *60*(5), 660–663.

Podesva, R. (2003). *The stylistic use of phonation type: Falsetto, fundamental frequency and the linguistic construction of personae*. Unpublished manuscript, Stanford University, Palo Alto, CA.

Podesva, R., Roberts, S., & Campbell-Kibler, K. (2002). Sharing resources and indexing meaning in the production of gay styles. In K. Campbell-Kibler, R. Podesva, S. Roberts, & A. Wong (Eds.), *Language and sexuality: Contesting meaning in theory and practice* (pp. 175–190). Palo Alto, CA: Stanford Center for the Study of Language and Information.

Polan, M. L., Desmond, J. E., Banner, L. L., Pryor, M. R., McCallum, S.W., et al. (2003). Female sexual arousal: A behavioral analysis. *Fertility and Sterility*, *80*(6), 1480–1487.

Provine, R. R. (2003). *Laughter: A scientific investigation*. New York: Penguin Books.

Rellini, A. H., McCall, K. M., Randall, P. K., & Meston, C. M. (2005). The relationship between women's subjective and physiological sexual arousal. *Psychophysiology*, *42*, 116–124.

Rogers, H., & Smyth, R. (2003). Phonetic differences between gay- and straight-sounding male speakers of North American English. In *Proceedings of the 15th International Congress of Phonetic Sciences* (pp. 1855–1858). Barcelona, Spain: Universitat Autònoma de Barcelona.

Rogers, H. H, Smyth, R., & Jacobs, G. (2000). *Vowel and sibilant duration in gay- and straight-sounding male speech*. Paper presented at IGALA 1, Stanford University, Stanford, CA.

Salt N Pepa. (n.d.). Sexy noises turn me on [Lyrics]. Available from http://www.sing365.com/music/Lyric.nsf/Sexy-Noises-Turn-Me-On-lyrics-Salt-N-Pepa/531AD985F0CB4A00482568A900252D18-17k

Savic, I., Berglund, H., & Lindstrom, P. (2005). Brain response to putative pheromones in homosexual men. *Proceedings of the*

National Academy of Science USA, *102*(20), 7356-7361.

Scherer, K. R. (1988). *Facets of emotion*. Mahweh, NJ: Lawrence Erlbaum Associates.

Schneider, B., Cohen, E., Stani, J., Kolbus, A., Rudas, M., et al. (2006). Towards the expression of sex hormone receptors in the human vocal fold. *Journal of Voice, 21*(4), 502-507.

Schroeder, M. (n.d.). Available from http://www.qub.ac.uk/en/isca/proceedings/pdfs/schroeder.pdf

Shenton, A. K. (n.d.). *A critical comparison of two works of British television drama: The unmutual prisoner. The projection room* (The prisoner compared . . .) "Cloud burst." Available from http://ww.theunmutual.co.uk/comparescloudburst.htm

Singer, J., & Singer, I. (1978). Types of female orgasm. In J. LoPiccolo & L. LoPiccolo (Eds.), *Handbook of sex therapy*. New York: Plenum Press.

Smyth, R., Jacobs, G., & Rogers, H. (2003). Male voices and perceived sexual orientation: An experimental and theoretical approach. *Language in Society, 32*(3), 329-350.

Stowers, L., Holy, T. E., Meister, M., Dulac, C., & Koentges, G. (2002). Loss of sex discrimination and male-male aggression in mice deficient for TRP2. *Science, 295*(5559), 1493-1500.

Syriana. (2005). Available from http://www.writings0tudio.co.za/page1087.html

Trinkl, A. (1999). Hormone involved I reproduction may have role in the maintenance of relationships. Retrieved July 14, 1999, from http://www.pub.ucsf.edu/newsservices/releases/2004010721

Villella, A., Ferri, S. L., Krystal, J. D., & Hall, J. C. (2005). Functional analysis of fruitless gene expression by transgenic manipulations of Drosophila courtship. *Proceedings of the National Academy of Science USA, 102*(46),16550-16557.

Walker, C. (2004, April 20). Ancient Egyptian love poems reveal a lust for life: The flower song. (M. V. Fox, Trans.). *National Geographic News*. Available from http://www.news.nationalgeographic.com/news/2004/04/0416

Warraq, I. (2002, January 12). Virgins? What virgins? *Guardian Unlimited*. Available from http://www.guardian.co.uk/saturday_review/story/0,3605,631332,00.html4

When Harry Met Sally. (1989). Available from http://www.greatestfilms.org

Whipple, B., Hartman, W. E., & Fithian, M. A. (1994). Good vibrations. In V. L. Bullough & B. Bullough (Eds.), *Human sexuality: An encyclopedia* (pp. 430-433). New York: Garland.

Whipple, B., Ogden, G., & Komisaruk, R. B. (1992). Physiological correlates of imagery induced orgasm in women. *Archives of Sexual Behavior, 21*, 121-133.

Wysocki, C. J., & Preti, G. (2004). Facts, fallacies, fears, and frustrations with human pheromones. *Anatomic Record, Part A: Discoveries in Molecular, Cellular, and Evolutionary Biology, 281*(1), 1201-1211.

APPENDIX A

Emotion and Language

In discussing the material for this chapter with my colleagues (both female and male), from all parts of the world, cultures, and religions, and who are all completely cosmopolitan, it became clear that speaking is a part of the initial part of the act of lovemaking, and that emotional speaking in general is felt best when it is executed in the language that is native to the person.

It is noted by many that, when partners speak to each other in the moments of high emotional load, both pleasant and unpleasant in content or context, they may automatically reverse to the primary language, even if that language may no longer be used on daily basis. When expressing emotions in the secondary language, the prosodic features associated with emotive states may suffer or be in a way "contorted" by the learned constraints of the new language, often because of the inherent prosodic pattern difference between the languages, and possibly because the familiarity of the other language affects the pitch level (see Chapter 14 in this volume). And this brings to my mind an interesting observation expressed in a single sentence that I read in a ladies' magazine at the beginning of January 2006 while on a trip in Warsaw, Poland. The article in question, "Na Swieta Wreszcie w Domu" by M. Gajewski (n.d.) ("Finally at Home for the Holidays"), was an interview with a Hollywood based but Polish born actress, Ms Joanna Pacula, most known for her Globe nominated role in the 1983 movie entitled *Gorky Park* (n.d.). Like many things in California, this movie creation seems to typify the cosmopolitan character of our life here. Ms. Pacula was born in Poland, and moved more or less involuntarily to the USA via France during the period of the marshall law in Poland. In the movie, she plays a Russian woman, as a matter of fact of Siberian origin. The name of her character she plays is Irina Asanova (sic), not to be confused with Dinara Asanova (a Soviet era cinematographer born in what is today known as Kyrgyztan). One of Pacula's lines in the movie is "The director of that film promised me a pair of new boots if I went to bed with him. Think I should?" spoken in my opinion rather unemotionally as with defiant intention and an apparent disgust for the interrogating police inspector. The actual director of *Gorky Park,* not the one in the movie, was British born Michael Apted, and most of the main character actors were either English or Scottish. The movie was filmed on location in Glasgow (Scotland), Stockholm (Sweden), and Helsinki (Suomi-Finland) and compiled in California. The writing credits go to a Pennsylvania born American novelist whose mother was a Pueblo Indian jazz singer and to an Englishman cowriter who once wanted to be a politician; when he discovered he was afflicted with cancer, he nick-named it "Rupert" to register his disdain for the Australian born media mogul Rupert Murdoch (Bordwell, 2006). (For more trivia on this see http://www.imdb.com/name/nm0693259/bio). In the piece of text I am referring to published by PANI monthly magazine (see page 33), this native Polish actress working in Hollywood for nearly 25 years and acting predominantly in the English language was discussing that she has been perceived by some of her countrymen (in fact, women) when she visits Poland as being no longer a fluent Polish language speaker because of her occasional insertions of English words and at times what I am interpreting as a mispronunciation of the Polish language. Ms. Pacula states in this interview to her defense (and I read it as a rather bitter remark) that she feels unjustly blamed for these linguistic problems, as she is subject (the same way I am, by the way) to a linguistic emigrant driven diaspora. She hence explains *"rozmawiam, denerwuje sie i ciesze w jezyku angielskim,"* roughly translated as "I converse, express my anger and my joy in the English language," meaning that she needs to use English on day-to-day basis because she lives in Southern California and lives there to the fullest extent of the meaning of this word. So what is my point? The point being, that it may be at times cumbersome to express spontaneously and verbally the emotions in other than the native language, and it may be easier to do so when the emotions are part of acting. This difficulty is not an uncommon experience in my own multilingual and multicultural international life, as I journeyed and grew up in at least four different cultural and linguistically diverse societies at different stages of my life, and I attempted to fit as best as I could into each sociolinguistic milieu with all the consequences. Though I considered myself fluent in many languages, two things remained constant. One was the fact that my deep emotions were always connected best to my primary language and prosody, and second, my dream to be a TV anchor in each of these strange languages is a proof to myself that I really got it. The furthest I ever got with the second one was a 3½ year career as a voluntary DJ at a college FM station in San Francisco.

The role of using a foreign language in acting, to portray realistically the character of a nonnative, is becoming nowadays a symbol of well-deserved acculturation and tolerance, even in Hollywood. In fact, what Hollywood tells us is not always bad (Bordwell, 2006). More on the role of international actors in the movies and the quest for linguistic accuracy and expressions can be learned from a Web site discussing how important it was to portray linguistic truth in the recent movie *Syriana* (2005).

CHAPTER 2

A Rationale for Exploring Vocal Pleasantness

Deryle Lonsdale, Matthew P. Spackman, and Bruce L. Brown

Abstract

This chapter addresses the notion of vocal pleasantness, a long-neglected aspect of the human voice. The pleasing qualities of a voice are somewhat related to vocal attractiveness and to vocal expressions of emotion. Possible research approaches for investigating the notion of vocal pleasantness are explored.

A Rationale for Exploring Vocal Pleasantness

Voices perceived as pleasant would be, according to the *Oxford English Dictionary* (online version http://www.oed.com/), "Agreeable to the mind, feelings, or senses." However, few studies in the literature examine vocal pleasantness directly, and when pleasantness is dis-

cussed, exact definitions are elusive. Still, there may be convergent concepts from other areas of nonverbal communication that help in defining the issues. In particular, there is need to distinguish vocal pleasantness from a number of other vocal characterizations that exist in the literature and to ask how they relate to vocal pleasantness. For example, as there are a number of studies of vocal attractiveness it may be productive to ask how vocal pleasantness and vocal attractiveness relate to one another. Can one imagine, for example, a voice that is attractive but not pleasant, or conversely a voice that is pleasant but not attractive?

Another question to be asked is how particular emotions in voice relate to the concept of pleasantness. Can anger be expressed in pleasant as well as unpleasant ways? If so, what would differentiate them acoustically? A similar question could be asked of happiness. Can it be expressed in a uniquely unpleasant way? On the other hand, it could be that there are some emotions that are inherently pleasant or unpleasant and examples could not be found that vary on the dimension of pleasantness.

One should differentiate between the ratings of vocal pleasantness—the topic of this chapter—and the ratings of perceived pleasantness (or attractiveness) of the speaker on the basis of his or her idiosyncratic vocal qualities. Although some scant literature exists on each of these issues, where it does exist, the variables are not well defined. Vocal pleasantness is almost never defined for the respondents—they are simply asked to rate voices for pleasantness.

Here, then, we attempt to explore vocal pleasantness from a theoretical viewpoint, and make suggestions for further research that could help provide insight into vocal pleasantness. This chapter will therefore focus on definitional and conceptual issues. Given the uneven coverage of previous literature on the topics of vocal attractiveness, pleasantness, and emotion, we begin by attempting to tease apart the relevant distinctions and what previous work has revealed in each of these areas.

Literature Review

Emotion and Pleasantness

There is a large body of research on the vocal and acoustical concomitants of various emotions and evidence of a fair degree of agreement as to the concomitants associated with particular emotions. The publication of Darwin's (1872) work on expressions of emotion in humans and animals not only legitimated emotions as a topic worthy of scientific inquiry but also introduced what has become an important area of investigation of itself, that is, the question of how emotions are communicated. Two major areas of research emerged from Darwin's work on communication of emotion. The first addresses how emotions are communicated via the face (see, for example, Ekman, 1972; Ekman, 1994). The second area of research is relevant to the issue of pleasantness of voice and addresses the question of how emotion is encoded by the voice.

The majority of research on vocal communication of emotions has addressed two primary questions: a) Can persons accurately identify emotions expressed by persons' voices? and b) What are the properties of the voice associated with particular emotions (Banse & Scherer, 1996)?[1] There seems to be agreement in the literature that persons can identify emotions from voice at better than chance levels of accuracy (Banse & Scherer, 1996; Murray & Arnott, 1993; Pittam & Scherer, 1993; Scherer, 1986; Scherer, Banse, Wallbott, & Goldbeck 1991; Van Bezooijan, 1984; Wallbott & Scherer, 1986). In addition, though the literature has not been as consistent, vocal and

---

[1]A third question has also received more recent attention: Are the vocal correlates for particular emotions similar across cultures (Elfenbein & Ambady, 2002; Scherer, 2003)?

acoustic profiles for particular emotions have become relatively well identified (Bacharowski & Owren, 2003; Banse & Scherer, 1996; Juslin & Laukka, 2003; Murray & Arnott, 1993; Pittam & Scherer, 1993; Scherer, 1986; Scherer et al., 1991; Wallbott & Scherer, 1986).

Given that particular emotions such as anger and happiness have been shown to have relatively stable and differentiated vocal and acoustic profiles, it may well be asked to what extent particular vocal expressions of emotions are associated with pleasantness of voice. At least two possible relationships between vocal expressions of emotion and vocal pleasantness may be suggested. It may be that particular emotional expressions are perceived as being relatively pleasant or unpleasant. For example, happiness is generally seen as an experientially pleasant emotion. It may be that persons' voices signaling happiness are also perceived as pleasant. Anger is often perceived as an experientially unpleasant emotion. It may be that vocal expressions of anger are perceived as being unpleasant.

A second relationship between vocal expressions of emotion and vocal pleasantness may, however, be suggested. That is, it may be that particular emotions are not themselves associated with pleasant or unpleasant voices, but that emotions may be encoded in a pleasant or unpleasant fashion. For example, happiness may be expressed vocally in such a way as to be perceived as pleasant but may also be encoded in an unpleasant fashion (e.g., the high-pitched, screaming happiness of young children). Anger could be vocally encoded in such a way as to be pleasant (e.g., the almost kindly angry threat one might imagine making with a smile) or unpleasant.

We are aware of no research on the relationship between the vocal or acoustic profiles of particular emotions and pleasantness of voice. In addition, and as discussed above, there is very little research on the vocal or acoustic profiles of a pleasant or unpleasant voice. What scant research we have found on the characteristics of vocal pleasantness involved ratings of vocal properties of voices (Buller & Burgoon, 1986; Burgoon, 1978; Burgoon, Birk, & Pfau, 1990; Deal & Oyer, 1991).

We have found no research on vocal pleasantness incorporating acoustical measures. The few studies on the properties of pleasant voices we have found indicate that vocal pleasantness is associated with voice qualities such as warmth, fluency, clarity, variability of pitch, and variability in tempo. Unpleasant voices, at least for English, have been associated with pauses, nasality, and lack of variability in pitch and tempo. Other languages and cultures may differ on the perceived pleasantness of these dimensions.

As the characteristics associated with pleasant and unpleasant voices in the literature are vocal ratings of voice quality, and not acoustic measures, matching these characteristics to the profiles of particular emotions found in the literature is difficult. Some of these voice characteristics are readily operationalized, such as variability of pitch and tempo, but the remaining characteristics are not easily operationalized and have not been employed in studies of vocal expressions of emotion. For example, pleasant voices have been found to have variability in pitch. Juslin and Laukka's (2003) extensive review of studies of vocal expressions of emotion indicates that both happiness and anger have also been found to have high variability of pitch.

It would, however, be premature to conclude that both happiness and anger may be associated with pleasant voice. Happiness and anger have been found to be differentiable on the basis of other vocal/acoustic characteristics and none of these include such dimensions as warmth, another characteristic associated with pleasant voice. At this point, the degree to which vocal pleasantness is associated with particular emotions or the degree to which particular emotions may be encoded in pleasant or unpleasant fashion is unclear.

Differentiating Vocal Pleasantness and Vocal Attractiveness

Researchers investigating vocal pleasantness are faced with the conceptual question of the relationship between vocal pleasantness and vocal attractiveness. Though there is some research that bears on the topic (see the Future Directions section below), it is a question that has not received sufficient attention. In addressing this issue, it may be helpful to draw some parallels to facial pleasantness and attractiveness. It is not difficult to imagine examples of attractive faces that are, in many senses, unpleasant—such as the cold and proud images of highly attractive fashion models. Conversely, one can imagine the visage of a kind and sweet-faced, but haggard and wrinkled, elderly woman. Are there vocal analogues of these two examples?

Studies may well be designed to differentiate between vocal pleasantness and attractiveness. One hypothesis is that vocal attractiveness is associated with perceptions of competence/dominance/ social attractiveness, and that vocal pleasantness is associated with perceptions of benevolence/kindness/altruism.

We might well ask whether pleasantness is positively correlated with attractiveness. The answer is most likely yes, and it is probably a fairly strong correlation. However, it may be more theoretically productive to ask whether one could identify or synthesize voices that are attractive but not pleasant, or pleasant but not attractive. Such a procedure would enable us to tease apart the divergence in meaning between vocal pleasantness and vocal attractiveness and to then examine carefully the acoustic and vocal properties of such voices.

An additional distinction important to differentiating vocal pleasantness and vocal attractiveness is that between perceptions of speakers' voices and of their personalities. There is a fairly large body of research from several decades ago on personality attributions associated with particular vocal and acoustical characteristics (Apple, Streeter, & Krauss, 1979; Brown, Strong, & Rencher, 1973; 1974; 1975; Scherer, 1979). These personality attributions are made for the speaker. It is important to separate the issues of ratings of speakers from ratings of speakers' voices, as personality ratings of speakers may well be independent of ratings of their voices. A likeable and pleasant person could conceivably have a very unpleasant voice and, conversely, a dour or churlish person could have a highly pleasant voice.

Vocal Attractiveness and Vocal/Acoustical Mediators

When we make judgments about others we evaluate their actions, their looks, and even their voices. Unfavorable first impressions may be due to a "weak voice" (Zuckerman, Miyake, & Hodgins,

1991), and voice-based negative impressions are difficult to overcome (Giles & Powesland, 1975). Certain personality characteristics are routinely inferred based on vocal characteristics, and people tend to agree on what types of personalities these characteristics imply (Kramer, 1964; Scherer, 1979). In this section, we explore the vocal/acoustical correlates of vocal attractiveness.

Though the literature exploring the acoustic and vocal correlates of attractive voice is scant, some research has addressed how the characteristics of a speaker's voice affect perception of the speaker's personality. Addington (1968) matched nine vocal characteristics to 40 personality traits via recordings of actors reading the same passage in a variety of different ways as stimuli. Among other findings, a faster rate of speech made both sexes sound more animated and extroverted. Increased intonational contour (i.e., variance of F_0) gave the impression that a male speaker was more dynamic, feminine, and aesthetically inclined than other males, and the impression that a female speaker was more dynamic and extroverted than other females. Other researchers have found that decreased variance of F_0 prompted judgments of less competence and benevolence, as does increasing average F_0 (Brown et al., 1973; 1974). Male speakers with high pitch were perceived in one study as less truthful, less empathetic, weaker, and more nervous (Apple et al., 1979). Another study found that listeners perceive male voices with higher variance of intensity, more exaggerated variance of F_0, and a faster speech rate to be more extroverted, confident, dominant, and bold (Aronovitch, 1976).

In summary, up to a certain threshold well within the "male pitch range," higher F_0 has resulted in greater judgments of extroversion, assertiveness, confidence, and competence (Scherer, 1979). Past this threshold, males have been perceived as weak, effeminate, and incompetent. Males with a high F_0 have also been perceived as less emotionally stable and as having more psychological tension. Scherer has noted consistency across studies concerning personality perception of different levels of pitch variation. High variation "is seen as indicative of a dynamic, extroverted and outgoing and benevolent person" (Scherer, 1979).

Interestingly, an attractive voice has a greater effect on overall positive personality perception than does physical attractiveness (Zuckerman & Driver, 1989). The attractiveness of the voice has even been shown to be as important as that of the face in determining overall attractiveness (Hart & Brown, 1974). It has been hypothesized that because people tend to agree on other voice perceptions, such as those mentioned previously, they are likely to agree on vocal attractiveness as well (Zuckerman & Driver, 1989). After asking subjects to rate voices on a scale of 1 to 7 (1—very unattractive, 7—very attractive), Zuckerman and Driver compared these judgments to personality judgments made by other listeners. Judges generally agreed on which voices were attractive, attributing more favorable personality traits to speakers with higher attractiveness ratings. High vocal attractiveness had a significant effect on how calm, good-natured, and conscientious a speaker was perceived to be. Vocal attractiveness affected perceived conscientiousness even more than facial attractiveness did. Persons with higher vocal attractiveness have also been perceived as more powerful, competent, warm, and honest (Berry,

1991; 1992). To learn more on the role of vocal attractiveness in sexual behavior and interaction.

So what does an attractive voice sound like? Researchers have found that it is generally mature (Zuckerman, Miyake, & Elkin, 1995) and submissive (Raines, Hechtman, & Rosenthal, 1990). In an attempt to determine the actual acoustical parameters of an attractive voice, Zuckerman and Miyake (1993) had judges rate voices on vocal attractiveness and then analyzed each voice according to a number of objective and subjective acoustical parameters. They found that male voices that rated high in vocal attractiveness were generally less monotonous, more articulate, lower in average F_0, medium to higher in variance of F_0, low in squeakiness, and intermediate in total pauses. Ray, Ray, and Zahn (1991) also showed that medium and high pitch variation is more attractive than low pitch variation. In one study, when subjects of either sex were asked to simulate a "sexy" voice, they typically lowered their voice an average of 20 to 25 Hz. Interestingly, these sexy voices were not actually rated by others as particularly sexy (Tuomi & Fisher, 1979). Instead, males and females have both rated mid-pitch voices of the opposite sex as "most sexy," whereas high-pitched male voices were rated as "least sexy" (Hall, 1991).

A recent study (Riding, 2002; Riding, Lonsdale, & Brown, 2006) focused on the question of which levels of pitch (high, medium, or low) and intonation (high, medium, or low) are the most attractive in the male voice, which of these factors is most important in determining vocal attractiveness, and how these ratings relate to what women assume they find attractive. With acoustically manipulated voices they were able to show that high-pitched voices are significantly less attractive to females. There was also a significant interaction on the benevolence factor: high or low pitch with flat intonation was rated particularly low on the attractiveness scale.

In this chapter we have so far tried to tease apart various issues that involve the voice: emotion, pleasantness, and attractiveness. These relationships are by no means orthogonal, but we believe that careful examination must be made concerning where they interact and where they do differ. Prior research, while rich in low-level data in some of these areas, has not provided a clear appreciation for vocal pleasantness in particular. On the other hand, research in other areas of perception (e.g., facial attractiveness and pleasantness) may provide helpful clues. In the next section we discuss possible directions that we suspect can be pursued to help clarify these issues.

Future Directions

In looking for possible strategies to explore vocal pleasantness in the context of vocal attractiveness and specific emotional content, three possible strategies are suggested. The first is the idea that perhaps the voices that are most pleasant and/or most attractive are in fact those that are most modal or average in terms of acoustic qualities and perceived vocal qualities.

The second idea is that perhaps all of the past literature on ratings of emotion and of personal attributes from voice is applicable to the questions of the acoustical and perceptual properties of pleasant voice and of attractive voice. That is, it may be that pleasantness and attractiveness can be effectively conceived as latent variables underlying specific judgments of such attributes as confident, active, ambitious, intelligent, strong, likeable, dependable, sincere, kind, just, compassionate, etc.

The third possible strategy is an experimental one. It may be illuminating to have persons actually try to create voices that fit each of the four possible combinations of high and low pleasantness and high and low attractiveness, and use the lens model to evaluate the extent to which various acoustic and vocal properties effectively mediate judging accuracy in identifying the intended fourfold classification of each voice. This same strategy could be used to compare ratings of the person as attractive or pleasant versus ratings of the voice as attractive or pleasant.

The *Attractiveness as Average* Hypothesis and the *Pleasantness as Average* Hypothesis

The question of attractiveness has been addressed from the perspective of facial attractiveness. Researchers have investigated indicators of facial attractiveness and found that "average" faces are rated most attractive (Langlois & Roggman, 1990; Langlois, Roggman, & Musselman, 1994). That is, if multiple persons' faces are digitized and then averaged, these modal composite faces are rated as more attractive than the original faces.

It could be asked whether vocal pleasantness is somehow comparable to vocal attractiveness in that the most pleasant voice is also the most modal voice. In future studies it may be profitable to tease apart and compare the two: when attractiveness is separated from pleasantness, is the modality hypothesis truer of attractiveness than it is of pleasantness, or vice versa?

Vocal Pleasantness as a Latent Variable

Brown and Gilman (1960) argued effectively for two underlying dimensions, power and solidarity, as the conceptual foundation for understanding the development of pronoun forms in European languages over the past two millennia. In his classic social psychology text, Roger Brown (1965) followed up on his earlier paper with Gilman and proposed that these two dimensions, status and solidarity, are the two underlying dimensions of all interpersonal relationships. On this basis, it might be expected that if one were to factor analyze a variety of person-rating adjectives, something akin to status and solidarity would emerge as the two underlying factors. In today's language, we would refer to them as *latent variables*.

Brown et al. (1975) in fact found two such underlying factors, which they labeled competence and benevolence, in their summary and review of a number of vocal rating studies. Similar factors were found by Burgoon (1978) in her analysis of newscaster voices. These are reflective of Roger Brown's status and solidarity dimension of interpersonal relationship. Competence is highly correlated with adjectives related to social attractiveness, and benevolence is highly correlated with those related to pleasantness. It is found that increasing speech rate leads to increases in ratings of competence and decreasing it leads to decreases in ratings of competence. In other words, it is a linearly increasing positive function. Ratings of benevolence, on the other hand, are found to have an inverted-U relationship with speech rate, with intermediate levels of rate being rated as most benevolent.

It could be hypothesized that vocal attractiveness is in fact synonymous with this competence latent variable, and that vocal pleasantness is synonymous with the benevolence latent variable. It would follow that vocal attractiveness would have a linearly increasing relationship with speech rate and that vocal pleasantness would have an inverted-U relationship with speech rate (that is, intermediate levels of rate would be most pleasant). However, there may be a separation between competence and attractiveness at the highest rates. A rapid-fire, staccato delivery may be evidence of competence, but not particularly attractive.

Ratings of emotion voices could also be seen as having similar latent structure. It might be possible in meta-analytic re-analyses of past emotion studies to find hypothesized relationships between various emotions and the latent variables of attractiveness and pleasantness.

Experimental Studies of Vocal Pleasantness and Vocal Attractiveness Using the Lens Model

In future studies it may be possible to uncover the properties of vocal pleasantness in relation to vocal attractiveness and specific vocal attributes with experimental studies that target some of the hypotheses suggested in this chapter. For example, one could replicate one of the standard experimental paradigms used to examine the effects of acoustical manipulations (see, for example, Brown, 1980; Riding et al., 2006), but with targeted instructions to respondents alerting them to the possible divergence of attractiveness and pleasantness and instructing them to directly rate each. Similar instructions could be used to separate pleasantness or attractiveness of the voice from perceived pleasantness or attractiveness of the person. These direct ratings of pleasantness and attractiveness could then be compared statistically with ratings of specific vocal and personality characteristics to test the hypotheses suggested in this chapter. A similar paradigm could also be used with experimental studies of emotion voices to uncover the relationship of vocal pleasantness and vocal attractiveness to each of the portrayed emotions.

Scherer (1979; 2003) has continued to advocate the use of the Brunswikian lens model for analyzing the mediation of the vocal communication of personality markers and emotion. The lens model, as originally conceived by Brunswik (1952, 1956), is a model of human perception, but it is particularly useful as an analytical method for quantifying the extent to which the vocal or acoustical basis for accuracy in identifying emotion or personal characteristics is understood (Beal, Gillis, & Stewart, 1978; Hammond, 1966; Hammond & Stewart, 2001). Given acoustic measurements or vocal ratings of the spoken utterances, the lens model can identify what percent of identification accuracy is mediated by those measurements or ratings. A lens model analysis of the data gathered from studies such as those described in the preceding paragraph would be particularly valuable in answering the questions and testing the hypotheses posed in this chapter.

References

Addington, D. W. (1968). The relationship of selected vocal characteristics to personality perception. *Speech Monographs, 35,* 492–503.

Apple, W., Streeter, L. A., & Krauss, R. M. (1979). Effects of pitch and speech rate on personal attributions. *Journal of Personality and Social Psychology*, *37*(5), 715–727.

Aronovitch, C. D. (1976). The voice of personality: Stereotyped judgments and their relation to voice quality and sex of speaker. *Journal of Social Psychology*, *99*, 207–220.

Bacharowski, J. A., & Owren, M. (2003). Sounds of emotion: Production and perception of affect-related vocal acoustics. *Annals of the New York Academy of Sciences*, *1000*, 244–265.

Banse, R., & Scherer, K. R. (1996). Acoustic profiles in vocal expression of emotion. *Journal of Personality and Social Psychology*, *70*, 614–636.

Beal, D., Gillis, J., & Stewart, T. (1978). The lens model: Computational procedures and applications. *Perceptual and Motor Skills*, *46*, 3–28.

Berry, D. S. (1991). Accuracy in social perception: Contributions of facial and vocal information. *Journal of Personality and Social Psychology*, *61*(2), 298–307.

Berry, D. S. (1992). Vocal types and stereotypes: Joint effects of vocal attractiveness and vocal maturity on person perception. *Journal of Nonverbal Behavior*, *16*(1), 41–54.

Brown, B. L. (1980). Effects of speech rate on personality attributions and competency evaluations. In H. Giles, W. P. Robinson, & P. M. Smith (Eds.), *Language: Social psychological perspectives* (pp. 293–300). Oxford, UK: Pergamon Press.

Brown, B. L., Strong, W. J., & Rencher, A. C. (1973). Perceptions of personality from speech: Effects of manipulations of acoustical parameters. *Journal of the Acoustical Society of America*, *54*, 29–35.

Brown, B. L., Strong, W. J., & Rencher, A. C. (1974). Fifty-four voices from two: The effects of simultaneous manipulations of rate, mean fundamental frequency, and variance of fundamental frequency on ratings of personality from speech. *Journal of the Acoustical Society of America*, *55*(2), 313–318.

Brown, B. L., Strong, W. J., & Rencher, A. C. (1975). Acoustic determinants of perceptions of personality from speech. *International Journal of the Sociology of Language*, *6*, 11–32.

Brown, R. (1965). *Social psychology*. New York: The Free Press.

Brown, R., & Gilman, A. (1960). The pronouns of power and solidarity. In T. A. Sebeok (Ed.), *Style in language* (pp. 253–276). Cambridge, MA: The Technology Press of MIT.

Brunswik, E. (1952). *The conceptual framework of psychology*. Chicago: Chicago University Press.

Brunswik, E. (1956). *Perception and the representative design of experiments*. Berkeley, CA: University of California Press.

Buller, D., & Burgoon, J. (1986). The effects of vocalics and nonverbal sensitivity on compliance: A replication and extension. *Human Communication Research*, *13*, 126–144.

Burgoon, J. (1978). Attributes of the newscaster's voice as predictors of his credibility. *Journalism Quarterly*, *55*, 276–281, 300.

Burgoon, J., Birk, T., & Pfau, M. (1990). Nonverbal behaviors, persuasion, and credibility. *Human Communication Research*, *17*, 140–169.

Darwin, C. (1872). *The expression of the emotions in man and animals*. London: John Murray.

Deal, L., & Oyer, H. (1991). Ratings of vocal pleasantness and the aging process. *Folia Phoniatrica*, *43*, 44–48.

Ekman, P. (1972). Universal and cultural differences in facial expressions of emotions. In J. K. Cole (Ed.), *Nebraska symposium on motivation, 1971* (pp. 207–283). Lincoln: University of Nebraska Press.

Ekman, P. (1994). Strong evidence for universals in facial expressions: A reply to Russell's mistaken critique. *Psychological Bulletin*, *115*(2), 268–287.

Elfenbein, H., & Ambady, N. (2002). On the universality and cultural specificity of emotion recognition: A meta-analysis. *Psychological Bulletin, 128*, 203–235.

Giles, H., & Powesland, P. F. (1975). *Speech style and social evaluation*. New York: Academic Press.

Hall, J. D. (1991). Are male and female homo sapiens selected for different auditory stimuli? In W. von Raffler-Engel, J. Wind, & A. Jonker (Eds.), *Studies in language origins* (Vol. 2, pp. 65–75). Amsterdam, Netherlands: John Benjamins.

Hammond, K. (1966). *The psychology of Egon Brunswik*. New York: Holt, Rinehart & Winston.

Hammond, K., & Stewart, T. (2001). *The essential Brunswik*. Oxford, UK: Oxford University Press.

Hart, R. J., & Brown, B. L. (1974). Interpersonal information conveyed by the content and vocal aspects of speech. *Speech Monographs, 41*(4), 371–380.

Juslin, P., & Laukka, P. (2003). Communication of emotions in vocal expression and music performance: Different channels, same code? *Psychological Bulletin, 129*, 770–814.

Kramer, E. (1964). Personality stereotypes in voice: A reconsideration. *The Journal of Social Psychology, 62*, 247–251.

Langlois, J., & Roggman, L. (1990). Attractive faces are only average. *Psychological Science, 1*, 115–121.

Langlois, J., Roggman, L., & Musselman, L. (1994). What is average and what is not average about attractive faces? *Psychological Science, 5*, 214–220.

Murray, I., & Arnott, J. (1993). Toward the simulation of emotion in synthetic speech: A review of the literature on human vocal emotion. *Journal of the Acoustical Society of America, 93*, 1097–1108.

Oxford English Dictionary Online. http://www.oed.com

Pittam, J., & Scherer, K. (1993). Vocal expression and communication of emotion. In M. Lewis & J. M. Haviland (Eds.), *Hand-book of emotions* (pp. 185–198). New York: Guilford Press.

Raines, R. S., Hechtman, S. B., & Rosenthal, R. R. (1990). Physical attractiveness of face and voice: Effects of positivity, dominance, and sex. *Journal of Applied Social Psychology, 20*, 1558–1578.

Ray, G. B., Ray, E. B., & Zahn, C. J. (1991). Speech behavior and social evaluation: An examination of medical messages. *Communication Quarterly, 2*, 47–57.

Riding, D. R. (2002). *The effects of pitch and intonation on male vocal attractiveness*. Honors thesis, Brigham Young University, Provo, Utah.

Riding, D. R., Lonsdale, D., & Brown, B. L. (2006). The effects of average fundamental frequency and variance of fundamental frequency on male vocal attractiveness to women. *Journal of Nonverbal Behavior, 30*(2), 55–61.

Scherer, K. R. (1979). Personality markers in speech. In K. R. Scherer & H. Giles (Eds.), *Social markers in speech* (pp. 147–210). Cambridge, UK: Cambridge University Press.

Scherer, K. (1986). Vocal affect expression: A review and a model for future research. *Psychological Bulletin, 99*, 143–165.

Scherer, K. (2003). Vocal communication of emotions: A review of research paradigms. *Speech Communication, 40*, 227–256.

Scherer, K., Banse, R., Wallbott, H., & Goldbeck, T. (1991). Vocal cues in emotion encoding and decoding. *Motivation and Emotion, 15*, 123–148.

Tuomi, S. K., & Fisher, J. E. (1979). Characteristics of a simulated sexy voice. *Folia Phoniatrica, 31*, 242–249.

Van Bezooijan, R. (1984). *The characteristics and recognizability of vocal expressions of emotions*. Dordrecht, Netherlands: Foris.

Wallbott, H., & Scherer, K. (1986). Cues and channels in emotion recognition. *Journal of Personality and Social Psychology, 51*, 690–699.

Zuckerman, M., & Driver, R. E. (1989). What sounds beautiful is good: The vocal attractiveness stereotype. *Journal of Nonverbal Behavior*, *13*(2), 67–82.

Zuckerman, M., & Miyake, K. (1993). The attractive voice: What makes it so? *Journal of Nonverbal Behavior 17*(2), 119–135.

Zuckerman, M., Miyake, K., & Elkin, C. S. (1995). Effects of attractiveness and maturity of face and voice on interpersonal impressions. *Journal of Research in Personality*, *29*(2), 253–272.

Zuckerman, M., Miyake, K., & Hodgins, H. S. (1991). Cross-channel effects of vocal and physical attractiveness and their implications for interpersonal perception. *Journal of Personality and Social Psychology*, *60*(4), 545–554.

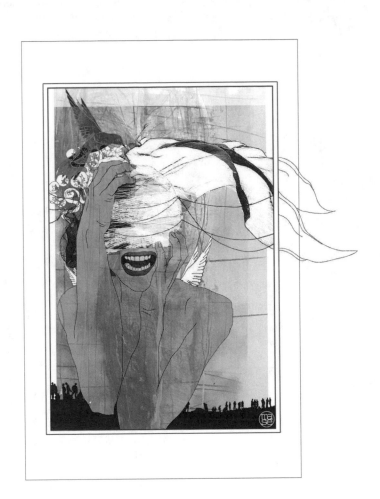

CHAPTER 3

A Unified Model of Cognition, Emotion, and Action and Its Relation to Vocally Encoded Cognitive-Affective States

Branka Zei Pollermann and Krzysztof Izdebski

Abstract

The unified model of cognition, emotion, and action suggests that cognitive processes that steer and organize adaptive behaviors evolve in what is commonly known as affective space. By combining insights from constructivist epistemology (Piaget, 1950) and cybernetics, the unified model explains how and why affect is inherent to cognitive processes involved in adaptive interaction with the environment. The functioning of adaptive behavior is explained within the framework of dynamic systems with self-organizing properties. Valence, arousal, and potency are considered as the system's control parameters—critical organizing factors underlying adaptive change, while the amplitude and speed of change in control parameter values are seen as generators of more or less stable states that can be subjectively felt as emotional. Each state can then be defined as a point in a three-dimensional space. Depending on their structure and stability over time, such states can be conceptualized as *motivations*, *emotions, moods,* or *personality traits.* The choice of valence, arousal, and potency as control parameters is explained from the cybernetic point of view enriched with *genetic* epistemology. After defining the semiological status of vocal indicators of affect, the results of a pilot study on vocally encoded interpersonal stance are presented.

Multiplicity of Emotion Theories—A Call for Integration

Over the past hundred years, emotion psychology has mainly concentrated on various constituents of the organism's emotional response such as: cognitive appraisals, physiological, neurological, and hormonal activations, motor, expressive, and behavioral reactions, linguistic "labeling," consciousness, and the subjective feelings, however without offering an integrative theoretical framework. One of the disturbing results of this gap is a remarkable diversity of emotion theories and consequently a lack of consensus on the definition of *emotion*—the main object of study.

In this chapter we shall suggest a theoretical framework that will allow the integration of several theories and suggest a definition of *emotion.* The epistemological orientation is that of *genetic* epistemology applied to open systems (Bertalanffy, 1968) with self-organizing properties (Carver & Scheier, 2002).

Theoretical Framework of the Unified Model

Be it in the works of art, in sports, in intellectual pursuits, or at peace or war times, emotional states are considered to be initiators, modulators, or terminators of actions. They appear to mediate adjustment to environmental conditions and improve the individual's chances of biological and social survival. In the construction of autonomous agents, emotions are viewed as determinants of action selection and behavior arbitration (Scheutz, 2002; Snaith & Holland, 1991; Tyrrell, 1993). Does this mean that affective processes—emotions in particular—are dedicated systems that serve an adaptive purpose and that one needs to be in an emotional state in order to engage in adaptive behavior?

We would say "No." We believe that affective aspects of cognitions are inherent to the functioning of dynamic systems. In such systems adaptive behavior results from organization through a limited number of interacting lower-order elements acting as control parameters. The output is then a coordinated response of the system's components. Shifts in values and the interactions between control parameters produce different behavioral outputs.

As the behavioral adjustments are made with regard to each parameter's value, we are then concerned with the identification of the control parameters that guide adaptive action and influence the emergence of processes and states that may be subjectively felt or externally recognized as emotional. We believe that the system's control space can be defined by three dimensions: valence, arousal, and potency. These dimensions have so far been considered as intrinsically *affective* (Bachorowski & Owren, 1995; Laukka, Juslin, & Bresin, 2005; Mehrabian & Russel, 1974; Osgood, May, & Miron, 1975; Russell, 2003; Russell & Barrett, 1999).

In Faith and Thayer's model of emotion, valence and arousal are conceptualized as the dynamic systems' control parameters (Faith & Thayer, 2001). We agree with these authors' convincing demonstration of valence and arousal acting as control parameters, but we do not share their opinion that they are specific to *emotion systems*. Hence, we defend the view that these control parameters per se are inherent to the organism's interaction with the environment and that it is only under certain conditions (explained below) that valence, arousal, and potency come to be conceptualized as dimensions of emotions.

This is close to Peter Lang's view that " . . . there is no clear demarcation between affective and non-affective behavior. However, popular consensus defines the terrain of emotion as including responses that vary in valence, arousal and control or dominance . . . " (Lang, 1990, p. 221).

Stating this allegiance to Lang, we can thus take a stand against theories based on specific *emotional mechanisms* (Plutchik, 1962; 1980) and agree with George Mandler (Mandler, 1975; 1982) who argues "against any theories of emotion that are independent of or different from a more general analysis of human processing systems" (Mandler, 1975, p. 84). In their recent theoretical work, Matthews and colleagues pointed out the nonexistence of an overarching model allowing discrimination of higher order complexes of affect, motivation, and cognition that may reflect different modes of self-regulation (Matthews et al., 2002). Much earlier, Howard Leventhal (Leventhal, 1970) suggested that emotion theories should be included into a more general systems approach to describe the mechanisms that control behavior (Carver & Scheier, 1981; 1982; Leventhal & Nerenz, 1985). According to his model, two parallel systems structure and control behavior: one controls problem-oriented behavior and the other affect-oriented behavior. Each of the systems follows three stages: representing the environment, responding to it, and evaluating the response outcomes. A similar model of the structure and the stages of basic behavioral units was provided by Miller and colleagues (Miller, Galanter, & Pribram, 1986). While we agree on the nature of the three "stages," we do not share Levethal's view of there being two distinct control systems.

Rooted in Jean Piaget's *genetic* epistemology, we are proposing a unified model where the very functioning of the subject's interaction with environment implies the construction and usage of schemata (of varying complexity) that necessarily include affective aspects (Piaget, 1954). For reasons explained later we shall use the term *reaction* to mean the organism's hardwired responses (like reflexes or innate releasing mechanisms producing preprogrammed stereotyped behaviors or fixed action patterns) and the term *behavior* to mean the organism's adaptive response guided by cognitive evaluations of both the environment and the ongoing interaction with it. Our model will be mainly concerned with the architecture and the functioning of the interaction processes which apply to organisms described as open systems with dynamic teleology (Bertalanffy, 1968).

Piaget's general model of interaction comprises two types of interactions (Piaget, 1975). The Type I interaction produces the knowledge of the relation between the properties of the object and the properties of the subject's action. The most elementary form of such a relation is covariation. For example, in a situation where a subject lifts an object, the object's perceived weight is relative to the muscular effort employed to lift it. It then follows that the knowledge of the object's characteristics is inseparable from the knowledge of the characteristics of the subject's action schemes used in the interaction. The knowledge thus constructed becomes a cognitive instrument for the subject's further cognitions and actions. The discovery of the role of mirror neurons in cognition (Gallese, Keysers, & Rizzolatti, 2004) can be seen as empirical evidence for Piaget's concept of assimilation as a *computational* principle underlying human cognition—a mechanism for the coordination of perceptual and motor actions. The coupling of perception with actions via mirror neurons can then explain the simultaneous construction of the internal representations of the world and the self (Gallese & Lakoff, 2005).

Type II interaction includes the properties of perceptual and sensorimotor schemata as elaborated in Type I interaction, to which are added inferential coordinations, consciousness, and retroactive regulation. It then follows that adaptive action implies the construction and coordination of three types of knowledge (Cellérier, 1979):

1. A set of empirical features of a situation associated with the anticipated set of features to be resulting from action. The latter set of features is the value the set will acquire as a result of action.

2. A set of pragmatic features of the transformations due to action associated with the set of empirical features.

3. A cognitive composite reflecting a tripartite structure of an instrumental act with the transformation having the status of a means, the result having the status of the end, and the situational features playing the role of the operand.

For Cellérier the first two types of knowledge are functionally subordinate to the third. Both early cybernetic models of self-organizing adaptive systems (Cellérier, 1968) and modern architectures of autonomous agents (Canamero, 2001; Orlando, Canamero, & te Boekhorst, 2003; Tyrell, 1993) agree that for a system to be adaptive, it should perform at least five tasks:

1. Sense the internal and external environment (including its own actions), interpret, and store the sensory input (perception, information processing, and memory).

2. Use the perceptual inputs and memory to decide which of its repertoire of actions is most appropriate (action selection and arbitration, decision making).

3. Regulate the internal resources for execution of action (in humans: neuroendocrine, somatic, and autonomic adjustments).

4. Transform the chosen action into patterns of overt behavior including (if necessary) communicative actions.

5. Evaluate the outcome (perception, information processing, and memory).

The unified model proposed here suggests that the control parameters that steer the execution of the five tasks are: valence, activation, and potency. Figure 3–1 is a schematic representation of the affective space defined by these three dimensions. Why valence, arousal, and potency are proposed as the control parameters is explained below.

Valence as Control Parameter

We consider the attribution of valence as inherent to tasks 1, 2, and 5, in which the subject assimilates internal and/or external stimuli into the already existing knowledge structures (perceptual, sensorimotor, and conceptual schemata). In the framework of these tasks, each knowledge structure is attributed a value related to the actual or potential hedonic valence of the stimulus and its beneficial or detrimental character. The value thus assigned can be conceived of as a *tag*[1] representing the subjective hedonic meaning attributed to the activated schemata (Piaget, 1954). Valence tagging is considered to be inherent to the subject's adaptive behavior, which aims at maintaining or achieving positively valenced states and/or avoiding negatively valenced states. The target states can concern any or all of the three dimensions of self, namely *intrapersonal self* (personal interests, including own body), *interpersonal self* (relational and social interests) (Hobson, 1993; Trevarthen, 1993), and *transpersonal self* (meta-cognitions, religious pursuits, or more global trans-societal interests).

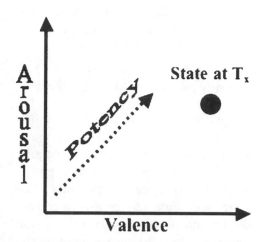

Affective Space Control Parameters

Figure 3–1. Schematic illustration of the dimensions of affective space with a the state of the organism marked as a point at t1 reflecting a possible configuration of valence, arousal, and potency values.

Affective neuroscience research suggests that primitive motivational subsystems based in subcortical neural structures subserve the attribution of valence by providing an evaluative outcome necessary to initiate an approach or withdrawal response (Davidson, 1992a; 1992b) (Lane et al., 1997; Lang, 1995). The function of valence tags would thus be to regulate approach-avoidance behaviors (Cacioppo, Klein, Bentson, & Hatfield, 1993). The attribution of valence is considered to occur unconsciously and automatically. The degree of valence can also be influenced by the contextual factors such as outcome expectancy and uncertainty (Mandler, 1997). It then follows

---

[1]Ohman (1999) uses the term *tagging* to denote the mainly unconscious process of assigning emotional meaning.

that the pleasure in relief would be different from that in satisfying an unhindered concern, because the former takes into account the past from which one has escaped, whereas the latter does not (Lambie & Marcel, 2002).

Potency as Control Parameter

Attribution of the *potency tag* is inherent to task 2 of an adaptive system, which involves: action selection and arbitration, decision making, and an appraisal of the subject's coping potential. The latter aspect refers to the estimated relative coping power, that is, the relation between available resources and the resources needed to cope with the situation. The subject's coping potential can be strongly influenced by stimulus ambiguity or restricted response action availability. The decision making and action selection can also be influenced by errors in the judgment of the likelihood of future outcomes and simplified heuristics that people use to cope with the complexity of decision making (Tversky & Kahneman, 1981).

While the potency dimension is seen as a scalar, one can conceptualize it in terms of three broad categories, each related to a type of behavioral response:

1. Very low potency with no decisional power and no choice prior to execution such as instinctive reactions, vital emergency responses, or phobias (Lang, 1990).
2. Medium level of potency with partial decisional power and a limited choice of alternatives (e.g., imitation, "forced choice," or pseudo-choice situations).
3. High level of potency with full decisional power.

Decision taking implies choice. From the cybernetic point of view, it is only if the machine has the possibility of reacting in different ways (Bertalanffy's equifinality principle, (1968) that its behavior can be regulatory (Ashby, 1961). Many scholars have emphasized the importance of choice and decisional power. For example, Dewey pointed out that deliberation takes place in ideas, not in overt behavior, and that it requires a rehearsal of alternative possible courses of action (Dewey, 1922), while Damasio suggested that eating and avoiding falling objects belong to the "animal spirit" while deciding is typically "human spirit" (Damasio, 1994). Prieto offers an original and powerful theoretical explanation of how decision taking and choice are related to the construction of the self as an *acting subject* (Prieto, 1975). He argues that in an instrumental act, the subject's body is the initiator of the action that the tool will exert upon a material object in order to transform it. The object's transformation is then seen as a "natural" result of the tool's action. Now the tool's action is also a natural result of the subject's action applied on it. At the end of such backward chaining of cause-effect relationships, one comes to the subject's action itself that does not have a natural cause. It is the feeling that one can be a cause without being an effect that generates the sense of agency and allows one to acquire self-identity. To quote Gallagher, "This is the feeling of identity, of being the perspectival origin of one's own experience, which is a basic component of the experienced differentiation of self from non-self" (Gallagher, 2005, p. 201).

It then follows that if the subject's action is imposed by an outside agency, he or she can only *react* and not *behave*.

Consistent with this view, Prieto defines *behavior* as the act of engaging in praxis by one's own decision in a situation of choice. He also adds that the transformations of material reality due to man's praxis constitute the historic aspect of the reality, which is not a natural and possibly predictable consequence of the preceding state (Prieto, 1991).

Activation as Control Parameter

Activation tag is inherent to tasks 3 and 4 of the cybernetic model. It denotes the afferent-feedback-based *on-line* percept of internal body tone as well as an estimate of the required task-relevant activation of resources. The *on-line* percept can be defined as a cognitive composite of feedback information from cardiovascular targets, gut, lungs, muscles, and electrocortical arousal and is conceptually close to Damasio's "somatic marker hypothesis" (Damasio, 1994). The *activation tag* thus carries the information about the amount of energy mobilization involved in autonomic, motor, physiological, and computational ongoing changes as well as those estimated as required to handle the stimulus and/or its consequences. In the latter case, it can be seen as schema activation before becoming overt energy engagement. Piaget considers bodily energy management to be an affective dimension of behavior involving the attribution of a *yield value* (*"valeur de rendement"*) which takes into account the actual or required investment of energy (Piaget, 1954). To the extent that activation mechanisms are *goal driven*, the behavior will tend to be oriented towards correcting disturbances in homeostatic variables of the internal milieu, rectifying undesirable external situations, and guiding the subject's actions towards his or her goals.

In summary, adaptive action involves the construction and usage of implicit and explicit knowledge of the environment, of the internal milieu, of one's own actions, and of the self as acting subject. We consider valence, arousal, and potency as the elementary parameters that control adaptive interaction with the environment. There is reason to believe that valence is primary in that it recruits and drives responses including the appraisal of potency and activation (Watt, 2001). From the neurological viewpoint, hemispheric specialization for valence is considered to represent the phylogenetic development of primitive networks that provide an evaluative outcome necessary to initiate an approach or withdrawal response (Davisdon, 1992a; 1992b; Lane et al., 1997). The interaction between control parameters produces complex schemata (perceptual-sensorimotor-conceptual) that tend to be assimilated into each other and serve as instruments for both adaptive action and further construction of knowledge.

Emotions as Specific Configurations of the Control Space

Inspired by the insightful works of Elisabeth Duffy (1941) in the physiology of behavior and more recent work on neurological aspects of emotions (Chapman & Nakamura, 2001), we suggest the following conceptual framework for distinguishing between emotional and nonemotional responses.

A relentless change in the configuration of the control parameter values assures a dynamic equilibrium of the system. As long as these variations are within a limited range, the equilibration processes are largely unconscious and the state of the organism is perceived as *normal*. If however, the amplitude and/or the speed of change of control-parameter values falls outside their normal range of variation, such a state becomes cognitively dominant. It is then likely to penetrate consciousness, be felt as *unusual*, and conceptualized as emotional. From the neurological point of view LeDoux explains that (at least in the domain of fear) this transformation of cognition into emotion—this hostile takeover of consciousness—occurs when the amygdala comes to dominate working memory (LeDoux, 2002). Sander and colleagues convincingly demonstrated the amygdala's pivotal role as a general relevance detector (Sander, Grafman, & Zalla, 2003), which in our view determines the focus and the content of the working memory that influences and modulates executive functions.

In summary, we suggest that when any or all of the control-parameter values falls outside a *normal* range of variation, such a configuration becomes cognitively dominant and lends itself to be subjectively known as a motivational or emotional state (see Figure 3–2).

The detection of deviations in control parameters is rooted in the fundamental physiological principle of *set-point* detection. As Douglas Watt writes:

> When internal physiological states are outside a desirable range, both visceral sensations and action dispositions (thirst and pursuit of fluids) are activated. But phenomenal states of rage, separation distress, fear must have similar mechanisms, that these are "not OK" departures from ideal organismic baselines, activating defensive responses, while play and affection, sexual stimuli etc., must encode or activate the opposite, setting in motion basic appetitive mechanisms. These are central and not peripheral aspects of affect. Events that

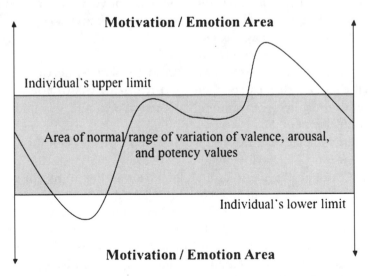

Figure 3–2. Schematic illustration of the position of motivation/emotion areas as zones situated ouside a *normal* range of control-parameter variations.

modify this crucial valence aspect alter the whole experiential picture, and not just pieces or fragments of affect. (Watt, 2001, p. 306).

The deviation from a set-point is implicit in Russel's two-dimensional model of emotion, where the center of the circumplex represents a neutral point on both bipolar dimensions, and "each emotion label can be thought of as a vector originating from the center of the circle with its length representing intensity (extremity or saturation)" (Russel, 1989, p. 87). The deviation principle is also conceptually close to Mandler's discrepancy detection mechanism (Mandler, 1997). Once triggered, an emotional response can then involve a resetting of procedural priorities and the regulation of the speed of task execution (which can be set to zero, as in the a case of a freeze-reaction). As evidenced by Watson and Tellegen (1999), avoidance gradients have steeper slopes than approach gradients.

It goes without saying that the sensitivity thresholds and ceiling values will vary from one person to the other depending on genetic, physiological, contextual, and social factors. Drawing on Van Geert's dynamic systems model of developmental mechanisms (Van Geert, 1998), we assume a weight update function to be applied each time the system has gone through an action/experience sequence. Such a mechanism would allow valence, potency, and activation tags to be updated. Stable reaction schemata, which include prototypical situational features with prototypical values for valence, activation, and potency, acquire a weight that can then give access precedence over less automatic schemata. In dynamic systems terminology, this behavioral mode is in *attractor state*.

Attractors may have varying degrees of stability and instability. Some attractor states are so stable that they appear inevitable. The concept of attractor states may correspond to what are usually referred to as *discrete emotions*; that is, when systems self-organize, they settle into a few modes of behavior that the system prefers over all the possible modes. Interestingly, Plutchik's theory of emotion assumes that a small number of types of adaptive behaviors are the prototypes that form the basis for emotions. The latter are then defined as behavioral adaptations that have been successful in increasing the chances of survival (Plutchik, 1962; 1980; Plutchik & Kellerman, 1986).

The effects of increase or decrease in control parameter *readouts* could be conveniently studied within the framework of nonlinear dynamic systems theory. Molenaar and Oppenheimer (Molenaar & Oppenheimer, 1985) have shown that models based on nonlinear dynamic systems theory transcend the dichotomy between the organismic and mechanistic paradigms.

The *catastrophe theory* models (Thom, 1974) are of particular interest as they consider discontinuities in behavioral variables as a function of continuous variation in the control variables. The original goal of catastrophe theory was the classification of all possible discontinuities in a series of elementary catastrophes. The *cusp* model is one of the elementary catastrophes that has been used in many fields. Applications have been made in social sciences (Zeeman, 1976), in perception research (Stewart & Peregoy, 1983), in phonetics (Noblitt, 1978), and more recently in appraisal processes of emotions (Scherer, 2000).

To conclude, the proposed *unified model of cognition, emotion,* and *action* suggests that in the context of adaptive interaction with environment, cognition steers the organism's response by assigning values to the activated perceptual-sensorimotor-conceptual schemata in terms of valence, potency, and activation. It then follows that such complex schemata necessarily include affective aspects. In addition, the activated schemata tend to be assimilated into each other and form new complex cognitive structures subserving both perception and action. An interesting example of a unitary action of complex schemata can be seen in the fact that the processing of information is facilitated if actions and thoughts are congruent—positively valenced thoughts with approach behavior and negatively valenced thoughts with avoidance behavior (Bargh, 1997; Förster & Strack 1997).

Representation of Affect and Language

Piaget's theory of knowledge posits that knowledge is constructed by means of assimilation of the object of cognition into the subject's own schemata (perceptual, sensorimotor, and conceptual), which are also continuously enriched and accommodated to new situations. Assimilation itself involves *thematization*—a process whereby different components of the object are selected, categorized, often translated into semiotic entities (e.g., words), and placed into a relational network of concepts. As pointed out by Karmiloff-Smith, the development of knowledge proceeds through a process called "representational re-description" (Karmiloff-Smith, 1992). This is consistent with the view that the way language is used to describe emotions modifies what one knows about emotions and how they are experienced consciously. Drawing on Piaget's theory of knowledge, Richard Lane's model of emotional consciousness links the different levels of consciousness to the levels of the complexity of representational schemata (Lane, 2001). A key assumption in the author's work on emotional awareness is that "language promotes the development of schemata for the processing of emotional information, whether that information comes from the internal or external world" (Lane & Zei Pollermann, 2002, p. 280). The verbal expression of emotional experiences can be considered as a process which elevates the procedural dimension of emotion onto a representational level, allowing for more flexible and more powerful handling of emotional contents. The shifting of sensorimotor contents onto a representational level requires conceptualization, which is facilitated by the use of language as a semiotic system that translates concepts into communicable entities.

Linguistic signs seem to facilitate the representational redescription of activated schemata through the mechanisms of thematization and generalization. Hans Kurath's work on the semantic sources of the words for emotions in Sanskrit, Greek, Latin, and the Germanic languages exemplifies how various components of complex perceptual-sensorimotor schemata are thematized and linguistically encoded (Kurath, 1921). Interestingly, one could draw a parallel between Kurath's classification of names of feelings and emotions and the foci of various emotion theories. Kurath reports the following semantic fields related to the words expressing emotions: (a) parts of the body and organs not subject to conscious control (the heart, the organs of respiration, the viscera, liver, spleen, gall), (b) physiological displays of vigor or weakness, gestures related to approach and avoidance behaviors, excitement and inhibition movements, (c) sense perceptions with kinesthetic and tactile perceptions having stronger affective tone than those of hearing and especially those of sight, (d) vocal gestures— inarticulate sounds, wailing, and grumbling. By this work Kurath provided evidence for a firmly established principle of semantics, that all the more complex processes (including both body and mind) are named according to their simpler and more tangible components (Wundt & Schaub, 1921). This also illustrates the observer-dependent character of our knowledge about emotions. The history of physics provides examples of how the same material phenomenon can be conceptualized in different ways. For instance, electromagnetic phenomena can be conceptualized either as waves or as particles (photons). The physicist knows that such different "realities" result from the differences in the measuring methods applied to the same material reality.

By analogy, Piaget suggests that the subject's perceptual-sensorimotor-conceptual schemata be conceived of as the measuring instruments that determine the nature of the object of cognition—be it external-world-object or self.

Vocal Indicators of the Speaker's Cognitive-Affective States and Processes

Speech communication, just as any other interactive behavior, necessarily reflects the configuration of the speaker's affec-tive space at two levels: (a) the underlying configuration extending over a longer period of time (moods, stable attitudes, and personality traits) and (b) each moment's *on-line* configuration (emotions, interpersonal stances, and communication strategies).

In natural settings the on-line configuration is influenced by ever-changing discursive context including the speaker's and the receiver's own nonverbal reactions, the discourse content, and the conversational interaction pattern itself. Vocal variations are manifest on three levels: suprasegmental (e.g., intonations, accentuation, speaking rate), segmental (e.g., format precision), and intrasegmental (voice quality).

Now, what is the cognitive mechanism involved in the attribution of emotional meaning to vocal variations? Piaget's concept of assimilation offers a model whereby vocal information is directly mapped onto the observer's analogous complex perceptual-sensorimotor-conceptual schemata elaborated in his previous experiences (with their respective valence, activation, and potency tags). This is also in agreement with Gallese and colleagues' findings that the fundamental mechanism, at the basis of the experiential understanding of others' emotions, involves activation of the corresponding viscero-motor centers in the observer (Gallese et al., 2004). Indeed, a great deal of emotion research is successfully done by exposing the subjects to emotion-inducing stimuli (visual, auditory, and imagery) in the laboratory (as an example, see Faith & Thayer, 2001). Given the fact that the subjects are aware of the artificiality of the situation, it appears that the induction of emotions is made possible in such conditions precisely because the stimuli are assimilated into the subject's cognitive-affective schemata.

Studying the manifestations of affect in speech communication poses the question of the semiological status of vocal signaling of affect, which in turn raises the issue of expression vs. communication of affect whereby *expression* has the status of an automatic external manifestation of an inner state (Darwin, 1872), while *communication* implies intentional signaling (Prieto, 1975).

To address these questions let us consider the three basic types of semiotic entities involved in the mechanism of indication:

1. *Spontaneous indicators* (Prieto, 1975) are semiotic entities where the link between the signifier and the signified is naturally given. It is said to be *motivated* because the link reflects relations such as spatial or temporal contiguity, causality, implication, or *pars pro toto* relationship, e.g., footprints in snow or temperature as a symptom of illness. In other words, spontaneous indicators have an informative value without having been produced to this purpose (Piaget, 1967).

2. *Falsely spontaneous indicators* (Buyssens, 1943; Prieto, 1975) are those that are purposely produced in order to appear as natural or spontaneous, e.g., a foreign accent produced by a speaker wanting to appear as a foreigner.

3. *Intentional indicators* are semiotic entities that are produced in order to provide information other than their own existence. These include:

   a. *Symbols*, where an originally natural link between the signifier and the signified has been conventionalized for purposes of communication, e.g., a picture of a snake symbolizing a pharmacy. In the course of history, a symbol may lose its previously motivated nature.

   b. *Icons,* where the link between the signifier and the signified is motivated by topological similarity between the two (Sebeok, 1985), e.g., maps, images, diagrams.

   c. *Signs,* where the relationship between the signifier and the signified is unmotivated and conventionalized for purposes of communication, e.g., words of a language (Saussure, 1972).

We believe that the semiological status of vocal affect signaling can be that of a spontaneous indicator (a symptom), a falsely spontaneous indicator, or a symbol, but never a sign as defined above. The nonarbitrary nature of vocal indicators of affect is supported by cross-cultural studies showing that the subjects can quite accurately infer emotional states from acoustic cues produced in other cultures and languages (Clynes & Nettheim, 1982; Juslin & Laukka, 2003). Parallelisms in animal affect signaling are of interest here as well. Scherer's model of vocal-affect signaling provides precise predictions for phonetic and macro-prosodic changes related to the outcome of each of the stages of the cognitive appraisal steering emotional processes (Scherer, 1986). It then follows that emotionally induced phonetic and prosodic variations primarily have a status of spontaneous indicators or symptoms of physiological reactions. They reflect the so called *push* force in affect signaling (Scherer, Helfrish, & Scherer, 1980). In the case of intense *primary emotions* (anger, fear, joy, sadness, and disgust), the push effects may be dominant and the speaker may have little freedom in influencing his vocal expression. A special case could be made for highly distressful situations where vocal characteristics are intentionally modified for purposes of better transmission over a distance and as cues for the sender's localization. In addition to the *push* force, speech communication is influenced by the norms or expectations imposed by the physical or social environment, which require production of specific acoustic features allowing the sender to achieve a particular effect. Such a *pull* force may restrict or enhance some of the surface features of the *push* effects (Scherer, Helfrish, & Scherer, 1980).

It then follows that, when *push* and *pull* factors are blended, vocal signals have a twofold status of symptoms and symbols. When *pull* effects dominate, vocal signals may have a status of falsely spontaneous indicators or symbols. An example would be the use of highly pitched voices in signaling submission and appeasement in friendly or submissive encounters.

The semiological status of affect signaling can thus vary from a symptom to a conventionalized or ritualized symbol. This also raises the issue of speaking *styles*. Is any speaking pattern a style? We link the answer to this question to the potency dimension of cognitive-affective states and suggest that a speaking pattern will be a style as long as it is a result of the speaker's choice. Vocal choice may thus be a psychologically important factor related to the speaker's identity.

In Table 3-1, we present the control-parameter features for five types of cognitive-affective states with the corresponding semiotic status of their vocal correlates. The five states correspond closely to Scherer's descriptions of major types of affect (Scherer, 2005).

Table 3–1. Predictions for control-parameter configurations for five types of cognitive-affective states and the semiotic status of their vocal correlates. *Open* = unpredicted

Type of cognitive-affective state	Position of control-parameter values	Rapidity of change of control-parameter values	Stability over time	Semiological status of vocal patterns
Emotions	Outside normal range	Very high	Low	Symptom
Moods	Within normal range or close to critical limits	Medium	Low to Medium	Mainly symptom
Attitudes	Within normal range	Low to medium	Medium to high	Symptom and/or symbol
Interpersonal stances	Within normal range	Medium to high	Short to medium	Mainly symbol
Personality	Within normal range	Open	Very high	Symptom

As the interpretation of the speech signal is probabilistic, we believe that affectively marked speech patterns function as parallel codes that provide contextual information, thus helping the receiver to disambiguate the meaning of the utterance (see Chapter 15).

Vocal Manifestations of Cognitive-Affective States and Processes

Within the framework of the unified model, vocal manifestations of cognitive affective states and processes can be studied in their continuity from the states traditionally regarded as purely cognitive (doubt, certainty) and unemotional, to emotionally *colored* interpersonal stances (friendly), up to full-fledged emotional reactions. While vocal correlates of discrete emotions have been amply studied in the past two decades, those of other affectively colored states have received less attention. Exceptions are relatively recent studies in assessing the emotional tone in spontaneous dialogues (Cowie, Douglas-Cowie, & Romano, 1999), those related to the acoustic indicators of attitudes (Wichmann, 2002), and various cognitive-affective dimensions (Kehrein, 2002). Both Wichmann's and Kehrein's work emphasize the importance of social and linguistic context for the interpretation of vocally encoded cognitive-affective states. In addition to the classical vocal parameters related to F_0, Nì Chasaide and Gobl (2002) found the association between voice quality and the perceived *affective coloring* of speech. Eric Keller's study (2003) provided evidence for vocal changes related to attitude and thematic coloration of speech. Research on vocal indicators of emotional dimensions has shown that listeners can consistently rate vocal expressions of emotions on the scales of activation, valence, and potency and that each dimension is correlated with a number of vocal parameters (Laukka et al., 2005).

Vocal Correlates of Interpersonal Stance in Medical Interviews

Zei Pollermann conducted a pilot study of vocal correlates of interpersonal stance in pre-anesthesia medical interviews. Interpersonal stance is defined as an affective stance taken toward another person in a specific interaction, coloring the interpersonal exchange in that situation as for example: distant, cold, warm, supportive, reassuring, calming, or contemptuous. As the pre-anesthesia medical interview has a well-defined structure (Wolff & Scemama-Clergue 2002), it allowed setting clear hypotheses about the type of affective stance appropriate for each of the two main phases of the interview. The aim of the first phase is to obtain anamnestic information and examine the patient, while the aim of the second phase is to decide on the type of anesthesia, to inform the patient about the risks without creating anxiety, and to obtain the patient's consent. It was hypothesized that the interpersonal stance appropriate for the examination phase could be described as encouraging, while that appropriate for the announcement of risks would be reassuring and calming. Our predictions regarding vocal correlates of such affective stances took into account discursive operations of topicalization, focalization, and comment. These operations use prosodic marking to attribute various degrees of informative salience to different topics (Caelen-Haumont, 1991) and signal the speaker's emotive involvement in the conversation (Selting, 1994).

Hypotheses

It was hypothesized that vocal signaling of an encouraging affective stance would follow the prosodic patterns congruent with higher informative salience, higher than neutral levels of positively valenced arousal, and a medium level of potency. By contrast a reassuring and calming affective stance would be characterized by prosodic patterns congruent with low informative salience, low level of arousal, neutral or slightly negatively valenced state, and a medium level of potency. We thus expected the acoustic configurations of the physicians' voices at the time of examining their patients (*exam-voices*) to be different from those at the time of informing them about anesthetic risks (*risk-voices*). Drawing on our previous work regarding acoustic patterns of affect (Scherer & Zei, 1988; Zei Pollermann & Archinard, 2002) and more recent studies (Juslin & Laukka 2003 ;), we expected the *exam-voices* to display higher values on F_0 parameters, close to neutral or low levels of mean vocal intensity and its range (the doctor being physically close to the patient), and a slower speaking rate. By contrast, the *risk-voices* (reflecting a reassuring affective stance) were expected to be characterized by lower values on F_0 parameters, unchanged levels of energy parameters, and a faster pace.

Subjects and Design

Twenty-six patients expected to undergo minor surgical operations were interviewed by six physicians (comprising 19 male-to-male dyads and 7 female-to-female dyads)[2]. The interviews were recorded in a noise-free room, on a professional CD recorder with head fitted microphones allowing mouth-to-microphone distance to be kept constant. Prior to the interview, the patients gave their written consent. The duration of the interview varied from 20 to 30 minutes. The physicians' voices were analyzed by using Praat (Boersma & Weenink, 1996). A classical set of vocal parameters was extracted: mean F_0, F_0 coefficient of variation, F_0 range, F_0 mean absolute slope, mean energy of voiced speech segments, voiced energy range, and the rate of delivery (expressed as the number of syllables uttered per second). The obtained values were normalized by dividing each value by that obtained from the acoustic analysis of the physicians' neutral speech samples recorded outside the hospital environment.

Three external judges assessed the interviews by using the Relational Communication Scale for Observational measurement (RCS-O) (Gallagher, Hartung, & Gregory, 2001), which measured six dimensions of doctor-patient interactions: affection, similarity/depth, receptivity/trust, composure, formality, and dominance.

Statistical Analyses

Paired Samples t-Test was applied to measure the difference between the vocal

---

[2]The authors thank the physicians of Anesthesiology Department of Geneva University Hospitals and specifically Dr. Alain Forster for their active involvement in this study.

parameters obtained in *exam-voices* vs. *risk-voices*. Table 3–2 presents the t-Test results and basic statistics for the normalized values of vocal parameters.

As shown in Table 3–2, the results confirm most of our predictions regarding the configuration of vocal parameters related to the change of affective stance from *encouraging* (in the examination phase) to *calming reassuring* (in the risk-announcing phase) of the interview. The *exam-voices* displayed higher mean F_0, more pitch variability, and a slower pace compared with *risk-voices*. The vocal pattern of the *risk-voices* could be described as *vocal minimization* and is congruent with the aim of informing the patient about the risks without making him or her anxious. The faster rate of delivery in the risk-announcing phase of the interview could also be interpreted as a cue that augments the speaker's credibility (Miller et al 1976).

Pearson correlation coefficients were computed between various dimensions of the RCS-O scale and the vocal parameters. The conversation partners' gender, age and age difference were controlled for when necessary. The results presented in Table 3–3, show that in both conditions *Affection* was negatively correlated with mean F_0, while it was positively correlated with voiced energy range. The *Similarity/depth* dimension was also related to the same parameters. On the *Trust/receptivity* dimension, the exam voices differed from those of *risk-voices* in that the former were correlated with the rate of delivery (r = .39; p = .05) and F_0 coefficient of variation (r = −.38; p = .05). No such correlations were found in *risk-voices* for this dimension. In the *exam-voices* the *Composure* dimension was negatively correlated with mean F_0 (r = −.74; p = .000), and mean absolute slope (r = −.40; p = .05), while it was positively related to the speaker's pace (r = .57; p = .000). In the *risk-voices* the *Composure* dimension was negatively correlated with mean F_0 (r = −.65; p = .000) while it showed a positive correlation with the voiced energy range (r = .43; p = .04). The *Dominance* dimension was found to be significantly related to F_0 coefficient of variation in *risk-voices* only.

Table 3–2. Paired Samples t-Test results for risk-voices vs. exam-voices, with basic statistics for the normalised values of vocal parameters.

Vocal parameter	Exam-voices		Risk-voices		Paired Samples t-Test		
	Mean	SD	Mean	SD	DF	T	Sig. (2-tailed)
Mean F_0	1.24	0.17	1.12	0.16	25	6.47	0.000
F_0 coef. of variation	0.15	0.04	0.12	0.03	25	3.33	0.003
F_0 range	2.48	0.59	2.24	0.53	25	1.73	0.095
F_0 mean absolute slope	1.16	0.22	1.07	0.21	25	2.40	0.024
Rate of delivery	0.87	0.12	0.98	0.12	25	-3.95	0.001
Mean voiced energy	1.06	0.93	1.08	0.11	25	-1.62	0.118
Voiced energy range	1.38	0.10	1.40	0.10	25	-1.10	0.283

Table 3–3. Pearson correlation coefficients with 2-tailed significance levels for the correlations between vocal parameters and five dimensions of the Relational Communication Scale for Observational measurement. Only the parameters significant for at least one dimension are noted for each condition.

Vocal parameter	Affection		Similarity		Trust		Composure		Dominance	
	r	Sig.	r	Sig.	r	Sig.	r	Sig.	r	Sig.
Whole Interview										
Mean F_0	-.68	.00	-.67	.00	-.74	.00	-.73	.00		ns
F_0 coef. of variation		ns	-.45	.02		ns	-.38	.05		ns
F_0 mean abs. slope		ns		ns	-.40	.05		ns		ns
Rate of delivery		ns		ns	.57	.00	.39	.05		ns
Voiced energy range	.44	.03	.43	.04		ns		ns		ns
Risk-voices										
Mean F_0	-.61	.00	-.55	.00	-.58	.00	-.65	.00		ns
F_0 coef. of variation		ns		ns		ns		ns	.43	.04
Voiced energy range	.63	.00	.48	.02		ns	.43	.04		ns
Exam-voices										
Mean F_0	-.66	.00	-.63	.01	-.65	.00	-.72	.00		ns
F_0 coef. of variation		ns	-.44	.03	-.44	.03	-.45	.03	.43	.04
F_0 mean abs. slope		ns		ns		ns		ns	.41	.04
Rate of delivery		ns		ns		ns	.40	.05		ns
Voiced energy range	.61	.00	.52	.01		ns		ns		ns

59

In summary, most of statistically significant correlations with the RCS-O scale are related to F_0 parameters. The results seem to confirm most of our hypotheses regarding the difference between vocal correlates of an encouraging affective stance and a reassuring and calming one. The two types of stances appear to follow the prosodic patterns congruent with the presumed configurations of the speakers' affective-cognitive states (the *push* force), and the interaction context (the *pull* force).

Final Remarks

The proposed unified model of cognition, emotion, and action suggests that cognitive processes that trigger and steer adaptive behavior necessarily evolve in a three-dimensional affective space—the dimensions being valence, arousal, and potency. As a result, the subject's perceptual-sensorimotor-conceptual schemata activated for purposes of goal driven action always include affective components. States and processes called *emotions, moods, attitudes, interpersonal stances,* or *personality traits* are then observer dependent conceptualizations of transitory and/or long-term configurations of the person's affective space. Seen from such a perspective, human voice necessarily reflects the ever-changing configurations of the speaker's affective space. The model needs further elaboration in terms of theoretical sophistication and empirical examination of (a) the interactions between the three control parameters, (b) retroactive influence of consciousness and learning on valence, activation, and potency tagging, and (c) the relations between intra-personal, interpersonal, and transpersonal dimensions of self as major sources of competing interests at stake in adaptive behavior.

References

Ashby, W. R. (1961). *An introduction to cybernetics*. London: Chapman & Hall.

Bachorowski, J. A., & Owren, M. J. (1995). Vocal expression of emotion: Acoustic properties of speech are associated with emotional intensity and context. *Psychological Science, 6*(4), 219–224.

Bargh, J. A. (1997). The automaticity of everyday life. In R. S. Wyer, Jr. (Ed.), *The automaticity of everyday life: Advances in social cognition* (Vol. 10, pp. 1–61). Mahwah, NJ: Erlbaum.

Bertalanffy, L. V. (1968). *General system theory: Foundations, development, applications*. New York: Braziller.

Boersma, P., & Weenink, D. J. M. (1996). Praat: Doing phonetics by computer, version 3.4. Amsterdam, Netherlands: Institute of Phonetic Sciences.

Buyssens, M. E. (1943). *Les langages et le discours*. Bruxelles: Lebègue

Cacioppo, J. T., Klein, D. J., Bentson, G. G., & Hatfield, E. (1993). The psychophysiology of emotions. In M. Lewis &. J. M. Haviland (Eds.), *Handbook of emotions* (pp. 119–142). New York: Guildford.

Caelen-Haumont, G. (1991). *Stratégies des locuteurs en réponse à des consignes de lecture d'un texte: Analyse des interactions entre modèles syntaxiques, sémantiques, pragmatique et paramètres prosodiques*. Unpublished doctoral thesis, University of Aix-en-Provence, France.

Canamero, L. (2001). Emotions and adaptation in autonomous agents: A design perspective. *Cybernetics and Systems, an International Journal, 32,* 507–529.

Carver, C. S., & Scheier, M. F. (1981). *Attention and self-regulation: A control-theory approach to human behavior*. New York: Springer-Verlag.

Carver, C. S., & Scheier, M. F. (1982). Control theory: A useful conceptual framework for personality-social, clinical, and health psychology. *Psychological Bulletin, 92*(1), 111–135.

Carver, C. S., & Scheier, M. F. (2002). Control processes and self-organization as complementary principles underlying behavior. *Personality and Social Psychology Review, 6*, 304–315.

Cellérier, G. (1968). Modèles cybernétiques et adaptation. In J. Piaget (Ed.), *Etudes d'épistémologie génétique* (Vol. XXII, pp. 6–90). Paris: Presses universitaires de France.

Cellérier, G. (1979). Structures cognitives et schèmes d'action I. *Archives de Psychologie, 180*, 87–106.

Chapman, C. R., & Nakamura, Y. (2001). The affective dimension of pain: Mechanisms and implications. In A. Kazniak (Ed.), *Emotions qualia and consciousness* (pp. 181–210). London: World Scientific.

Clynes, M., & Nettheim, M. (1982). The living quality of music: Neurobiologic basis of communicating feeling. In M. Clynes (Ed.), *Music, mind, and brain* (pp. 47–82). New York: Plenum.

Cowie, R, Douglas-Cowie, E. & Romano, A. (1999). Changing emotional tone in dialogue and its prosodic correlates. In *Proceedings of the European Speech Communication Association Workshop on Dialogue and Prosody*, September 1–3, 1999, Eindhoven, The Netherlands, pp. 41–46.

Damasio, A. R. (1994). *Descartes' error: Emotion, reason, and the human brain*. New York: Putnam.

Darwin, C. (1872). *The expression of the emotions in man and animals*. London: Murray.

Davidson, R. J. (1992). Emotion and affective style: Hemispheric differences. *Psychological Science 3*, 39–43.

Davidson, R. J. (1992). Prolegomenon to the structure of emotion: Gleanings from neu-ropsychology. *Cognition and Emotion, 6*, 245–268.

Dewey, J. (1922). Human nature and conduct. In *The Collected Works of John Dewey; Middle Works: Vol. 14 Habits and Will* (pp. 21–32). Carbondale, IL: Southern Illinois University Press.

Duffy, E. (1941). An explanation of "emotional" phenomena without the use of the concept of emotion. *The Journal of General Psychology, 25*, 283–293.

Faith, M., & Thayer, J. F. (2001). A dynamical systems interpretation of a dimensional model of emotion. *Scandinavian Journal of Psychology, 42*(2), 121–133.

Förster, J., & Strack F. (1997). Motor actions in retrieval of valenced information: a motor congruency effect. *Perceptual and Motor Skills, 85*, 1419–1427.

Gallagher, S. (2005). *How the body shapes the mind*. Oxford, UK: Clarendon Press.

Gallagher, T.-J., Hartung, P. J., & Gregory, S. W., Jr. (2001). Assessment of a measure of relational communication for doctor-patient interactions. *Patient Education and Counseling, 45*, 211–218.

Gallese, V., Keysers, C., & Rizzolatti, G. (2004). A unifying view of the basis of social cognition. *Trends in Cognitive Science, 8*(9), 396–403.

Gallese, V. & Lakoff, G. (2005). The brain's concepts: The role of the sensory-motor system in conceptual knowledge. *Cognitive Neuropsychology, 22*(3/4), 455–479.

Hobson, R. P. (1993). Through feeling and sight to self and symbol. In U. Neisser (Ed.), *The perceived self: Ecological and interpersonal sources of self-knowledge* (pp. 254–279). New York: Cambridge University Press.

Juslin, P. N., & Laukka, P. (2003). Communication of emotions in vocal expression and music performance: Different channels, same code? *Psychological Bulletin, 129*(5), 770–814.

Karmiloff-Smith, A. (1992). Beyond modularity: A developmental perspective on cognitive science. Cambridge, MA: MIT Press.

Kehrein, R. (2002). *The prosody of authentic emotions*. Paper given at the 1st International Conference on Speech Prosody, Aix-en-Provence, France.

Keller, E. (2003, August). *Voice characteristics of MARSEC speakers*. Paper given at the VOQUAL: Voice Quality: Functions, Analysis and Synthesis conference, Geneva, Switzerland.

Kurath, H. (1921). *The semantic sources of the words for the emotions in Sanskrit, Greek, Latin, and the Germanic languages*. Chicago: Chicago.

Lambie, J. A., & Marcel, A. J. (2002). Consciousness and the varieties of emotion experience: A theoretical framework. *Psychological Review, 109*(2), 219-259.

Lane, R. (2001). Hierarchical organisation of emotional experience and its neural substrates. In A. Kazniak (Ed.), *Emotions qualia and consciousness* (Vol. 10, pp. 247-270). London: World Scientific.

Lane, R. D., Reiman, E. M., Bradley, M. M., Lang, P. J., Ahern, G. L., Davidson, R. J., et al. (1997). Neuroanatomical correlates of pleasant and unpleasant emotion. *Neuropsychologia, 35*(11), 1437-1444.

Lane, R., & Zei Pollermann, B. (2002). Complexity of emotion representations. In L. Feldman Barrett & P. Salovey (Eds.), *The wisdom in feeling, psychological processes in emotional intelligence* (pp. 271-293). New York: Guilford.

Lang, P. (1990). Cognition in emotion: Concept and action. In C. E. Izard, J. Kagan, & R. B. Zajonc (Eds.), *Emotions, cognition and behavior* (pp. 193-226). Cambridge: Cambridge University Press.

Lang, P. (1995). The emotion probe: Studies of motivation and attention. *American Psychologist, 50*(5), 372-385.

Laukka, P., Juslin, P. N., & Bresin, R. (2005). A dimensional approach to vocal expression of emotion. *Cognition and Emotion, 19*(5), 633-653.

LeDoux, J. (2002). *Synaptic self*. Harmondworth, UK: Penguin Books.

Leventhal, H. (1970). Findings and theory in the study of fear communications. In L. Berkowitz (Ed.), *Advances in experimental social psychology* (Vol. 5, pp. 119-186). New York: Academic Press.

Leventhal, H., & Nerenz, D. (1985). The assessment of illness cognition. In P. Karoly (Ed.), *Measurement strategies in health* (pp. 517-554). New York: John Wiley & Sons.

Mandler, G. (1975). *Mind and emotion*. New York: Wiley.

Mandler, G. (1982). *Mind and emotion* (2nd ed.). Malabar, FL: R. E. Krieger.

Mandler, G. (1997). *Human nature explored*. New York: Oxford University Press.

Matthews, G., Campbell, S. E., Falconer, S., Joyner, L. A., Huggins, J., Gilliland, K., et al. (2002). Fundamental dimensions of subjective state in performance settings: Task engagement, distress, and worry. *Emotion, 2*(4), 315-340.

Mehrabian, A., & Russel, J. (1974). *An approach to environmental psychology*. Cambridge, MA: MIT Press.

Miller, G. A., Galanter, E., & Pribram, K. H. (1986). *Plans and the structure of behavior*. New York: Adams-Bannister-Cox.

Miller, N., Maruyama, G., Beaber, R. J., & Valone, I. C. (1976). Speed of speech and persuasion. *Journal of Personality and Social Psychology, 34*, 615-624.

Molenaar, P. C. M., & Oppenheimer, L. (1985). Dynamic models of development and the mechanistic organismic controversy. *New Ideas in Psychology, 3*, 233-242.

Nì Chasaide, A., & Gobl, C. (2002). Voice quality and the synthesis of affect. In E. Keller, G. Bailly, A. Monaghan, J. Terken, & M. Huckvale (Eds.), *Improvements in speech synthesis* (pp. 252-263). London: Wiley.

Noblitt, J. S. (1978, December). *Compensation and catastrophe: Motor equivalence in vowel production*. Paper presented at the First Conference of AAAL, Boston, MA.

Ohman, A. 1999. Distinguishing unconscious from conscious emotional processes: Methodological considerations and theoretic implications. In T. Dalgleish and M. Power (Eds.), *Handbook of cognition and emotion* (pp. 321-352). Chichester, UK: Wiley.

Orlando, A. G., Canamero, L., & te Boekhorst, R. (2003). *Analyzing the performance of "winner-take-all" and "voting-based" action selection policies within the two-resource problem*. ECAL 2003: 733-742. Paper presented at AISB 05, Agents that want and like. Hatfield, UK.

Osgood, C. H., May, W. H., & Miron, M. S. (1975). *Cross-cultural universals of affective meaning*. Urbana, IL: University of Illinois Press.

Piaget, J. (1950). *Introduction à l'épistémologie génétique. 3 La pensée biologique, la pensée psychologique et la pensée sociale* (1st ed., Vol. 3). Paris: Presses universitaires de France.

Piaget, J. (1954). *Les relations entre l'affectivité et l'intelligence dans le développement mental de l'enfant*. Paris: Centre de documentation universitaire.

Piaget, J. (1967). *La psychologie de l'intelligence*. Paris: A. Colin.

Piaget, J. (1975). *L'équilibration des structures cognitives: Problème central du développement* (1st ed.). Paris: Presses universitaires de France.

Plutchik, R. (1962). *The emotions: Facts, theories, and a new model*. New York: Random House.

Plutchik, R. (1980). *Emotion, a psychoevolutionary synthesis*. New York: Harper & Row.

Plutchik, R., & Kellerman, H. (1986). *Biological foundations of emotion*. Orlando, FL: Academic Press.

Prieto, L. J. (1975). *Pertinence et pratique: Essai de sémiologie*. Paris: Editions dc Minuit.

Prieto, L. J. (1991). *Sull'arte e sul soggetto*. Parma, Italy: Pratiche Editrice.

Russel, J. (1989). Measures of emotion. In R. Plutchik & H. Kellerman (Eds.), *The measurement of emotions* (pp. 83-111). San Diego, CA: Academic Press.

Russell, J. A. (2003). Core affect and the psychological construction of emotion. *Psychological Review,110*(1), 145-172.

Russell, J. A., & Barrett, L. F. (1999). Core affect, prototypical emotional episodes, and other things called emotion: Dissecting the elephant. *Journal of Personality and Social Psychology, 76*, 805-819.

Sander, D., Grafman, J., & Zalla, T. (2003). The human amygdala: An evolved system for relevance detection. *Reviews in the Neurosciences, 14*(4), 303-316.

Selting, M. (1994). Emphatic speech style—with special focus on the prosodic signalling of heightened emotive involvement in conversation. *Journal of Pragmatics, 22*, 375-408.

Saussure, F. D., (1972). *Cours de linguistique générale*. Paris: Payot.

Scheutz, M. (2002). Agents with or without emotions? In S. Haller & G. Simmons (Eds.), *Proceedings of FLAIRS 2002* (pp. 89-94). Menlo Park, CA: AAAI Press.

Scherer, K. R. (1986). Vocal affect expression: A review and a model for future research. *Psychological Bulletin, 99*(2), 143-165.

Scherer, K. R. (2000). Emotions as episodes of subsystem synchronization driven by nonlinear appraisal processes. In M. D. Lewis & I. Granic (Eds.), *Emotion, development, and self-organization: Dynamic systems approaches to emotional development* (pp. 70-99). New York: Cambridge University Press.

Scherer, K. R. (2005). Unconscious processes in emotion. In P. Niedenthal, L. Feldman-Barret, & P. Winkielman (Eds.), *The unconscious in emotion* (pp. 312-334). New York: Guilford.

Scherer, U., Helfrish, H., & Scherer, K. R. (1980). Internal push or external pull? Determinants of paralinguistic behavior. In H. Giles, P. Robinson, & P. Smith (Eds.), *Language: Social psychological perspectives* (pp. 279-282). Oxford: Pergamon.

Scherer, K. R., & Zei, B. (1988). Vocal indicators of affective disorders. *Psychotherapy and Psychosomatics, 49*, 179-186.

Sebeok, T. A. (1985). *Contributions to the doctrine of signs*. Lanham, MD: University Press of America.

Selting, M. (1994). Emphatic speech style with special focus on the prosodic signaling of heightened emotive involvement in conversation. *Journal of Pragmatics*, *22*, 375-408.

Snaith, M., & Holland, O. (1991). An investigation of two mediation strategies for behavioral control in animals and animats. In J.-A. Meyer & S. W. Wilson (Eds.), *Proceedings of the first international conference on simulation of adaptive behavior on From animals to animats* (pp. 255-262). Cambridge, MA: MIT Press.

Stewart, I. N., & Peregoy, P. L. (1983). Catastrophe theory modeling in psychology. *Psychological Bulletin*, *94*(1), 336-362.

Thom, R. (1974). *Modèles mathématiques de la morphogenèse*. Paris: Christian Bourgois.

Trevarthen, C. (1993). The self born in intersubjectivity: The psychology of an infant communicating. In U. Neisser (Ed.), *The perceived self: Ecological and interpersonal sources of the self-knowledge* (pp. 121-173). New York: Cambridge University Press.

Tversky, A., & Kahneman, D. (1981). The framing of decisions and the psychology of choice. *Science*, *211*(4481), 453-458.

Tyrrell, T. (1993). *Computational mechanisms for action selection*. Unpublished doctoral dissertation, University of Edinburgh.

Van Geert, P. (1998). A dynamic systems model of basic developmental mechanisms: Piaget, Vygotsky, and beyond. *Psychological Review*, *105*(4), 634-677.

Watson, D., & Tellegen, A. (1999). Issues in the dimensional structure of affect—Effects of descriptors, measurement error, and response formats: Comment on Russell and Carroll (1999). *Psychological Bulletin*, *125*, 601-610.

Watt, D. F. (2001). Affective neuroscience and extended reticular thalamic activating system (ERTAS) theories of consciousness. In A. Kazniak (Ed.), *Emotions qualia and consciousness* (pp. 290-320). London: World Scientific.

Wichmann, A. (2002, April). *Attitudinal intonation and the inferential process*. Paper given at the 1st International Conference on Speech Prosody, Aix-en-Provence, France.

Wolff, A., & Scemama-Clergue, J. (2002). La consultation d'anesthésie: Que dire et comment le dire, *Médecine et Hygiène*, *60*, 2397-4000.

Wundt, W. M., & Schaub, E. L. (1921). *Elements of folk psychology: Outlines of a psychological history of the development of mankind*. London: G. Allen and Unwin.

Zeeman, E. C. (1976). Catastrophe theory. *Scientific American*, *234*, 65-83.

Zei Pollermann, B., & Archinard, M. (2002). Acoustic patterns of emotions. In E. Keller, G. Bailly, A. Monaghan, J. Terken, & M. Huckvale (Eds.), *Improvements in speech synthesis* (pp. 237-245). London: J. Wiley.

CHAPTER 4

Anger or Fear? Cross-Cultural Multimodal Interpretations of Emotional Expressions

Åsa Abelin

Introduction

Speech and communication are basically multimodal, with emotions expressed with body and face to a higher degree than vocally. The present investigation focuses on the interaction between non-verbal and vocal expression of emotions in a specific cross-linguistic setting, Swedish and Spanish. Though many cross-linguistic studies of emotional prosody have demonstrated that some emotional expressions are well interpreted (for example, anger), other emotions (for example, joy) are less well interpreted (Abelin & Allwood, 2000; Massaro, 2000). One possible explanation for this discrepancy is that the expressions of some emotions vary more than the expressions of other emotions.

Another possibility is that some emotions are expressed more in the gestural than in verbal dimensions. Although it is thought that speakers are generally better at interpreting the prosody of their native language, there could be evolutionary reasons for this (Darwin, 1872/1965).

In the field of multimodal emotional communication, studies show that judges are almost as accurate in inferring different emotions from vocal as from facial expression (for an overview, see overview in Scherer, 2003). Massaro (2000; 2002), working under the assumption that multiple sources of information are used to perceive a person's emotion, made experiments with an animated talking head expressing four emotions in auditory, visual, bimodal consistent, and bimodal inconsistent conditions. Overall performance was more accurate with

65

two sources of consistent information than with either source of information alone. In another study de Gelder and Vroomen (2000) asked the participants to identify an emotion from a photograph and/or a spoken sentence. They found that identification judgments were influenced by both sources of information, even when judges were instructed to base their decisions on just the single source.

Matsumoto, Franklin, Choi, Rogers, and Tatani (2002) and Matsumoto and Ekman (1989) review many studies on the cultural influence on the perception of emotions, and found both universality and culture specificity in the perception of emotions. Universality in combination with display rules is generally accepted in psychology (i.e., culture-specific rules for how much certain feelings are displayed when other people are present).

Assuming that there is interaction between the senses, and that facial expression of emotion is more universal than prosody, then the cross-linguistic interpretation of emotions should be more successful in a multimodal setting than in a single modality only.

With this idea in mind we conducted the study reported here. The aim was to investigate how the speakers of Spanish and Swedish interpret vocally and multimodally expressed emotions in Spanish. Specifically, the following questions were asked:

1. Can Swedish as well as Spanish speakers accurately interpret Spanish emotional prosody?
2. Is there an influence between the auditive and visual channels in a cross-linguistic interpretation of emotional expressions?

Methods

A method of elicitation was used, with speakers enacting emotional speech from a set of stimuli of drawings of selected facial expressions. The verbal emotional expressions to the stimuli were elicited and audio recorded. Thereafter, the recorded audio data were presented to listeners for interpretation of the emotions expressed. The listeners first attended to the voice signals alone, and then they listened to voice in combination with looking at the facial expressions of the corresponding drawings, but were told to judge voice only.

Recordings were made of a male speaker of Spanish expressing eight different emotions. The emotions were (a) sad and tired, (b) angry, (c) sad, (d) skeptical, (e) delighted, (f) afraid, (g) depressed, and (h) very happy. The method of elicitation was the following: (a) The speaker was presented with the stimuli of schematic drawings of faces expressing emotions. (b) The speaker was instructed to try to experience emotionally what the face was expressing. (c) The speaker was instructed to try to express this emotion with the voice, while uttering the name "Amanda."

The expression was recorded into the software Praat (Boersma & Weenink, 2005). After each recording of an emotion, the speaker named just the emotion expressed, and this label was used as the correct answer in listening experiments that followed. In this way the facial stimuli were used for the speakers of several languages and hence were not culture specific.

The emotions expressed by the Spanish speaker were (a) sad and tired, (b) angry,

(c) sad, (d) skeptical, (e) delighted, (f) afraid, (g) depressed, and (h) very happy.

Elicitation of Listeners' Responses

The listener group consisted of 15 Swedish adult native speakers, 8 men and 7 women, and 10 Spanish adult native speakers, all male. The listeners were first presented with the speech material over a computer's speakers and were told to name the different emotions they heard, one by one. The speech material was presented once. Later, the listeners were presented with the speech material at the same time as they watched the faces presented on a computer screen, and they were asked to name the different emotions as they heard and saw each expression.[1] In this later subexperiment, the faces were presented with the emotional expression that was produced for each particular face. Listeners were told that the emotions expressed could be partly different from in the first experiment.

Results

The results for the Swedish interpretations of the Spanish speakers' prosodic expressions of the emotions are shown in Figure 4–1. There are clear differences in how well the Swedes interpreted the different emotions of the Spanish speaker, in comparison with the Spanish listeners. The two expressions of sadness were interpreted much more accurately by the Swedes than the other emotions—but only with 53% accuracy. The other emotions were interpreted quite poorly by the Swedes.

The results shown in Figure 4–1 are presented in comparison with the results of the "face only" and multimodal stimuli in Figure 4–2. Figure 4–2 demonstrates six interesting findings. These are: (a) Prosody alone is more difficult to interpret than multimodal stimuli. (b) Prosody with simultaneous facial expression produces a much better interpretation for all but one emotion (very happy). (c) Some emotions were easier to interpret than others. (d) The face alone is often easier to interpret than voice plus face; adding the voice makes the interpretation less accurate for four of the emotions. (e) There were some emotions that were more difficult to interpret in all modalities, while others were easier in all modalities (sad, happy, afraid, depressed). (f) The emotion that is recognized relatively well in vocal expression alone is sadness.

Finally, when we can add to Figure 4–2 the Spanish interpretations of Spanish vocal and multimodal stimuli, the following is noted (see Figure 4–3). Interpretation of emotional expressions was always more successful when the stimuli were multimodal for the Spanish listeners also. The Swedish listeners, who were poor at interpreting the Spanish voice, seemed to be greatly aided by the visual data. This made the difference larger between the oral and multimodal interpretations for the Swedish than for the Spanish listeners. Neither of the language groups was generally better at interpreting the multimodal stimuli.

---

[1]Utilizing Psyscope software.

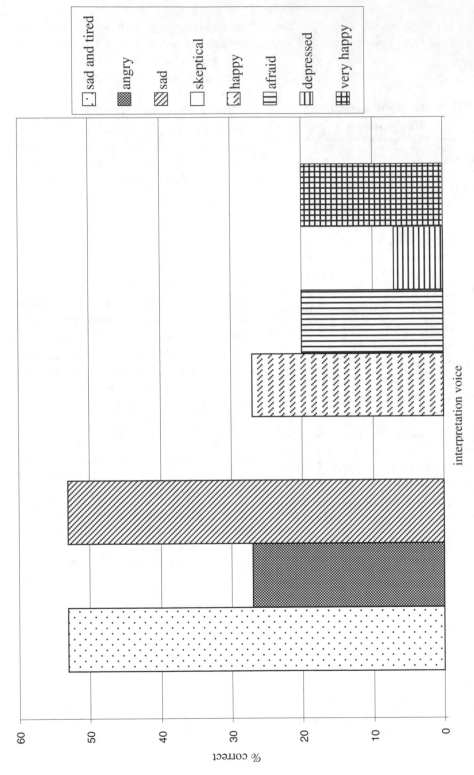

Figure 4–1. Swedish listeners interpretations Spanish speaker's prosody. The intended emotions of the speaker were, from left to right: sad and tired, angry, sad, skeptical, happy, afraid, depressed, and very happy.

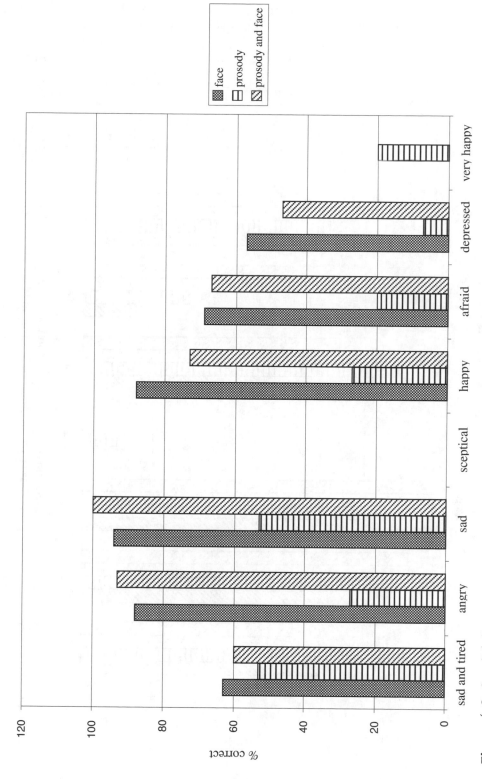

Figure 4–2. Swedish listeners' interpretations of (a) the eight faces, (b) emotional prosody expressed by the Spanish speaker, and (c) simultaneous emotional prosody expressed by the Spanish speaker and facial expression.

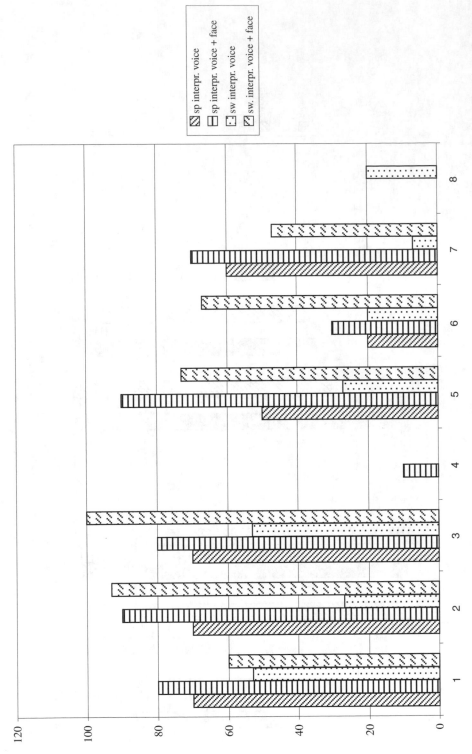

Figure 4–3. Percent correct interpretations of Spanish voice and voice + face of the eight different emotions: sad and tired, angry, sad, skeptical, happy, afraid, depressed, very happy, for both Spanish and Swedish listeners.

F_0 Analysis

An F_0 analysis of the stimuli showed that the speaker's F_0 was generally very high. Almost all of the listeners also interpreted the male speaker as a woman. The emotion with the highest maximum F_0 was fear, and thereafter skeptical and the two variants of happy. The emotion with the lowest minimum F_0 was anger. The ones with the lowest maximum F_0 were sad, depressed, and angry. In general, high maximum F_0 was accompanied by high minimum F_0 and vice versa. The exception was the skeptical emotion. The emotion with the highest F_0 was afraid, which is in agreement with many other studies (see Laukka, 2004).

The F_0 data are presented in Figure 4-4. The F_0 values could be related to the interpretations in the following way: the least successfully interpreted emotion (by both language groups)—skeptical— is the one with the largest F_0 variation. The sad and tired emotions, which were the emotions with the least F_0 variation, were interpreted best from the voice signal alone, by both language groups.

Gender Comparisons

The interpretations of 8 Swedish men and 7 women were contrasted to see if either gender group was generally better at interpreting the intended emotions. No gender tendencies were found. The Spanish group consisted of mainly men and therefore no gender comparison was made.

Another gender comparison could be made because the speaker, who was a male, had a very high F_0. One group of listeners was told that the speaker was a man, while another all female group of listeners was told that the speaker was a woman . The results showed no clear differences between the listener groups.

Discussion

The results of this study show that perception of emotional expressions in this cross-linguistic setting were more successful when the stimuli were multimodal, even though the facial stimuli were very schematic. The present study also shows that certain emotions (happy and afraid) are more difficult to interpret from prosody, by both language groups.

There are a number of inherent problems involved in studying cross-cultural interpretation of linguistic phenomena, specifically the expression of emotions. There are translation problems due to different categorizations of the emotional spectrum, different display rules for different emotions, listeners' differing knowledge of different display rules, word finding problems, and so on. This study has attempted to handle the translation problem by evoking prosodic expressions directly from facial stimuli. Expectations on different display rules were avoided by listeners not knowing the native language of the speaker.

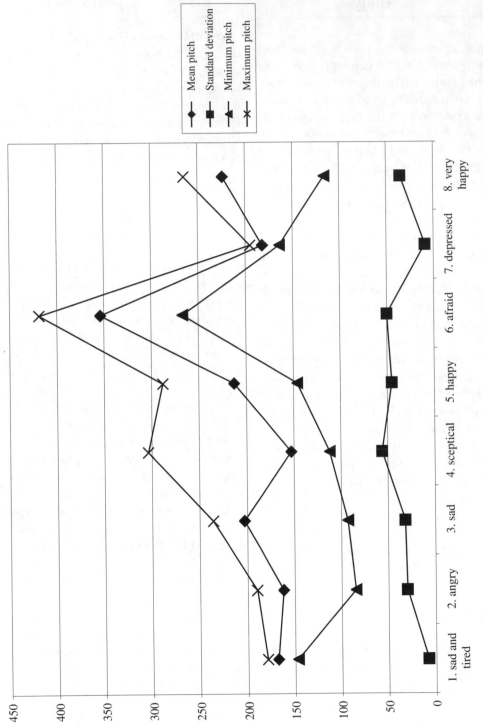

Figure 4–4. F0 mean, F_0 variation, F_0 maxima and minima for the eight different emotions.

Conclusions

Emotions are more appropriately interpreted intra- and cross-linguistically when both the visual and auditory signals are present than when only the auditory signal is present. Visual stimuli alone give the best interpretations. Some emotions are more easily interpreted, both intra- and cross-linguistically, prosodically and multimodally, e.g., sadness.

There is the possibility that the facial expression of emotion is more universal than prosodic expression. The prosodic production of emotional expressions per se could be universal, at least for certain emotions, but the emotional prosody is never heard in isolation, but always in combination with the speech prosody of each particular language. Another possibility, which will need further studies, is the question of whether certain emotions are more dependent on prosodic information and other emotions more dependent on facial expression.

References

Abelin, Å., & Allwood, J. (2000). Cross linguistic interpretation of emotional prosody. In R. Cowie, E. Douglas-Cowie, & M. Schröder (Eds.), *ISCA Workshop on speech and emotion* (pp. 110–113). Belfast, Northern Ireland: Textflow.

Boersma, P., & Weenink, D. (2005). Praat: Doing phonetics by computer (Version 4.3.01) [Computer program]. Retrieved September 2, 2005, from http://www.praat.org/

Darwin, C. (1872/1965). *The expression of the emotions in man and animals.* Chicago: University of Chicago Press.

de Gelder, B., & Vroomen, J. (2000). The perception of emotions by ear and eye. *Cognition and Emotion, 14*, 289–311.

Laukka, P. (2004). *Vocal expression of emotion—Discrete-emotions and dimensional accounts.* Uppsala, Finland: Acta Universitatis Upsaliensis.

Massaro, D. W. (2000). Multimodal emotion perception: Analogous to speech processes. In R. Cowie, E. Douglas-Cowie, & M. Schröder (Eds.), *Proceedings of the ISCA workshop on speech and emotion* (pp. 114–121). Belfast, Northern Ireland: Textflow.

Massaro, D. W. (2002). Multimodal speech perception. In B. Granström, D. House, & I. Karlsson (Eds.), *Multimodality in language and speech systems* (pp. 45–71). Dordrecht, Netherlands: Kluwer Academic Publishers.

Matsumoto, D., & Ekman, P. (1989). American-Japanese differences in intensity ratings of facial expressions of emotion. *Motivation and Emotion, 13*, 143–157.

Matsumoto, D., Franklin, B., Choi, J.-W., Rogers, D., & Tatani, H. (2002). Cultural influences on the expression and perception of emotion. In W. B. Gudykunst & B. Mody (Eds.), *Handbook of international and intercultural communication* (pp. 107–125). Thousand Oaks, CA: Sage.

Scherer, K. (2003). Vocal communication of emotion: A review of research paradigms. *Speech Communication, 40*(1), 227–256.

Scherer, K. R., Banse, R., & Wallbott, H. G. (2001). Emotion inferences from vocal expression correlate across languages and cultures. *Journal of Cross-Cultural Psychology, 32*(1), 76–92.

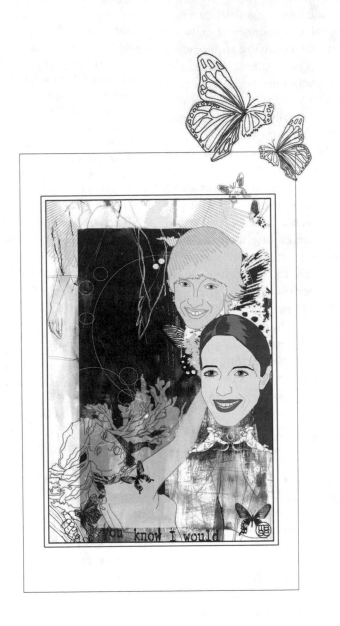

you know I would.

CHAPTER 5

Brain Correlates of Vocal Emotional Processing in Men and Women

Annett Schirmer and Elizabeth Simpson

The expression of emotions plays a key role in human communication. Besides language, humans use nonverbal cues such as facial and vocal expressions to convey emotions. The voice is especially important as an emotional medium because it is a carrier for spoken language production. Additionally, listeners can perceive vocal expressions across long distances and in situations where facial or gestural information is not available (e.g., telephone). It is commonly believed that women are better than men in recognizing emotional tone of voice and this belief has been confirmed in behavioral studies. Unfortunately, it is not until recently that gender has been considered as a modulating factor of the brain mechanisms underlying vocal emotion comprehension. Here we present work that sheds some light on the neuro-anatomical and temporal underpinnings of these mechanisms as they occur in men and women. Respective findings not only enhance our understanding of vocal emotional comprehension, they also make it clear that research on gender differences in emotion recognition provides useful insight into gender specific interaction patterns that may help explain some of the difficulties that arise when men and women communicate.

The Sounds of Emotions

Being happy or sad not only affects our state of mind; it also affects our body. For example, arousing emotions are correlated with an increase in heart rate, muscle tension, and rate and depth of breathing. These physiological changes, among other responses, affect how we interact with our environment and, more specifically, they influence the bodily systems we use for interpersonal communication. The vocal production system in particular is highly dependent on the physiological parameters modulated by emotional state (Scherer, 1989). For example, increased subglottal pressure (Ps) and greater laryngeal tension, which depend on respiration and laryngeal muscle actions, are correlated with an increase in a speaker's *loudness*. Ps and laryngeal tension also mediate the vibration of the vocal folds with increased vibration frequency being associated with a higher *pitch* (Van den Berg, Zantema, & Doornenbal, 1957). These and other acoustic changes such as increased *tempo* of vocal production are perceived by listeners as reflecting an increase in emotional arousal. Abnormally elevated Ps in habitual voice production by patients with adductor spasmodic dysphonia—a form of laryngeal dystonia— evokes a perception of their voice as being emotionally affected and produces a perception of speaking with undue stress or of being strangulated (Shipp, Izdebski, Schutte, & Morrissey, 1988).

Brain Regions Mediating Vocal Emotional Processing in Men and Women

Early work that investigated how listeners infer a speaker's emotional state based on vocal expressions employed emotional identification tasks. In these tasks, participants heard vocal expressions and indicated the perceived emotional state (e.g., happy, sad, angry, afraid). When summa-

rizing this work, Hall (1978) found that there was a small but consistent gender difference. Moreover, emotion identification accuracy was higher in women than in men.

Subsequent research on the brain correlates of vocal emotional perception failed to implement these findings. One approach that researchers took in this context was to compare the emotional identification accuracy of patients with brain lesions to the left or right hemisphere while averaging across gender. This work revealed that right hemisphere lesions impaired emotion recognition skills to a greater extent than left hemisphere lesions did (Blonder, Bowers, & Heilman, 1991; Van Lancker & Fromkin, 1973; Van Lancker, 1980). Based on these observations, it was concluded that the right hemisphere is specialized for the processing of vocal emotional information. Analysis of the emotion identification errors made by patients with left and right hemisphere lesions furthermore suggested that both groups of patients were differently impaired with respect to the acoustic parameters that convey emotions (Van Lancker & Sidtis, 1992). Specifically, the errors of right hemisphere patients seemed to be due to deficient processing of pitch information, whereas the errors of left hemisphere patients were associated with deficient temporal processing. Based on this it has been concluded that the two hemispheres are differently engaged in processing acoustic information (for a review see Schirmer, 2004).

Neuroimaging research that investigated the brain regions activated when listening to vocal emotional expressions provided evidence for the assumptions that the right hemisphere is specialized for emotional processing, and that the acoustic cues that convey emotional information are differently lateralized in the brain. Contrasting vocal emotional identification tasks with a resting baseline or a linguistic task consistently activated the right hemisphere to a greater extent than the left hemisphere (Wildgruber, Pihan, Ackermann, Erb, & Grodd, 2002; Wildgruber et al., 2005; Gandour et al., 2003; George et al., 1996; Buchanan et al., 2000). Moreover, within the right hemisphere, inferior and middle frontal gyrus (see Figure 5-1) were most frequently implicated, suggesting that these regions are crucial for emotional identification tasks. Furthermore, acoustic specialization of the two hemispheres was investigated by modulating spectral (i.e., frequency) properties and temporal properties of auditory stimuli. Modula-

tions in spectral properties elicited a right hemisphere lateralization, whereas modulations in temporal properties elicited a left hemisphere lateralization (Zatorre & Belin, 2001).

Taken together these results suggest that different brain structures mediate the processing steps that lead to the identification of a speaker's emotional state. Moreover, analysis of the acoustic cues that convey emotional information is mediated by the auditory cortex in both hemispheres. The right auditory cortex seems specialized in analyzing spectral information such as the melodic contour of an utterance; the left auditory cortex seems specialized in analyzing temporal information. The results of this analysis are forwarded to higher order processes such as emotional identification mediated

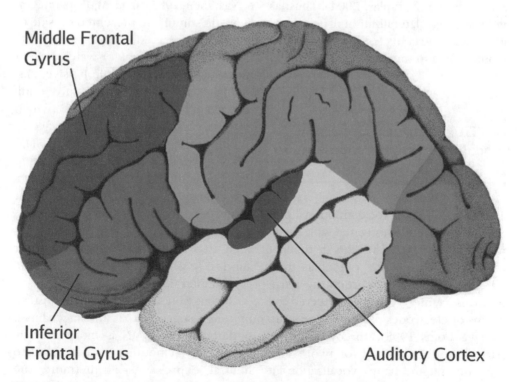

Figure 5–1. View of one cortical hemisphere. The shaded areas indicated by pointing lines represent middle frontal gyrus, inferior frontal gyrus and auditory cortex, respectively.

by right frontal cortex. Given that gender differences in hemispheric lateralization have been reported in other domains such as language processing (Hiscock, Inch, Jacek, Hiscock-Kalil, & Kalil, 1994; Hiscock, Israelian, Inch, Jacek, & Hiscock-Kalil, 1995; McGlone, 1980), one might speculate that similar gender differences may be observed for emotional identification. Evidence in favor of this assumption comes from a study by Wildgruber and colleagues (Wildgruber et al., 2002), who found that listening to vocal emotional expressions activated the right middle frontal gyrus more strongly in men than in women. Additionally, emotional identification studies that used facial expressions revealed activation in the right inferior and left middle frontal gyrus in women, but only right inferior frontal gyrus in men (Hall, Witelson, Szechtman, & Nahmias, 2004). Thus, as with language, lateralization of emotional identification seems less pronounced in women than in men.

The Temporal Course of Vocal Emotional Processing in Men and Women

The time course of vocal emotional processing has been investigated with event-related potentials (ERPs). ERPs are thought to reflect postsynaptic potentials from a large number of synchronously active neurons, which can be detected by means of electrodes placed on the scalp (Rugg & Coles, 1995). Moreover, by comparing the ERP elicited for two events (e.g., neutral and happy vocalization), it is possible to determine when in time the "brain response" elicited by both

events differed. Based on this, one can conclude that the critical information that differentiated both events has been processed. Frequently, the point of differentiation between two experimental conditions has been associated with specific negative or positive deflections in the ERP wave form. These deflections are referred to as components and are characterized by their polarity (i.e., positive or negative), peak latency (i.e., time between stimulus onset and component maxima), scalp topography, and dependency on a particular experimental manipulation.

The mismatch negativity (MMN) is an example of such components. It has a negative polarity, peaks approximately 200 ms following stimulus onset with a fronto-central scalp topography, and is elicited in response to acoustic deviants (Näätänen, 1995; Sams, Paavilainen, Alho, & Näätänen, 1985). In an MMN paradigm, acoustic stimuli are presented outside of attentional focus. Moreover, participants frequently read a book or watch a silent movie with subtitles while passively listening to a sequence of repetitive auditory events (e.g., 1000 Hz tones), which are occasionally interrupted by an acoustic deviant (e.g., 1500 Hz tone). The MMN elicited in response to acoustic deviants is thought to reflect a preattentive change detection mechanism that allows listeners to quickly react to relevant events in their environment. As such, it is believed to be important for survival (e.g., Tiitinen, May, Reinikainen, & Näätänen, 1994).

Recent work using vocalizations instead of tones suggests that the mechanism underlying the MMN is more strongly engaged for emotional, as compared to neutral, expressions. Furthermore, the influence of emotionality on the MMN seems to be gender specific (Schirmer,

Striano, & Friederici, 2005). In women, the MMN elicited to emotionally spoken syllables (i.e., happily or angrily spoken "dada") presented among neutral standards (i.e., neutrally spoken "dada") is larger than the MMN elicited to neutrally spoken syllables presented among emotional standards. In contrast, men show no difference between the MMN for emotional and neutral vocalizations (see Figure 5–2). Given that these gender differences appear both when participants watch a silent movie, and when they perform odd/even number judgments, it seems that they are independent of the primary task or occupation (Schirmer & Li, 2007). Moreover, given that men and women perform the primary task with comparable speed and accuracy, gender differences in vocal emotional processing cannot be explained by women attending more than men to the task-irrelevant vocalizations. Rather, they seem to reflect differential *preattentive* processing of emotional expressions in men and women. Further evidence for this assumption comes from research

showing that directing women's attention toward the auditory syllables by asking them to count deviants reduces MMN amplitude differences between emotional and neutral deviants such that gender differences in vocal emotional processing are no longer significant (Schirmer & Li, 2007). Larger MMN amplitudes to attended as compared to unattended neutral and emotional deviants furthermore suggests that attention enhances the significance of an acoustic event and may overwrite processing differences associated with emotionality.

Taken together these findings indicate that listeners have access to the emotional significance of vocal expressions within the first 200 ms following stimulus onset. Women but not men seem to discriminate between emotional and neutral vocal expressions when their attention is engaged elsewhere. Moreover, women seem to recruit more processing resources in response to emotional, as compared to neutral, vocalizations, which may increase the likelihood that these vocalizations capture attention.

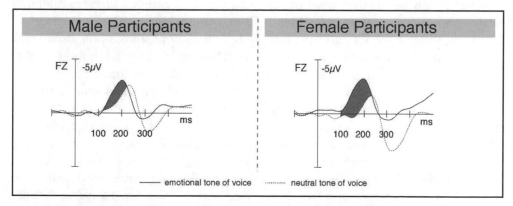

Figure 5–2. Mismatch negativity (MMN) elicited to emotionally (i.e., angry, happy) and neutrally spoken deviants presented in an auditory oddball paradigm. The area shaded in grey indicates the MMN for emotional deviants, which is significantly larger than the MMN for neutral deviants in women but not in men.

Gender Differences in the Influence of Vocal Emotional Information on Higher Order Cognitive Processes

One might speculate that gender differences in the preattentive processing of vocal emotional expressions affect the subsequent use of vocal emotional information for higher order cognitive processes. For example, when focusing on what is said during a conversation, women may be more likely than men to integrate vocal emotional information with verbal information. Whether this is true has been investigated in a series of ERP studies that used verbal stimulus material in order to elicit an N400 (Schirmer, Kotz, & Friederici, 2002; Schirmer & Kotz, 2003; Schirmer, Kotz, & Friederici, 2005). The N400 is a negativity that peaks approximately 400 ms following word onset and that is thought to reflect the retrieval of word information from the mental lexicon (for a review see Kutas & Federmeier, 2000). To study the influence of vocal emotional information on semantic retrieval, participants were presented with words that were either congruous or incongruous to the speaker's emotional tone of voice (e.g., "success" spoken with a happy or angry voice). Congruous words elicited a smaller N400 than incongruous words, suggesting that the retrieval of word information from the mental lexicon is less effortful when a word matches a speaker's vocal emotional expression (Schirmer et al., 2002; Schirmer & Kotz, 2003; Schirmer et al., 2005). Furthermore, in accordance with the above predictions, the influence of vocal emotional information on word processing differed as a function of attention and gender. Women showed an N400 effect regardless of whether the task required them to ignore vocal emotional information (e.g., verbal emotional identification task) or to attend to both vocal and verbal emotional information (e.g., voice-word congruency judgment). In contrast, men showed an N400 effect only when asked to attend to both vocal and verbal emotional information (Schirmer et al., in 2005; Schirmer, Lui, Maess, Chan, & Penney, 2006) or when there was a longer delay between the onset of vocal and verbal information (e.g., when a spoken utterance preceded a visual target word; Schirmer et al., 2002). A more automatized use of vocal emotional information for language processing in women, as compared to men, has also been demonstrated with functional magnetic resonance imaging. Women showed larger activity in the left inferior frontal gyrus in response to words spoken with incongruous as compared to congruous emotional tone when emotional tone was task-irrelevant (Figure 5-3; Schirmer, Zysset, Kotz, & von Cramon, 2004). Given that the left inferior frontal gyrus has been implicated in semantic retrieval (Wagner, Paré-Blagoev, Clark, & Poldrack, 2001), these findings provide further evidence that, depending upon attentional focus and gender, vocal emotional information may decrease or increase semantic retrieval effort. Interestingly, a more recent study indicated that the differential effort men and women direct at encoding words spoken with congruous and incongruous emotional tone affects their memory for these words (Mecklinger, Gaebel, Schirmer, Treese, & Johansson, 2007). In accordance with the more automatized processing and use of vocal emotional expressions in women,

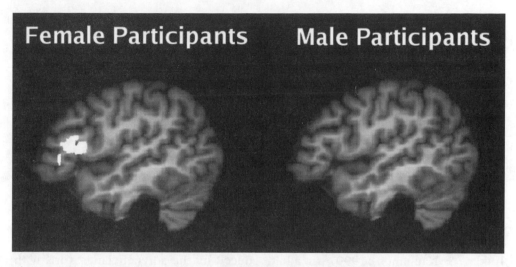

Figure 5–3. Brain activity associated with the perception of emotional words spoken with congruous and incongruous emotional tone of voice. Women show increased brain activity in the inferior frontal gyrus bilaterally for incongruous as compared to congruous trials. Men fail to show differences in brain activity between incongruous and congruous trials.

as compared to men, women are significantly better than men in remembering how a word was spoken. Furthermore, ERPs indicate that in women, but not in men, a word's recollection is facilitated when it was spoken with a congruous as compared to an incongruous emotional tone.

Taken together, these findings suggest that gender differences in the preattentive processing of vocal emotional information carry forward to the use of this information for higher order cognitive processes. More specifically, women seem more likely than men to integrate unattended vocal information during language processing, which enhances their sensitivity to incongruities between verbal and vocal information, as is the case for banter and sarcasm. Additionally, women show a better memory for the emotional tone of social interactions.

Biological and Environmental Modulators of Emotional Processing in Men and Women

Vocal emotional processing represents only one aspect of interpersonal communication that differs between men and women. Gender differences have been reported in the recognition of emotions from faces and gestures (Hall, 1978). As with vocal recognition, women are more accurate than men. Furthermore, men and women differ in their emotional evaluation of verbal material. In general, women perceive words as more emotional than men do (Grunwald et al., 1999), and they make faster emotional judgments (Schirmer & Kotz, 2003). A recent neuroimaging study additionally suggests that across different emotional media (e.g., words, faces, pictures) men engage the same network of brain structures for emotional processing. In contrast, the brain structures employed by women during emotional processing seem to be more adapted to the type of media (Lee, Liu, Chan, Fang, & Gao, 2005).

In addition to gender differences in perception, men and women differ in emotional expression. Moreover, these gender differences seem to emerge during development; girls have been found to increase emotional expressiveness as they mature, whereas boys show a decrease (Salminen, Saarijarvi, Aarela, Toikka, & Kauhanen, 1999). In adulthood, men talk less than women about feelings and men's risk of suffering from alexithymia—a deficit in verbalizing emotional sentiments and feelings—is almost twice as high as it is in women (Salminen et al., 1999). Women's spontaneous facial expressions elicited by emotional stimuli are more accurately recognized than men's facial expressions (for a review see Manstead, 1992). Furthermore, women are more likely than men to react with and show sadness in response to negative life events (Hess et al., 2000). In accordance with this, psychological health surveys indicate that women suffer approximately two times more frequently than men from emotional disorders such as depression or anxiety (Simonds & Whiffen, 2003).

Given these findings, it seems that women are generally more receptive to the emotions conveyed in communication and that they use verbal and nonverbal emotional expressions to a greater extent than men do. Different views have been proposed as to what causes these gender differences. Some researchers argue that they are the result of cultural norms and expectations. In line with this, parents have been found to talk less about feelings with boys than with girls and to restrict the expression of sadness in boys more than in girls (for a review see Maccoby, 1998). Parents have also been shown to influence the toy preference in boys and girls differently. However, research with girls suffering from congenital adrenal hyperplasia (CAH) suggests that these parental influences are insufficient to override biologically mediated toy preferences (Pasterski et al., 2005). CAH is a disorder that increases the concentration of androgens produced by the adrenal glands. Girls with CAH show more male-typical toy choices despite their parents' encouragement to use female-typical toys. Moreover, the toy selection of boys and girls seems to reflect their interest in social interactions. Specifically, only the female-typical toys included items that elicited social play (e.g. dolls), and these items were most preferred by normal girls. In contrast, male-typical toys included nonsocial items such building blocks as well as a gun, the latter being most preferred among boys (Pasterski et al., 2005). Interestingly, gender differences in toy preferences can be observed in nonhuman primates also, reinforcing the idea that they are biologically mediated (Alexander & Hines, 2002).

Additional evidence for biologically mediated gender differences comes from investigations of the size of brain structures implicated in emotional processing. For example, the medial frontal cortex, the hypothalamus, and the amygdala are larger in men, whereas cingulate cortex, nucleus accumbens, thalamus, auditory cortex, orbito-frontal, and lateral frontal cortex among other structures are larger in women (Goldstein et al., 2001). Some of these structures (e.g., orbito-frontal and auditory cortex) are more asymmetric in men than in women (Kovalev, Kruggel, & Cramon, 2003). Moreover, all of these structures show a high density of estrogen and androgen receptors early in life, suggesting an early onset of the observed gender differences (Goldstein et al., 2001).

Gender differences in emotional communication have also been associated with the action of neuropeptides, such as oxytocin. Oxytocin is synthesized in the hypothalamus and, apart from its peripheral role in parturition and lactation, has influence on pro-social behavior (Insel & Young, 2001) and stress-induced activity of the hypothalamic-pituitary-adrenal axis (Uvnas-Moberg, Ahlenius, Hillegaart, & Alster, 1994). For example, there is evidence that the number of oxytocin pulses in breastfeeding women correlates with their openness to social interactions (Uvnas-Moberg, 1998). Furthermore, administration of oxytocin to both men and women before a stressful situation has been shown to reduce blood cortisol concentration and perceived anxiety similarly to social support (Heinrichs, Baumgartner, Kirschbaum, & Ehlert, 2003). The reason these effects are of interest is that, although oxytocin can be found in either gender, it is more important in females than in males (Taylor et al., 2000; Young & Wang, 2004). Furthermore, females are more likely than males to affiliate in stressful situations and to establish long-term bonds to cope with potential stressors (e.g., male aggression, child care). These gender differences are believed to be mediated by oxytocin and female reproductive hormones (Taylor et al., 2000), which may enhance the processing of sensory information rele-vant for social recognition (i.e., emotional expressions) and make social interactions rewarding via modulations of the mesolimbic dopamine circuitry (Young & Wang, 2004).

Conclusions

The work reviewed here illustrates that women are not simply better than men at recognizing vocally expressed emotions. Rather, women and men seem to employ somewhat different processing mechanisms. Compared to men, women show a more bilateral brain activation in response to emotional vocalizations. Additionally, women process emotional vocalizations more automatically than men, which facilitates their memory for these vocalizations as well as their understanding of banter and sarcasm. Thus, it seems that processing in women is somewhat better adapted for engaging in social interactions. This gender difference has been linked to both environmental and biological influences. Furthermore, it has been shown that although environmental influences act upon the development of emotion recognition skills they do so in concert with biological influences. Moreover, for some aspects of social development it is now clear that biological influences can override environmental effects.

This demonstration calls for further research on the biological basis of gender differences in emotion recognition. One question that has to be addressed in this regard is at what time during child development these gender differences appear. Additionally, the phylogenetic development must be examined. The human brain is a product of not only the environment in which we currently live, but also the environments of our ancestors. To determine where gender differences arose in our evolutionary past, future research should investigate whether similar gender differences in emotion processing and socialization exist in closely related primate species.

References

Alexander, G. M., & Hines, M. (2002). Sex differences in response to children's toys in nonhuman primates (*Cercopithecus aethiops sabaeus*). *Evolution and Human Behavior, 23*, 467–479.

Blonder, L. X., Bowers D., & Heilman, K. M. (1991). The role of the right hemisphere in emotional communication. *Brain, 114*, 1115–1127.

Buchanan, T. W., Lutz, K., Mirzazade, S., Specht, K., Shah, N. J., Zilles, K., et al. (2000). Recognition of emotional prosody and verbal components of spoken language: An fMRI study. *Cognitive Brain Research, 9*, 227–238.

Gandour, J., Wong, D., Dzemidzic, M., Lowe, M., Tong, Y., & Li, X. (2003). A cross-linguistic fMRI study of perception of intonation and emotion in Chinese. *Human Brain Mapping, 18*, 149–157.

George, M. S., Parekh, P. I., Rosinsky, N., Ketter, K. A., Kimbrell, T. A., Heilman, K. M., et al. (1996). Understanding emotional prosody activates right hemisphere regions. *Archives of Neurology, 53*, 665–670.

Goldstein, J. M., Seidman, J. L., Horton, N. J., Kennedy, D. N., Caviness, V. S., Jr., Faraone, S. V., et al. (2001). Normal sexual dimorphism of the adult human brain assessed by in vivo magnetic resonance imaging. *Cerebral Cortex, 11*, 490–497.

Grunwald, S. I., Borod, J. C., Obler, L. K., Erhan, H. M., Pick, L. H., Welkowitz, J., et al.

(1999). The effects of age and gender on the perception of lexical emotion. *Applied Neuropsychology, 6*, 226–238.

Hall, G. B., Witelson, S. F., Szechtman, H., & Nahmias, C. (2004). Sex differences in functional activation patterns revealed by increased emotion processing demands. *Neuroreport, 15*, 219–223.

Hall, J. A. (1978). Gender effects in decoding nonverbal cues. *Psychological Bulletin, 4*, 845–857.

Heinrichs, M., Baumgartner, T., Kirschbaum, C., & Ehlert, U. (2003). Social support and oxytocin interact to suppress cortisol and subjective responses to psychosocial stress. *Biological Psychiatry, 54*, 1389–1398.

Hess, U., Senécal, S., Kirouac, G., Herrera, P., Philippot, P., & Kleck, R. E. (2000). Emotional expressivity in men and women: Stereotypes and self-perceptions. *Cognition and Emotion, 14*, 609–642.

Hiscock, M., Inch, R., Jacek, C., Hiscock-Kalil, C., & Kalil, K. M. (1994). Is there a sex difference in human laterality? I. An exhaustive survey of auditory laterality studies from six neuropsychological journals. *Journal of Clinical and Experimental Neuropsychology, 16*, 423–435.

Hiscock, M., Israelian, M., Inch, R., Jacek, C., & Hiscock-Kalil, C. (1995). Is there a sex difference in human laterality? II. An exhaustive survey of visual laterality studies from six neuropsychological journals. *Journal of Clinical and Experimental Neuropsychology, 17*, 590–610.

Insel, T. R., & Young, L. J. (2001). The neurobiology of attachment. *National Review of Neuroscience, 2*, 129–136.

Kovalev, V. A., Kruggel, F., & Cramon, D. Y. (2003). Gender and age effects in structural brain asymmetry as measured by MRI texture analysis. *NeuroImage, 19*, 895–905.

Kutas, M., & Federmeier, K. D. (2000). Electrophysiology reveals semantic memory use in language comprehension. *Trends in Cognitive Sciences, 4*, 463–470.

Lee, T. M. C., Liu, H. L , Chan, C. C. H., Fang, S. Y., & Gao, J. H. (2005). Neural activities associated with emotion recognition observed in men and women. *Molecular Psychiatry, 10*, 450-455.

Maccoby, E. E. (1998). The socialization component. In E. E. Maccoby (Ed.), *Growing up apart, coming together* (pp. 118-152). London: Harvard University Press.

Manstead, A. S. R. (1992). Gender differences in emotion. In A. Gale & M. W. Eysenck (Eds.), *Handbook of individual differences: Biological perspectives* (pp. 355-387). Oxford, UK: John Wiley & Sons.

McGlone, J. (1980). Sex differences in human brain asymmetry: A critical survey. *Behavioral and Brain Sciences, 3*, 215-263.

Mecklinger, A., Gäbel, A., Schirmer, A., Treese, A. C., & Johansson, M. (2007). *Memory for word-prosody associations: Event-related potentials reveal gender differences for emotional source.* Manuscript in preparation.

Näätänen, R. (1995, February). The mismatch negativity: A powerful tool for cognitive neuroscience. *Ear and Hearing, 16*, 6-18.

Pasterski, V. L., Geffner, M. E., Brain, C., Hindmarsh, P., Brook, C., & Hines, M. (2005). Prenatal hormones and postnatal socialization by parents as determinants of male-typical toy play in girls with congenital adrenal hyperplasia. *Child Development, 76*, 264-278.

Polce-Lynch, M., Myers, B. J., Kilmartin, C. T., Forssmann-Falck, R., & Kliewer, W. (1998). Gender and age patterns in emotional expression, body image, and self-esteem: A qualitative analysis. *Sex Roles, 38*, 1025-1049.

Rugg, M. D., & Coles, M. G. H. (1995). *Electrophysiology of mind.* Oxford, UK: Oxford University Press.

Salminen, J. K., Saarijarvi, S., Aarela, E., Toikka, T., & Kauhanen, J. (1999). Prevalence of alexithymia and its association with sociodemographic variables in the general population of Finland. *Journal of Psychosomatic Research, 46*, 75-82.

Sams, M., Paavilainen, P., Alho, K., & Näätänen, R. (1985). Auditory frequency discrimination and event-related potentials. *Electroencephalography and Clinical Neurophysiology, 62*, 437-448.

Scherer, K. R. (1989). Vocal correlates of emotional arousal and affective disturbance. In H. Wagner & A. Manstead (Eds.), *Handbook of social psychophysiology* (pp. 165-197). Oxford, UK: Wiley & Sons.

Schirmer, A. (2004). Timing speech: A review of lesion and neuroimaging findings. *Cognitive Brain Research, 21*, 269-287.

Schirmer, A. & Li, Q. (2007). *Preattentive and attentive processing of vocal emotional expressions in men and women.* Manuscript in preparation.

Schirmer, A., & Kotz, S. A. (2003). ERP evidence for a gender specific Stroop effect in emotional speech. *Journal of Cognitive Neuroscience, 15*, 1135-1148.

Schirmer, A., Kotz, S. A., & Friederici, A. D. (2002). Sex differentiates the role of emotional prosody during word processing. *Cognitive Brain Research, 14*, 228-233.

Schirmer, A., Kotz, S. A., & Friederici, A. D. (2005). On the role of attention for the processing of emotions in speech: Sex differences revisited. *Cognitive Brain Research, 24*, 442-452.

Schirmer, A., Lui, M., Maess, B., Chan, M., & Penney, T. B. (2006). On the influence of emotional prosody on speech processing in Cantonese male and female listeners. *Emotion, 6*, 406-417.

Schirmer, A., Striano, T., & Friederici, A. D. (2005). Sex differences in the pre-attentive processing of vocal emotional expressions. *Neuroreport, 16*, 635-639.

Schirmer, A., Zysset, S., Kotz, S. A., & von Cramon, D. Y. (2004). Gender differences in the activation of inferior frontal cortex during emotional speech perception. *NeuroImage, 21*, 1114-1123.

Shipp, T., Izdebski, K., Schutte, H., & Morrissey, P. (1988). Subglottal air pressure in spastic dysphonia speech. *Folia Phoniatrica, 40*, 105-110.

Simonds, V. M., & Whiffen, V. E. (2003). Are sex differences in depression explained by sex differences in co-morbid anxiety? *Journal of Affective Disorders, 77,* 197–202.

Taylor, S. E., Klein, L. C., Lewis, B. P., Gruenewald, T. L., Gurung, R. A., & Updegraff, J. A. (2000). Biobehavioral responses to stress in females: Tend-and-befriend, not fight-or-flight. *Psychological Review, 107,* 411–429.

Tiitinen, H., May, K., Reinikainen, K., & Näätänen, R. (1994). Attentive novelty detection in humans is governed by pre-attentive sensory memory. *Nature, 372,* 90–92.

Uvnas-Moberg, K. (1998). Oxytocin may mediate the benefits of positive social interaction and emotions. *Psychoneuroendocrinology, 23,* 819–835.

Uvnas-Moberg, K., Ahlenius, S., HiYoung, L. J., & Wang, Z. (1994). High doses of oxytocin cause sedation and low doses cause an anxiolytic-like effect in male rats. *Pharmacology, Biochemistry, and Behavior, 49,* 101–106.

Van den Berg, J. W., Zantema, J. T., Doornenbal, P. (1957). On the air resistance and the Bernoulli effect of the human larynx. *Journal of the Acoustical Society of America, 29*(5), 626–631.

Van Lancker, D. (1980). Cerebral lateralization of pitch cues in the linguistic signal. *International Journal of Human Communication, 13,* 227–277.

Van Lancker, D., & Fromkin, V. A. (1973). Hemispheric specialization for pitch and 'tone': Evidence from Thai. *Journal of Phonetics, 1,* 101–109.

Van Lancker, D., & Sidtis, J. J. (1992). The identification of affective-prosodic stimuli by left- and right-hemisphere-damaged subjects: All errors are not created equal. *Journal of Speech and Hearing Research, 35,* 963–970.

Wagner, A. D., Paré-Blagoev, E. J., Clark, J., & Poldrack, R. A. (2001). Recovering meaning: Left prefrontal cortex guides controlled semantic retrieval. *Neuron, 31,* 329–338.

Wildgruber, D., Pihan, H., Ackermann, H., Erb, M., & Grodd, W. (2002). Dynamic brain activation during processing of emotional intonation: Influence of acoustic parameters, emotional valence, and sex. *Neuroimage, 15,* 856–869.

Wildgruber, D., Riecker, A., Hertrich, I., Erb, M., Grodd, W., Ethofer, T., et al. (2005). Identification of emotional intonation evaluated by fMRI. *Neuroimage, 24,* 1233–1241.

Young, L. J., & Wang, Z. (2004). The neurobiology of pair bonding. *Nature Neuroscience, 7,* 1048–1054.

Zatorre, R. J., & Belin, P. (2001). Spectral and temporal processing in human auditory cortex. *Cerebral Cortex, 11*(10), 946–953.

CHAPTER 6

Emotion-Related Vocal Acoustics

Cue-Configuration, Dimensional, and Affect-Induction Perspectives

Jo-Anne Bachorowski and Michael J. Owren

Overview

The most common theoretical approach to understanding affect-related vocal acoustics has been to argue that these signals reflect the occurrence of discrete emotional states in the vocalizer. The key alternative view holds that the acoustics associated with underlying states are better described by a small number of continuous dimensions such as arousal (or activation) and a valenced dimension such as pleasantness. A review of the available evidence suggests, however, that neither approach is correct. Data from speech-related research provides little support for a cue-configuration view, with emotion-related aspects of the acoustics seeming to largely reflect

vocalizer arousal. However, links to an emotional valence dimension have also been difficult to demonstrate, suggesting a need for interpretations outside this traditional dichotomy. We therefore suggest a different perspective in which the key function of signaling is not to express emotion per se, but instead to impact listener affect and thereby influence the behavior of these individuals. In this view, the nuances of signaler states are not expected to be highly correlated with particular features of the sounds produced, but rather that vocalizers use acoustics to affect listener arousal and emotion. Attributions concerning signaler states thus become a secondary rather than primary outcome, reflecting inferences that listeners base on their own affective responses to the sounds, their past experience with such signals, and the context in which signaling is occurring. This approach has found recent support in laughter research, with the bigger picture being that affect-related vocal signals—be they carried in speech, laughter, or other species-typical signals—are not informative beacons on vocalizer states so much as tools of social influence used to capitalize on listener sensitivities.

Vocal Expression of Emotion in Speech

The best-known theoretical position regarding vocal expression of emotion in speech is that discrete affective states experienced by the vocalizer are reflected in specific patterns of acoustic cues in the speech being produced. This *cue-configuration* perspective is best exemplified by the work of Scherer and colleagues (e.g., Scherer, 1986; 1989; Banse & Scherer, 1996; Johnstone & Scherer, 2000). In contrast, the *dimensional* perspective argues that emotional cues in speech acoustics reflect continuous arousal and pleasure dimensions rather than discrete emotional states (e.g., Bachorowski, 1999; Kappas, Hess, & Scherer, 1991; Pakosz, 1983). While there has been lively debate among the advocates of these two positions, few if any empirical studies have been conducted to compare them directly.

Such testing is in fact difficult to engineer, and most studies have therefore examined smaller sets of predictions derived from one or the other of the two perspectives. An influential example is the work of Banse and Scherer (1996), who tested vocalizations produced by 12 professional actors asked to portray each of 14 different emotions. One key outcome was that, of the 29 acoustic properties measured, F_0 and mean acoustic amplitude were found to show the strongest connections to the emotions being portrayed. We consider these findings to be important because, regardless of theoretical position, researchers widely agree that these features likely index talker arousal rather than any specifically valenced state. While other acoustic measures also showed significant statistical links to particular emotional portrayals, they accounted for much smaller proportions of the variance involved.

Banse and Scherer found classification accuracy to be roughly 40% when differentiating the various emotions being portrayed using a subset of 16 of their acoustic measures. On the one hand, this classification success might be expected based on findings about other kinds of indexical cueing in speech (e.g., Bachorowski & Owren, 1999). On the other hand, Banse and Scherer had also carefully screened their recordings before attempting statistical classification, using only 224 of the 1324 originally recorded samples. As a result, the relatively modest level of classification success reported may have been inflated. When Banse and Scherer examined 40 hypothesized links between emotion and vocal acoustics (Scherer, 1986), 23 predictions were supported, evidence was tenuous in 6 other cases, and there were 11 instances in which results showed statistically significant deviations from the expected magnitude and/or direction of effect.

Other studies have produced a similar mix of supportive and contrary outcomes (e.g., Scherer, Banse, Wallbott, & Goldbeck, 1991; Sobin & Alpert, 1999), suggesting a need for further theoretical work and possible alternative approaches (e.g., Kappas et al., 1991; Kappas & Hess, 1995; Scherer et al., 1991). In addition, using stimuli based on simulated emotion produced by actors and then carefully screening the resulting stimuli rather than using representative samples may produce results that are more relevant to emblematic portrayals of affect than cueing that occurs under natural occurring circumstances.

Comparing Cue-Configuration and Dimensional Approaches

The most reliable empirical outcomes in testing the acoustics of emotional speech have been arousal-related. Numerous studies have, for example, shown that anger and joy are each associated with both increased F_0 and higher amplitude. Associations between valence and vocal acoustics are less clear-cut. This point was brought home in Bachorowski and Owren's (1995) study of vocal acoustics in which 120 naïve participants were individually recorded as they performed a lexical-decision task. As part of the procedure, each participant uttered a stock phrase just after receiving affect-inducing success or failure feedback. The three most prominent acoustic changes from baseline to on-task performance were F_0-related, and most plausibly reflected simple increases in vocalizer arousal. Valence-related differences emerged only in complex interactions among variables such as talker sex, the relative proportion of positive and negative feedback each participant received, and trait differences in emotional intensity.

A more exacting comparison was conducted with recordings of 24 naïve participants who each described the thoughts and feelings evoked by affect-inducing slides (Bachorowski & Owren, 1996). Again, acoustic outcomes were strongly associated with self-reported arousal and to a lesser extent with valence. Further analyses tested whether acoustic outcomes could be linked to discrete emotional states, but statistical outcomes were by and large nonsignificant.

Two conclusions that can be drawn from this work are that arousal plays a noticeably more important role in shaping speech acoustics than does valence, and that ready links to discrete emotional states are difficult to demonstrate. However, it would be premature to conclude that the acoustics of emotional speech only reflect arousal, or can be fully accounted for by a dimensional approach alone. Any such conclusion must be preceded by tests of alternative predictions derived from the two perspectives within the same empirical framework. The strongest conclusion to draw at this point may simply be that the acoustics of emotional speech are influenced by a variety of factors, not all of which are neatly aligned with the polarized theoretical positions that have been important in the field to date. The data suggest that arousal and valence effects, however construed, are not sufficient to account for the available data concerning vocal emotion effects. Other important factors appear to include talker sex and emotional traits, strategic shaping of vocal acoustics that a talker might show in pursuit of social goals, and the particular social context in which the speech is being produced (Bachorowski, 1999). Nonetheless, in now moving to the perceptual side of the equation, it is the acoustic cues associated with vocalizer arousal that again emerge as being the most important.

Vocal Perception of Emotion from Speech

Theoretical approaches and empirical outcomes associated with perception of emotion from speech acoustics generally parallel those we have reviewed for production. Specifically, some researchers adopt a cue-configuration perspective whereas others emphasize a dimensional view. When listeners are asked to identify the intended emotion in utterances produced by actors, accuracy is again relatively modest—about 55% across studies (reviewed by Johnstone & Scherer, 2000). Similar outcomes and confusions are observed across different cultures and language groups, although identification errors also reflect the degree of disparity between vocalizer and listener language (Scherer, Banse, & Wallbott, 2001). The standard strategy in these experiments has been to use a forced-choice identification paradigm in which listeners select a single emotion word deemed to best describe the affect being conveyed. Stimulus sets usually include only a small number of talkers and emotions, and are often selected to include presumably prototypical instances of the emotions in question (e.g., Banse & Scherer, 1996; Leinonen, Hiltunen, Linnankoski, & Laakso, 1997; Sobin & Alpert, 1999). As noted earlier, this strategy of using acted emotional samples and then testing only a screened subset may in and of itself be accounting for some of the evidence of differentiated perception of emotion.

When Pereira (2000) had listeners rate vocal samples of various discrete emotions using dimensional scales, by far the strongest associations between the ratings and vocal acoustics were arousal-related (see also Green & Cliff, 1975). F_0 and amplitude were again primary, as they were in a study by Streeter and colleagues (1983) in which participants evaluated talker stress levels from speech. Here, listeners reported that vocalizers were stressed when hearing significant variation in talker F_0 and amplitude, but otherwise usually failed to perceive stress. The link between speech acoustics and perceived valence is generally weaker, which again parallels outcomes observed on the production side. Ladd and colleagues (1985), for example, systematically varied several acoustic parameters as listeners rated vocalizer affect and attitude. A central finding in this study was that listeners' responses did not reveal categorical responses associated with discrete emotions, but rather varied continuously in accordance with continuous changes in F_0. Results are similar when cue-configuration and dimensional perspectives are compared within the same experimental setting, although only a few such studies have been conducted. Overall, listeners are found to be most likely to make errors when stimuli reflect similar arousal levels (e.g., Pakosz, 1983; Pereira, 2000) and among similarly valenced members of emotion families (e.g., Banse & Scherer, 1996; see also Breitenstein, Van Lancker, & Daum, 2001; Ladd, Silverman, Tolkmitt, Bergmann, & Scherer, 1985).

Taken together, the perceptual evidence shows that overall listener accuracy is quite moderate. Many investigators argue that the generally observed outcome of about 55% correct indicates both that vocalizer emotion is associated with differentiated acoustics and that listeners can in turn perceive these cues (e.g., Banse & Scherer, 1996; Johnstone & Scherer,

2000). However, we suggest that if dis-crete emotional cues are in fact present, the use of screened stimuli based on pro-fessional portrayals of emotional state should produce significantly better per-formance. Acoustic variability in these carefully constructed stimulus sets has likely been much lower than in naturally occurring speech, yet listeners judge them incorrectly a good proportion of the time. This kind of outcome does not mean that perceivers are similarly inaccurate under natural circumstances as well, as the emo-tional speech that humans typically hear is likely embedded in a rich social con-text and coming from familiar talkers. Both factors are likely to significantly boost lis-tener accuracy in inferring vocalizer emo-tion in real life compared to these labo-ratory circumstances, particularly with arousal-related variation providing rea-sonable cues to the occurrence of affect (Bachorowski, 1999; Pakosz, 1983).

From a methodological point of view, it becomes essential to recognize that when listeners are able to accurately perceive emotion in others, they may be depend-ing more on their own psychological processing and powers of inference than veridical acoustic cues provided by the vocalizers. This possibility is elaborated in the next section, which shifts the focus from hypothesized links between emotional states and vocalizer acoustics to the effects that sounds have on listener affect. While compatible with various aspects of both dimensional- and discrete-emotions views, this perspective suggests that emotion-related cueing by vocalizers is actually a secondary outcome of the communication process. The primary function of emotional vocal acoustics is instead proposed to be to influence the listener's state and behavior.

An Affect-Induction Account of Vocal Signaling

A central theme of the preceding discus-sion is that researchers have generally expected to find veridical links between vocalizer affect, associated vocal acous-tics, and listener perception. From this perspective, the function of emotion-related signaling is for vocalizers to con-vey to listeners that particular affective states are occurring. Of course, simply informing listeners about such states is not beneficial per se—the evolution of signaling is necessarily primarily shaped by the effect that signals have on listener behavior (see also Dawkins, 1989; Daw-kins & Krebs, 1978). There is for instance no guarantee that listeners will behave in ways that benefit vocalizers who are pro-viding veridical cues to internal state. The most fundamental selection pressure act-ing on signalers must therefore be mod-ulation of others' behavior in ways that are beneficial to themselves. This logic leads to viewing affect-related acoustics as a means of influencing rather than informing listeners. We suggest that such influence can occur via the impact of sig-nal acoustics on the emotional systems of listeners, thereby shaping the way these individuals behave towards vocalizers (Owren & Rendall, 1997; 2001). Here, we apply this perspective to the specific case of human laughter, a seemingly ubiquitous affect-related vocal signal.

Affect-Induction through Sound

Everyday experience shows that auditory stimuli routinely induce emotion-related reactions in listeners, with sounds as dramatic as a booming thunderstorm or

as subtle as a dripping faucet readily eliciting attention, arousal, and valenced
responses. Laughter and infant crying are
two examples of potent, affect-inducing
auditory signals, but speech acoustics
have also been shown to elicit emotion
in listeners (Hatfield, Hsee, Costello,
Weisman, & Denney, 1995; Neumann &
Strack, 2000; Siegman & Boyle, 1993).
This affect-induction property of sound
has had little influence on work examining vocal expression of emotion. Instead,
both the cue-configuration and dimensional perspectives approach the issue
from the standpoint that vocalizers
encode affect-related meaning in their
signals and listeners subsequently *decode*
that information (e.g., Laukka, 2005;
Scherer, 1988). Emotional expression is
thus treated as a kind of code that vocalizers use to represent their emotional
states in almost linguistic-like fashion.

The *affect-induction* model is an alternative to this general view. Originally
proposed for nonhuman primate vocalizations (Owren & Rendall, 1997, 2001;
Rendall & Owren, 2002), the approach
may also be applicable to human affective signaling (Owren, Rendall, & Bachorowski, 2003). Rather than viewing
emotional communication as a process
of encoding and decoding, the model
argues that the primary function of nonlinguistic vocal signals is to influence listeners' affect and thereby also modulate
their behavior. Whereas representational
accounts of communication implicitly rest
on rather sophisticated but undescribed
processes of information encoding and
decoding, the affect-induction approach
argues that vocal signals can be effective
by eliciting low-level affective responses
that then influence listeners' behavioral
decisions. The effects can be *direct*,
meaning that the signal acoustics themselves have an impact, or *indirect*, mean-

ing that listeners experience a learned
affective response to a sound as a result
of previous experience. For the former,
acoustic salience is critical, with aspects
like frequency modulation, amplitude
level, duration, and variability being primary. For the latter, learning occurs
through social interactions in which individually distinctive sounds produced by
a particular vocalizer are paired with
affect being experienced by the listener
as the interaction unfolds.

Differences between the affect-induction
and representational perspectives might
be best explained by noting critical similarities and differences between them.
One important point of contact is that
both approaches assume an association
between the signaler's internal state and
the signal being produced. The representational approach argues that this is a
strong association, with the connection
between a particular internal state and
corresponding vocal signal being sufficiently specific as to allow the listener to
accurately infer that it is occurring. The
affect-induction approach also proposes
that the vocalizer's internal state is critical in triggering signal production, but
that the function of signaling is to induce
rather than to convey emotion. As a
result, particular signal features are not
expected to be tightly linked to differentiated vocalizer states, as it may benefit
the signaler to induce similar responses
in the listener across a variety of situations. Conversely, a diverse set of acoustic properties in sounds produced in a
given situation might serve a common
function in modulating listener arousal
and valenced emotion. In this view, relationships between signaler state and
physical signal are probabilistic rather
than highly specific.

A second point of contact is that listeners are able to draw inferences about

vocalizer states or likely upcoming behaviors. From a representational perspective, such inferences are part and parcel of why communication evolves— listeners receive encoded information about vocalizer state and act on that content. The affect-induction perspective instead views listener inference as a secondary outcome. In this approach, the primary function of vocal behavior is to benefit the vocalizer by influencing perceiver affect and behavior, regardless of what particular mechanism may be involved. Vocal behavior is therefore expected to show substantial variability, which will nonetheless also show more general patterning. Listeners that attend to those patterns will therefore be able to draw some conclusions about vocalizer states and likely behavior, but only probabilistically. The difference between the two approaches is that the listener's ability to draw such inferences is the primary function of signaling from the representational perspective, but is a secondary outcome in the affect-induction view.

Affect-induction proposes that while emotion-related signals do not have representational value, they are still meaningful in the sense that listeners often draw inferences about their significance. Those inferences are based on a host of factors, however, including acoustic attributes of the sound, listener affective state and familiarity with both the signal and the vocalizer, and the overarching context in which signaling is occurring (see also Bachorowski & Owren, 2002; Hess & Kirouac, 2000; Kappas et al., 1991). A corollary is that affective responses to highly similar sounds may be quite variable. The same high-pitched shriek might for example induce positive affect when heard while attending a party but elicit a strong negative response when heard while walking down a dark,

isolated street. In both cases, the acoustics of a loud shriek make it likely to involuntarily draw the listener's attention, increase arousal, and thereby exacerbate whatever positive or negative affective state is already being experienced. In addition, if the sound has distinctive acoustic features that have previously been paired with either positive or negative affect in the listener, the sound will also activate corresponding learned responses. Finally, sounds can trigger more complex inferences, for instance, when the significance of a loud shriek at a party is that the vocalizer is tipsy and will have to be driven home.

While thus fundamentally different from a representational view of emotional expression, the affect-induction perspective has parallels to Scherer's *appeal* and *pull* functions of vocal expression of emotion (Scherer, 1988; 1992; see also Johnstone & Scherer, 2000), and with the construct of *emotion contagion*. Hatfield and colleagues' (1992) notion of primitive emotional contagion is somewhat similar in that this process was described as either unconditioned or conditioned, and occurring outside the realm of conscious awareness. However, the affect-induction perspective takes mechanism further than in the notions of appeal, pull, or contagion by also emphasizing links between the acoustics of vocal expressions of emotion and low-level neural responses in listeners.

An Affect-Induction Approach to Laughter

Human laughter provides a good example of representational interpretation of emotion-related vocalizations, with laughter typically being viewed as a means by which vocalizers provide information about their emotional states to listeners. Laugh acoustics are therefore expected to change in accordance with variation in those emotions, which have been proposed to include states as diverse as joy, amusement, nervousness, embarrassment, aggression, and submissiveness. To our knowledge, there are as yet no data that specifically test this hypothesis. Data that are available do show that substantial variability occurring in laugh acoustics, but in a situation involving only a single, positive state (Bachorowski, Smoski, & Owren, 2001). This work indicated that rather than being differentially associated with vocalizer state, laugh acoustics were better predicted by the sex and familiarity of the laugher's social partner (Bachorowski, Smoski, Tomarken, & Owren, 2005; see also Devereux & Ginsburg, 2001; Grammer & Eibl-Eibesfeldt, 1990). Males for instance laughed most and used acoustics likely to have the greatest direct impact on the listener when paired with a friend—especially a male friend. Females, on the other hand, were more likely to produce these kinds of high-impact sounds when paired with a male than with a female. A variety of other interactions occurred between acoustics, laugher sex, and social context, the interpretation of which is elaborated elsewhere (e.g., Owren & Bachorowski, 2003; Bachorowski et al., 2005). However, the gist is that both males and females were laughing strategically, producing high-impact sounds when the likely effect on listeners would be positively toned arousal, and using laughter rich in identity cues specifically with friends who would have pre-existing learned positive affective associations with these sounds.

In both cases, F_0 emerges as a critical component of laugher's affect-induction strategy. Grammer and Eibl-Eibesfeldt (1990), in their analysis of male-female stranger dyads, have for instance shown that males reported being more interested in female strangers when those women had produced more laughter during a 10-minute testing interval. More specifically, however, the laughter having this effect was voiced, meaning sounds produced using regular vocal-fold vibration, prominent F_0 (heard as vocal pitch), and concomitant harmonic structure. Noisy, unvoiced laughter that lacked vocal-fold vibration, F_0, and harmonic structure did not influence listener responses (see also Keltner & Bonanno, 1997), even though this kind of laughter is in fact extremely common (Bachorowski et al., 2001). Bachorowski and Owren (2001) later had listeners listen to and rate both voiced and unvoiced laughs, and participants were found to be very consistent in rating voiced sounds much more positively than unvoiced versions. More recent work has found that unvoiced laughter may even elicit slightly negative affect in listeners (Owren, Trivedi, Schulman, & Bachorowski, 2007).

Thus, as has been well documented with emotional speech, F_0-related acoustics play a crucial role in shaping listener responses to laughter (although tests of amplitude have not yet been conducted with laughter, it should also prove to be a high-impact acoustic feature). In the affect-induction view, vocal-fold vibration and F_0 characteristics exert their impact in at least two key ways. First, the F_0 component of voiced sounds is an extremely salient auditory feature, with high or strongly modulated F_0 having direct impact on listener attention and arousal. These features were in fact prominent among those that laughers were found to produce in a situationally dependent fashion when paired with same- or different-sex partners that were either friends or strangers (Bachorowski et al., 2005), and were also likely important in the effects uncovered in Grammer and Eibl-Eibesfeldt's (1990) study of males and females meeting for the first time. Work testing for indirect, learned responses to laughter has also highlighted the importance of voicing, which is also critical in conveying cues to the individual identity of the vocalizer (e.g., Owren & Cardillo, in press). As noted earlier, indirect, learned affective responses should emerge in listeners hearing particular vocalizers producing laugh sounds as they themselves are experiencing affect. However, the specificity of this kind of learning will be importantly dependent on individual distinctiveness of the sounds, suggesting that voiced laughter should be most important. While indirect, evidence from Smoski and Bachorowski's (2003a, 2003b) studies of temporal coordination in the laughter of friends versus strangers suggests both that hearing laughter from friends has particular affect-inducing potency, and that this effect is significantly more prominent for voiced than for unvoiced sounds.

Conclusions: Vocal Expressions of Emotion as Social Tools

Compared to speech, there is much yet to be learned about the acoustics and functions of laughter. Nonetheless, laughter resembles speech in being an inherently social event (Provine & Fischer, 1989) and a critical part of the communicative processes that are central to human social relationships. There also appear to be some telling commonalities in how acoustic features of both speech and laughter function in emotional aspects of this communication. A central conclusion for speech is that F_0- and amplitude-related features play a primary role. On the one hand, speech produced while experiencing salient emotion shows significant changes in these particular characteristics, which also clearly impact listener perception and attributions of emotion. On the other hand, there is little indication that these or other acoustic features of speech can be linked to either discrete emotional states or valenced affect, and when listeners are asked to gauge vocalizer states, performance based on speech acoustics alone is modest. While less information is available for laughter, outcomes are similar. For example, the degree of variability occurring in laugh sounds produced during positive states alone argues against the possibility of emotion-specific acoustics. Laugh sounds nonetheless have unambiguous impact on listener emotion, and voicing and F_0 in particular have been found to play a central role.

It has thus been difficult to demonstrate differentiated, state-specific acoustic effects for either speech or laughter, but quite easy to show that acoustics nonetheless have general and robust effects on listener emotions and evaluation of vocalizers. To us, these results raise substantial questions about the adequacy of representational approaches, and are instead more compatible with the view that vocalizers are using relatively undifferentiated acoustics that have potent effects on listener affect. The evidence is far from definitive, particularly as much of the work conducted on human vocal expression of emotion has assumed rather than tested the proposition that representational signaling is involved. However, it is therefore also noteworthy that this research has largely failed to support this assumption either for production or for perception. While readily hearing emotional "content," listeners' judgments about vocalizer states are highly constrained and context-dependent. Our interpretation is that these inferences primarily reflect the listeners' own arousal and valenced responses, which are richly interpreted when taking other information about the vocalizer and context into account. Affective communication in both speech and laughter thus becomes a process of attributing emotion to vocalizers, rather than one of recovering encoded information.

A larger implication of this view is that emotional expressions in general function most importantly as nonconscious strategies of social influence rather than as veridical representations of internal state (see also Bargh & Chartrand, 1999; Zajonc, 1980). Rather than informing per se, both kinds of signals function to sway or shape the perceiver's affect and attitude, promoting behavioral effects that ultimately benefit the signaler. The "information value" of a signal is thus critically dependent on a perceiver's previous general experience, particular history with the signaler, and ability to take signaling context into account (Hess & Kirouac, 2000; Owren & Rendall, 2001). These are difficult distinctions to make, however, and illustrate the need to significantly improve on the data that are currently available concerning vocal emotion expression. We suggest that it will be useful to focus on vocalizations acquired under controlled but naturalistic circumstances where vocalizers are experiencing actual rather than simu-

lated emotions. Further, alternative interpretations should be contrasted as directly as possible, including comparing cue-configuration versus dimensional approaches and representational versus affect-induction perspectives within the same experimental framework. Finally, it will be important to broaden the scope of inquiry so that the inferential processes that listeners use to make attributions about vocalizer states can be uncovered. With these desiderata as a framework, a deeper understanding of how humans use emotion-related vocal acoustics in their communicative endeavors should be within reach.

Author Note. Correspondence can be addressed to either Jo-Anne Bachorowski, Department of Psychology, Wilson Hall, Vanderbilt University, Nashville, TN, 37240, j.a.bachorowski@vanderbilt.edu, or Michael J. Owren, Department of Psychology, Georgia State University, P.O. Box 5010, Atlanta, GA, 30302-5010, owren@gsu.edu

References

Bachorowski, J.-A. (1999). Vocal expression and perception of emotion. *Current Directions in Psychological Science*, *8*, 53–57.

Bachorowski, J.-A., & Owren, M. J. (1995). Vocal expression of emotion: Acoustic properties of speech are associated with emotional intensity and context. *Psychological Science*, *6*, 219–224.

Bachorowski, J.-A., & Owren, M. J. (1996). Vocal expression of emotion is associated with vocal fold vibration and vocal tract resonance. *Psychophysiology*, *33*(Suppl. 1), S20.

Bachorowski, J.-A., & Owren, M. J. (1999). Acoustic correlates of talker sex and individual talker identity are present in a short vowel segment produced in running speech. *Journal of the Acoustical Society of America, 106,* 1054-1063.

Bachorowski, J.-A., & Owren, M. J. (2001). Not all laughs are alike: Voiced but not unvoiced laughter readily elicits positive affect. *Psychological Science, 12,* 252-257.

Bachorowski, J.-A, & Owren, M. J. (2002). The role of vocal acoustics in emotional intelligence. In L. F. Barrett & P. Salovey (Eds.), *The wisdom of feelings: Processes underlying emotional intelligence* (pp. 11-36). New York: Guilford.

Bachorowski, J.-A., Smoski, M. J., & Owren, M. J. (2001). The acoustic features of human laughter. *Journal of the Acoustical Society of America, 110,* 1581-1597.

Bachorowski, J.-A., Smoski, M. J., Tomarken, A. J., & Owren, M. J. (2007). *Laugh rate and acoustics are associated with social context.* Manuscript under revision.

Banse, R., & Scherer, K. R. (1996). Acoustic profiles in vocal emotion expression. *Journal of Personality and Social Psychology, 70,* 614-636.

Bargh, J. A., & Chartrand, T. L. (1999). The unbearable automaticity of being. *American Psychologist, 54,* 462-479.

Breitenstein, C., Van Lancker, D., & Daum, I. (2001). The contribution of speech rate and pitch variation to the perception of vocal emotions in a German and an American sample. *Cognition & Emotion, 15,* 57-79.

Dawkins, R. (1989). *The selfish gene* (2nd ed.). Oxford, UK: Oxford University.

Dawkins, R., & Krebs, J. R. (1978). Animal signals: Information or manipulation? In J. R. Krebs & N. B. Davies (Eds.), *Behavioral ecology: An evolutionary approach* (pp. 282-309). London: Blackwell Scientific.

Devereaux, P. G., & Ginsburg, G. P. (2001). Sociality effects on the production of laughter. *Journal of General Psychology, 128,* 227-240.

Grammer, K., & Eibl-Eibesfeldt, I. (1990). The ritualization of laughter. In W. Koch (Ed.), *Naturlichkeit der Sprache und der Kultur: Acta colloquii* (pp. 192-214). Bochum, Germany: Brockmeyer.

Green, R. S, & Cliff, N. (1975). Multidimensional comparisons of structures of vocally and facially expressed emotion. *Perception and Psychophysics, 17,* 429-438.

Hatfield, E., Cacioppo, J. T., & Rapson, R. L. (1992). Primitive emotional contagion. In M. S. Clark (Ed.), *Emotion and social behavior* (pp. 151-177). London: Sage.

Hatfield, E., Hsee, C. K., Costello, J., Weisman, M. S., & Denney, C. (1995). The impact of vocal feedback on emotional experience and expression. *Journal of Social Behavior and Personality, 10,* 293-312.

Hess, U., & Kirouac, G. (2000). Emotion expression in groups. In M. Lewis & J. Haviland-Jones (Eds.), *Handbook of emotions* (2nd ed., pp. 368-381). New York: Guilford.

Johnstone, T., & Scherer, K. R. (2000). Vocal communication of emotion. In M. Lewis & J. Haviland (Eds.), *Handbook of emotions* (1st ed., pp. 220-235). New York: Guilford.

Kappas, A., & Hess, U. (1995). Nonverbal aspects of oral communication. In D. U. M. Quasthoff (Ed.), *Aspects of oral communication* (pp. 169-180). Berlin, Germany: De Gruyter.

Kappas, A., Hess, U., & Scherer, K. R. (1991). Voice and emotion. In B. Rime & R. Feldman (Eds.), *Fundamentals of nonverbal behavior* (pp. 200-238). Cambridge, UK: Cambridge University.

Keltner, D., & Bonanno, G. (1997). A study of laughter and dissociation: Distinct correlates of laughter and smiling during bereavement. *Journal of Personality and Social Psychology, 73,* 687-702.

Ladd, D. R., Silverman, K. E. A, Tolkmitt, F., Bergmann, G., & Scherer, K. R. (1985). Evidence for the independence of intonation contour type, voice quality, and F_0 range in signaling speaker affect. *Journal of the Acoustical Society of America, 78,* 435-444.

Laukka, P. (2005). Categorical perception of vocal emotion expressions. *Emotion, 5,* 277-295.

Leinonen, L., Hiltunen, T., Linnankoski, I., & Laakso, M.-L. (1997). Expression of emotional-motivational connotations with a one-word utterance. *Journal of the Acoustical Society of America, 102*, 1853–1863.

Neumann, R., & Strack, F. (2000). "Mood contagion": The automatic transfer of mood between persons. *Journal of Personality and Social Psychology, 79*, 211–223.

Owren, M. J., & Bachorowski, J.-A. (2001). The evolution of emotional expression: A "selfish-gene" account of smiling and laughter in early hominids and humans. In T. J. Mayne & G. A. Bonanno (Eds.), *Emotion: Current issues and future directions* (pp. 152–191). New York: Guilford.

Owren, M. J., & Bachorowski, J.-A. (2003). Reconsidering the evolution of nonlinguistic communication: The case of laughter. *Journal of Nonverbal Behavior, 27*, 183–200.

Owren, M. J., & Cardillo, G. C. (in press). The relative roles of vowels and consonants in discriminating talker identity versus word meaning. *Journal of the Acoustical Society of America.*

Owren, M. J, & Rendall, D. (1997). An affect-conditioning model of nonhuman primate signaling. In D. H. Owings, M. D. Beecher, & N. S. Thompson (Eds.), *Perspectives in ethology: Vol. 12. Communication* (pp. 299–346). New York: Plenum.

Owren, M. J., & Rendall, D. (2001). Sound on the rebound: Bringing form and function back to the forefront in understanding nonhuman primate vocal signaling. *Evolutionary Anthropology, 10*, 58–71.

Owren, M. J., Rendall, D., & Bachorowski, J.-A. (2003). Nonlinguistic vocal communication. In D. Maestripieri (Ed.), *Primate psychology* (pp. 359–394). Cambridge, MA: Harvard University.

Owren, M. J., Schulman, A., Trivedi, N., & Bachorowski, J.-A. (2007). Laughter produced in positive circumstances can elicit both positive and negative responses in listeners. Manuscript under revision.

Pakosz, M. (1983). Attitudinal judgments in intonation: Some evidence for a theory. *Journal of Psycholinguistic Research, 12*, 311–326.

Pereira, C. (2000). Dimensions of emotional meaning in speech. In R. Cowie, E. Douglas-Cowie, & M. Schröder (Eds.), *Proceedings of the International Speech Communication Association Workshop on Speech and Emotion* (pp. 25–28). Belfast, UK: Textflow.

Provine, R. R., & Fischer, K. R. (1989). Laughing, smiling, and talking: Relation to sleeping and social context in humans. *Ethology, 83*, 295–305.

Rendall, D., & Owren, M. J. (2002). Animal vocal communication: Say what? In M. Bekoff, C. Allen, & G. Burghardt (Eds.), *The cognitive animal* (pp. 307–314). Cambridge, MA: MIT.

Scherer, K. R. (1986). Vocal affect expression: A review and model for future research. *Psychological Bulletin, 99*, 143–165.

Scherer, K. R. (1988). On the symbolic functions of vocal affect expression. *Journal of Language and Social Psychology, 7*, 79–100.

Scherer, K. R. (1989). Vocal measurement of emotion. In R. Plutchik & H. Kellerman (Eds.), *Emotion: Theory, research, and experience: Vol. 4. The measurement of emotions* (pp. 233–259). New York: Academic.

Scherer, K. R. (1992). Vocal affect expression as symptom, symbol, and appeal. In H. Papoucek, U. Jürgens, & M. Papoucek (Eds.), *Nonverbal vocal communication: Comparative and developmental approaches* (pp. 43–60). Cambridge, UK: Cambridge University.

Scherer, K. R., Banse, R., & Wallbott, H. G. (2001). Emotion inferences from vocal expression correlate across languages and cultures. *Journal of Cross-Cultural Psychology, 32*, 76–92.

Scherer, K. R., Banse, R., Wallbott, H. G., & Goldbeck, T. (1991). Vocal cues in emotion encoding and decoding. *Motivation and Emotion, 15*, 123–148.

Siegman, A. W., & Boyle, S. (1993). Voices of fear and anxiety and sadness and depression: The effects of speech rate and loudness on fear and anxiety and sadness and depression. *Journal of Abnormal Psychology, 102,* 430–437.

Smoski, M. J., & Bachorowski, J.-A. (2003). Antiphonal laughter between friends and strangers. *Cognition & Emotion, 17,* 327–340.

Smoski, M. J., & Bachorowski, J. A. (2003). Antiphonal laughter in developing friendships. *Annals of the New York Academy of Sciences, 1000,* 300–303.

Sobin, C., & Alpert, M. (1999). Emotion in speech: The acoustic attributes of fear, anger, sadness, and joy. *Journal of Psycholinguistic Research, 28,* 347–365.

Streeter, L. A., Macdonald, N. H., Apple, W., Krauss, R. M., & Galotti, K. M. (1983). Acoustic and perceptual indicators of emotional stress. *Journal of the Acoustical Society of America, 73,* 1354–1360.

Zajonc, R. B. (1980). Feeling and thinking: Preferences need no inferences. *American Psychologist, 35,* 151–175.

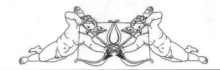

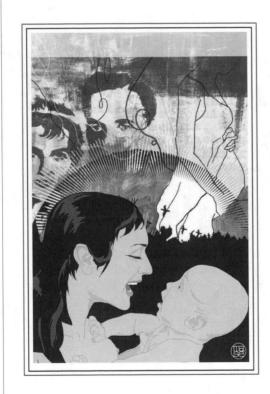

CHAPTER 7

Emotions in Spoken Finnish: Cues for the Human Listener and the Computer

Juhani Toivanen, Tapio Seppänen, and
Eero Väyrynen

Introduction

Finnish belongs to the Uralic language family; the two main branches are the Finno-Ugric languages and the Samoyedic languages. Thus, Finnish is not part of the Indo-European language family. The peoples speaking Hungarian and Finnish are the largest groups in the Finno-Ugric branch. Finnish (5.2 million speakers) and Estonian (1.1 million speakers) are the biggest groups of the Baltic-Finnic languages within the Finno-Ugric group. A hallmark of the Finnish language is the extremely rich (and complicated) case system: 12 cases are productive, i.e., any Finnish noun can be followed by 12 case suffixes. This entails, however, that the word order is relatively free because the case system takes care of many of the functions handled by prepositions and articles in languages such as English.

Prosodically, Finnish has been said to be a somewhat monotonous language: pitch range is narrow and average pitch is low (Hakulinen, 1979). The basic pitch pattern in non-emphatic, non-affective utterances is a falling intonation contour (F_0 contour) with rising-falling peaks on accented words (semantically important content words). The basic pattern is very common with statements and questions; in utterance-final position, creak voicing is common. An important point is that F_0 rises are relatively rare, even with questions—the rules of final rise signaling interrogativity in French, English, and

German, for example, are not relevant in spoken Finnish (Iivonen, 1998). However, to express interrogativity, prosody can be used in Finnish, too. Questions usually involve a high initial pitch in spoken Finnish; the high initial pitch is followed by falling F_0 as with statements. Rising F_0 contours are possible (but relatively rare) in echo questions, involving a request for repetition of the previous piece of information. In emotional speech, however, rising pitch is possible, and the trends described above do not necessarily hold (we shall return to this issue below).

Three degrees of accentual classes can be distinguished in Finnish (Iivonen, 1998). Accent for *rheme* (new information) is often (but not always) accompanied by a higher F_0 peak on the first syllable of the accented word. The thematic parts of the utterance (containing old information) do not contain such F_0 peaks. Accent for contrast involves an extra high F_0 peak in the accented syllable; additional cues are increased intensity and duration. Emphatic accent is achieved by making two syllables, instead of only one, accented: thus, with monosyllabic words, an extra syllable is created for emphatic accent. It is also possible that, in a multisyllabic word, every syllable gets the intensified accent if the word carries emphatic accent.

In spoken Finnish, as in other languages, prosody is used to signal syntactic functions and the information structure of discourse, but, on the whole, it can be said that, at least from the viewpoint of non-affective speech, Finnish is less melodious than many other languages (Niemi, 1984). For example, accent (as described above) is less melodic or tonal in Finnish than in English (Niemi, 1984); duration has a more important role in the accent system of

Finnish than in English. To take one example, in so-called compound words, the first element is strongly accented in English: *black bird*, referring to a type of bird (*Turdus merula*), gets a prominent F_0 peak on *black*. In Finnish, in the word *mustarastas* (*Turdus merula*), the element *musta* involves a more gradual F_0 declension instead of a high F_0 peak followed by a steep fall—in clear contrast with the corresponding prosodic structure (on *black*) in English.

There is also the stereotype that Finns do not express affect in speech as freely and intensively as speakers of some other languages (e.g., Italians). It has been assumed that Finns tolerate long silences in conversation and are reluctant to engage in spontaneous small talk with strangers in communicative situations. On the other hand, the evidence concerning the purely affective aspects of spoken Finnish is very fragmentary. While there is empirical evidence on the syntactic prosodic aspects of spoken Finnish, the literature on the affective prosody is limited. There has been very little research on the vocal parameters of affective content in continuous spoken Finnish. For example, Laukkanen, Vilkman, Alku, and Oksanen (1996; 1997) focus on very short units (nonsense syllables with Finnish phonotactic structure) in their investigation of the vocal expression of emotion.

Here we present results of a recent research project on the vocal parameters of emotions in continuous spoken Finnish; to our knowledge, this is the first systematic study of the prosodic features of emotions in connected Finnish speech. The data were analyzed from the viewpoint of the perception of emotions (i.e., from the viewpoint of listeners analyzing the emotional content and utilizing prosodic cues to aid the inference process). In addition, the data were utilized with the aim of the automatic classification/discrimination of emotions from speech: a statistical classifier was developed that uses prosodic cues to classify the emotions into predetermined categories. Thus we looked at the way in which emotions are expressed in continuous Finnish speech, and how human listeners and the computer can classify the emotions with the help of a number of acoustic/prosodic cues. We also present the speech corpus on which the research was based: in classification experiments, it is always necessary to collect a representative database, preferably as large as possible, and to systematically base the experiments on the corpus.

Speech Data: MediaTeam Emotional Speech Corpus

The *MediaTeam Emotional Speech Corpus* is currently the largest existing emotional speech corpus for continuous Finnish language (Seppänen, Toivanen, & Väyrynen, 2003). The corpus is used to investigate in detail the phonetic and phonological correlates of basic emotions in Finnish, and the results are used in developing speech corpus search engines (Toivanen & Seppänen, 2002). The speech material was produced by 14 professional actors (eight men, six women) from Oulu City Theater in Finland. The subjects were aged between 26 and 50, and all were speakers of the same northern Finnish dialect. The speakers simulated the following basic emotions while reading out a phonetically rich text of 120 words adapted from a newspaper article: neutral, sadness, anger, and happiness.

The speakers were allowed to repeat the reading if they were not satisfied with the first rendition. Semantically, the text was as neutral as possible, describing features of a berry that grows in the northern parts of Finland. In addition to the monologue text, the speakers acted out two prewritten dialogues containing specific emotional lines of varying length. Thus the corpus contained linguistic units with specific emotional content ranging from short exclamations to monologues of approximately 1 minute in length.

The audio recordings were made in an anechoic chamber using a high quality condenser microphone and a DAT recorder, resulting in a 48 kHz, 16-bit recording. The data were stored in a PC as WAV format files. The acoustic analysis was carried out with F_0Tool (developed by MediaTeam Language and Audio Technology Group). F_0Tool is a speech analysis software implemented in the MATLAB language; F_0Tool is a cepstrum-based voiced/unvoiced segmentation and time domain F_0 extraction algorithm using waveform-matching. The performance of the tool was tested with challenging speech material from radio conversations involving Finnish fighter pilots, and the accuracy of the tool was found to be quite comparable to the performance level of the existing standard speech analysis algorithms. The tool and the verification of its performance level are described in detail in Toivanen, Väyrynen, and Seppänen (2004).

Currently, F_0Tool is capable of analyzing over 40 acoustic/prosodic parameters fully automatically from a speech sample of basically any length; the input required by F_0Tool is an audio waveform file (Toivanen et al., 2004). The parameters are F_0-related, intensity-related, temporal, and spectral features—see the other article by our group in *Voice & Emotion* (Toivanen, Seppänen & Väyrynen, 2006) for a discussion of these parameters. Note that the term *segment* refers to a part of the signal of varying duration, which may be realized as silence or as voiced or voiceless speech (the term does not designate any phonological unit).

Some examples of the general F_0-based parameters were the following: mean F_0, median F_0, maximum F_0, minimum F_0, F_0 range, 5th fractile of F_0, and 95th fractile of F_0. The parameters describing the dynamics of F_0 were, for example, the following: average F_0 fall/rise during a continuous voiced segment, average steepness of F_0 fall/rise, maximum F_0 fall/rise during a continuous voiced segment, and maximum steepness of F_0 fall/rise. The intensity-related parameters were, for example, the following: mean RMS intensity, median RMS intensity, intensity range, 5th fractile of intensity, 95th fractile of intensity, and the range between the fractiles. Some of the temporal parameters were the following: average duration of voiced segments, average duration of unvoiced segments shorter than 300 ms, maximum duration of voiced segments, and maximum duration of silence segments. Some of the ratio parameters were the following: ratio of speech to long unvoiced segments and ratio of silence/speech segments. The spectral features concerned the proportion of low-frequency energy (below 500/1000 Hz). Additional parameters were jitter and shimmer.

The speech corpus was complemented with more focused and ecologically valid (i.e., more "emotion-prone") material with multiple repetitions featuring the following simulated emotions: neutral, sadness, happiness, anger, and tenderness. The speech data were produced by nine professional actors (five men and four women). Some of these speakers had participated in the first data production sessions. The emotional states were simulated when reading out a passage of some 80 words from a well-known and topical Finnish novel. Each speaker produced, in a random order, 10 renditions of each emotional state while reading out the passage. The material could be convincingly interpreted with many emotions, and multiple repetitions allowed the speakers to use their emotional expression repertoire to the full. The data collection procedure was technically similar to that used in the first data set, but the calibration for intensity measurements was obtained from a standard voice source (93.6 dB).

Classification Experiments

Speaker-independent classification was performed using the k-Nearest-Neighbor classifier (kNN), which is applied as a standard nonparametric method in statistical pattern recognition; leave-one-out was used for evaluating classifier performance (see the other article by our group in *Voice & Emotion* (Toivanen, Väyrynen & Seppänen, 2004) for a discussion of kNN and other classifiers). The level of automatic classification of emotions reached a level of just below 70% with the following prosodic parameters representing seven dimensions in the classification procedure: intensity range, maximum F_0 rise during a continuous voiced segment, ratio of silence segments, 5–95% F_0 range, shimmer, jitter, and intensity variation.

Human classification experiments were performed in the form of listening tests. The listeners were students in a junior high school, aged between 14 and 15: 51 subjects (27 males, 24 females) participated as volunteers. All listeners were speakers of the same northern variety of Finnish as the actors. The emotional labels to choose between were limited to the intended emotions; distracters were not used. The average emotion discrimination performance of the listeners was 77%. The exact performance levels of the classification and the full list of the best parameters for the first data set can be found in Toivanen et al. (2004). The classification is performed with two kinds of truth data; both the intended emotions and the perceived emotions are used as the basis for classification.

The automatic classification experiments and the listening tests have been carried out only for the first data set (involving the reading out of the newspaper text). The second data set (involving the fiction passage) is yet to be tested, but our hypothesis based on preliminary data analysis is that significantly better results (for both the human listeners and the computer) can be expected with the second data set, which involves a more intense and natural emotion expression scenario.

Discussion: Cues for the Computer and the Human Listener

The existing literature suggests that the computer achieved quite a good discrimination rate. It has been argued that, in a speaker-independent classification task, as in our experiment, the performance level can reach 60–70% for three basic emotions (ten Bosch, 2003). Looking at the best feature vector in the classification task, it was observed that, to express emotion vocally, the speakers used cues largely similar to those reported for other languages, that is, variations in energy, speech rate, and pitch. The optimal set of parameters in the classification procedure including intensity range, maximum F_0 rise during a continuous voiced segment, ratio of silence segments, 5–95% F_0 range, shimmer, jitter, and intensity variation clearly reflects the "liveliness" of the speech: intensity range, F_0 range, the dynamics of F_0 change, as well as the amount of speech within a speaking turn obviously correlate with the activity level of the speech situation and the speaker. It can thus be concluded that Finns use prosody to express affect in speech in a way that must be essentially similar to the vocal expression of emotion reported for major languages such as English and French. Showing that the same prosodic parameters are utilized in the emotion portrayals through voice, and demonstrating that emotional spoken Finnish is not qualitatively different from other languages, our research finding dispels a prior understanding about the characteristics of Finnish speech.

An interesting product of our experiment is the 7% difference between the performance levels for the computer and the human listeners, demonstrating that the human listeners utilized acoustic/prosodic parameters unavailable to the computer. The computer can utilize only automatically computable prosodic primitives, while the human listener also pays attention to the linguistically relevant prosodic phenomena. As was pointed out above, in spoken Finnish, the basic non-affective utterance contains a descending F_0 curve with rising-falling peaks in the syllables of the accentuated words. These peaks represent moderate accent mainly accompanying rhematic information.

According to Suomi, Toivanen, and Ylitalo (2003), in spoken Finnish, three degrees of accentuation can be distinguished: word stress (no accent), moderate accent (with rhematic information), and strong accent (with contrastive information or strong emotional content). Mere word stress is not signaled tonally (i.e., with F_0), while accents (containing rising-falling F_0 movements) are signaled mainly tonally in such a way that strong accent has a more extensive F_0 movement than moderate accent (a higher peak value after the F_0 rise and a lower end point after the F_0 fall).

Our point here is that accents that are signaled tonally tend to co-occur with special emotional content in speech. The human listener will hear these accents as discrete phonological phenomena, but the classifier (the computer) is not capable of this—in its current form (see our remark on future directions of research below). Thus the human listener has access to more information than the computer in evaluating the affective dimensions of speech–as the observed performance level difference in our data suggests. In emotional Finnish, the dynamic aspects of F_0 variation (e.g., maximum F_0 rise) thus probably have an important role from the perceptual viewpoint. In addition to signaling the beginning of (strong) accent, F_0 rises occur in utterances which are "globally emotional": they do not just contain single accentuated words with contrastive and/ or emotional content, but they represent speaking turns which are emotional throughout. As was pointed out above, a rising intonation is rare in standard Finnish unless an emotional dimension is intended. Utterances with high-rising tones can be assumed to convey strong emotional meanings (annoyance, incredulity, etc.) in spoken Finnish. Again, it must be noted that the current classifier does not "hear" these syntactic features of rising F_0 movements (in final position) in an utterance. By contrast, the human listeners can be expected to be fully aware of this kind of "marked" prosody in a speaking turn. It should also be noted that these phonological (emotion-related) F_0 features certainly exist in spoken Finnish regardless of the observations that Finnish is not, phonologically, as tonal as some other languages. The degree of tonality may be small only in comparison with other languages: the language-specific tonal features are quite distinct in Finnish to separate strong accents from moderate ones, and emotional speech from non-emotional speech.

The results of the classification experiments offer (indirect) support for the hypothesis that discrete nongradable phonological features also convey affective content in Finnish. This has implications for the development of classification methods. It will not be enough to concentrate on the automatically measurable phonetic variables; at some point, the classifier must tackle the more abstract prosodic patterns if the aim is to ultimately improve the emotion discrimination performance level. An important future direction in the development of classification methods would be to model the abstract F_0 phenomena in a computable (computer-interpretable) way. There is no reason to assume that this would be an impossible task in the long run. Essentially, what is needed is the gradual development of language-specific models of legitimate phonological F_0 features, which the classifier must be trained to recognize. Eventually, in the classification procedure, the constantly varying prosodic features and the more abstract features must be combined.

categorization of emotions is promising, and that, in the near future, computer recognition of human vocal emotions may approach a natural state, yielding access to new exciting product applications.

Conclusion

Our research project on the human and automatic classification of emotion in spoken Finnish, which is the first such research on this minority language, has yielded very interesting results. First, features of F_0 and intensity have been found to accompany emotional Finnish speech—this is probably a universal phenomenon in the expression of emotion. Second, the performance level of the human emotion classification exceeds that of the automatic classification. Although this is not surprising in itself, we suggest that phonological features of F_0 variation, especially rising F_0, are emotion-carrying features in spoken Finnish, in addition to the global constantly varying average features of F_0, intensity, duration, etc. Also in this respect, it can be argued that Finnish, a minority language in a minority language group, is not qualitatively different from major Indo-European languages. This finding contradicts prior notions of "emotionality" of the Finnish language. In languages in general, prosodic parameters are hierarchically organized as concrete (phonetic or paralinguistic) and as more abstract (phonological or linguistic) phenomena, and there is no reason to assume that some of these levels would be irrelevant from the viewpoint of the vocal communication of emotion. Finally, the results suggest that contrastive research on human vs. computer

References

Hakulinen, L. (1979). *Suomen kielen rakenne ja kehitys (The structure and development of the Finnish language)*. Helsinki: Otava.

Iivonen, A. (1998). Intonation in Finnish. In D. Hirst & A. Di Cristo (Eds.), *Intonation systems: A survey of twenty languages* (pp. 311–327). Cambridge, UK: Cambridge University Press.

Laukkanen, A.-M., Vilkman, E., Alku, P., & Oksanen, H. (1996). Physical variations related to stress and emotional state: A preliminary study. *Journal of Phonetics, 24*, 313–335.

Laukkanen, A.-M., Vilkman, E., Alku, P., & Oksanen, H. (1997). On the perception of emotions in speech: The role of voice quality. *Logopedics Phoniatrics Vocology, 22*, 157–168.

Niemi, J. (1984). *Word level stress and prominence in Finnish and English. Acoustic experiments on production and perception*. Joensuu, Finland: Publications in the Humanities 1, University of Joensuu.

Seppänen, T., Toivanen, J., & Väyrynen, E. (2003). MediaTeam Speech Corpus: A first large Finnish emotional speech database. In (Ed.), *Proceedings of the 15th International Congress of Phonetic Sciences* (Barcelona): *Vol. 3* (pp. 2469–2472).

Suomi, K., Toivanen, J., & Ylitalo, R. (2003). Durational and tonal correlates of accent in Finnish. *Journal of Phonetics, 31*, 113–138.

ten Bosch, L. (2003). Emotions, speech and the ASR framework. *Speech Communication, 40*, 213–225.

Toivanen, J., & Seppänen, T. (2002). Prosody-based search features in information retrieval. In (Ed.), *Proceedings of FONETIK 2002* (Stockholm) (pp. 105–108).

Toivanen, J., Väyrynen, E., & Seppänen, T. (2004). Automatic discrimination of emotion from spoken Finnish. *Language and Speech*, *47*, 383–412.

Toivanen, J., Seppänen, T. & Väyrynen, E. (2006). Automatic discrimination of emotion from voice: A review of research paradigms. In K. Izdebski (Ed.), *Voice & Emotion*. San Diego, CA: Plural.

CHAPTER 8

Judgments of the Affective Valence of Spontaneous Vocalizations

The Influence of Situational Context

Arvid Kappas and Natalia Poliakova

Abstract

The present study demonstrates for the first time a context effect for ratings of affective valence of spontaneous vocalizations. Sixteen spontaneous vocal one-word samples were taken from recordings of a voice-controlled video game. Depending on whether judges believed the stimuli were taken from a situation that was pleasant or unpleasant for the encoder, they rated the affective state of the encoders as more pleasant or unpleasant, respectively. The impact of the context information was a function of stimulus strength and ambiguity as assessed in a separate sample of judges who did not possess context information. The strength of the context information was also assessed in an independent sample. We conclude that decoding of affective expressions is not simply based on the recognition of specific features or configurations, but instead an active construction based on expectations, beliefs, and biases.

Judgments of the Affective Valence of Spontaneous Vocalizations: The Influence of Situational Context

In recent years, it has become very clear that judgments of emotional facial expressions are not only based on observable patterns of facial activation, but also on the contextual information that judges possess. Demonstrations of such effects range from the classic film experiment by Kuleshov (cited for example in Russell, 1997; see also Wallbott, 1988) to more recent experimental studies (e.g., Wallbott, 1988; Carroll & Russell, 1996; Fernández-Dols, Wallbott, & Sanchez, 1991). In most of these recent studies still photos or video recordings of facial expressions were presented together with a verbal description of the situation in which the expression was supposedly taken (the so-called person-scenario approach or Goodenough-Tinker paradigm, named after the methodology first used by Goodenough & Tinker, 1931; see also Fernández-Dols & Carroll, 1997, for an extended critique). A majority of studies on the influence of situational context has been trying to answer the question whether the context is *more important* than the face or vice versa for the decoding of specific emotions. However, this question as such might not be very meaningful. Ekman, Friesen, and Ellsworth (1982) already pointed out that there are many different facets to the complexity of both facial expressions and of situational context. In particular they suggested that the relative clarity of the two sources of information would likely contribute to the importance of each of them. Specifically, they distinguished three components of source clarity: ambiguity, message complexity, and strength. Ekman et al. argued that unless the source clarity of context and faces to be judged were perfectly matched, no meaningful test of the relative contribution of both channels could be conducted—in effect a condition that might be impossible to achieve. To some degree the question of relative importance of voice and context is reminiscent of other "which channel is more important" debates, e.g., in the context of studies on the relative importance of facial and vocal cues (see Hess, Kappas, & Scherer, 1988; also de Gelder, 2000). With hindsight it appears naïve to assume the relative importance of channels or cues could be static and constant. Instead, it is highly likely that the meaning analysis of context and facial expression is integrated in a dynamic fashion. For example, it has been suggested that the context might change the accessibility of emotion categories, which would facilitate or focus the attribution of a particular label to a pattern of facial changes (e.g., Fernández-Dols et al., 1991; see also Wallbott, 1988). Obviously, there are boundary conditions in which a very strong context might lead to a complete discounting of facial information and vice versa, but these are not typical situations. However, in most cases it is likely that the attribution of an emotion label, the judgment of the intensity of an emotion, or similar affective decoding processes rely on a complex interplay of conscious and automatic information processing. This interplay might be characterized as an affective bias or priming process (see Pell, 2005).

One of the rare *process models* regarding how context and *facial* information might interact has been proposed by Russell (e.g., 1997). He suggests that we obtain "easily" and "automatically" two kinds of information from the face. The primary information regards an automatic estimate of the "overall level of pleasure (pleased vs. displeased) and arousal (agitated vs. sleepy)" (1997, p. 298) from observing an expresser. This information is then combined with other information, such as situational context and information about the expresser that yields then a perception of a *specific emotion*.

This process model has the advantage that it is not only large in scope, but it appears to make testable assumptions about two elements of the decoding process, (a) it suggests that the role of context is limited to the attribution of emotion labels once an automatic judgment has occurred regarding the "quasi-physical features" and the attribution of the psychological state of the interaction partner in a two-dimensional pleasure-arousal space, and (b) it is explicit concerning how, in Russell's view, dimensional representations and emotion categories are related. Based on these assumptions we can deduce that judgments in a pleasure-arousal space should not be affected by contextual information. Thus, the first goal of the current study is to test whether affective dimensional judgments regarding spontaneous vocalizations are affected by contextual information.

While there is a growing body of research on judgments of *facial* expressions in situational context, little is known regarding the role of context for the decoding of *affective vocalizations*. Specifically, to our knowledge, there are no studies on contextual influences on judgments of spontaneous affective vocalizations. While there have been studies that looked at the effects of mixed messages in which facial and vocal channels encode discrepant affective information

(e.g., Hess et al., 1988; de Gelder, 2000), we are aware of only one study that investigated children's reliance on the vocal and situational cues presented in vignette form (Hortaçsu & Ekinci, 1992; see van den Stock, Righart, & de Gelder, 2007 for a recent study in which bodily expressions provide a context for the perception of facial expressions or tone of voice). However, in the latter study only one encoder was used who was portraying happy, angry, or neutral endings to the vignettes presented. This study showed a certain reliance on situational cues, particularly with increases in age (preschool, second grade, fifth grade).

There appear to be several reasons for a lack of studies on context effects for the decoding of affect from voice. By their very nature, there is usually a "context" accompanying vocalizations in that they are the carrier of speech, which frequently contains information about the affective state of the encoder as well as the relation between the partners in an interaction or their attitudes towards some object. Often researchers have tried to control for content in judgment studies by using either nonsense syllables, or standardized neutral phrases (see Kappas, Hess, & Scherer, 1991; Johnstone & Scherer, 2000). Obviously, these types of standardized vocalizations are difficult to obtain spontaneously during various affective states and, in consequence, researchers have relied on portrayals by professional actors or simply asked encoders to pronounce a standardized phrase "as if they were," for example, angry. However, the use of actors to portray vocal affective changes has been criticized mainly on two grounds (see Kappas et al., 1991; Kappas & Hess, 1995; Bachorowski & Owren, 1995; but also Wallbott & Scherer, 1986). First, there is a risk that professional actors and naïve encoders alike will tend to create highly stereotypical portrayals. The problem here is that high inter-rater agreement in judgment studies is not an indicator of the validity of the portrayals but might simply reflect shared stereotypes in a given culture (see also Kappas, 2003). If actors in Bali, for example, were instructed to communicate emotion through posture and gestures they might use rather ritualized forms, which would be indeed recognized well by members of the same culture. Yet, their portrayals would be difficult to decode by Western observers, and likely would bear little resemblance to spontaneous emotional reactions. Second, there is ample reason to believe that various acoustic changes considered to be associated with affective vocalizations are not under voluntary control (see Scherer, 1986; Jürgens, 1996). Thus, it becomes apparent that decoding studies require the use of spontaneous vocalizations while encoders are indeed in particular affective states or in ongoing interaction. This necessity to rely on spontaneous vocalizations and yet use standardized content (i.e., words) constitutes the conundrum that has led to a shortage of studies in this area. The second goal of the current study tries to address this scarcity and attempts to establish whether there are context effects on the decoding of spontaneous affective vocalizations.

Recently, we have developed a paradigm in which highly standardized yet spontaneous affective vocalizations could be recorded (Kappas, 1997). In this paradigm, participants played a Pacman-type video game using vocal commands (up, down, left, right[1]). We have used the same video game in previous research with participants interacting with the game using a joystick (e.g., Kappas, 1995; Pecchinenda & Kappas, 1995; Kappas & Pecchinenda, 1996; Pecchinenda, Kappas, & Smith, 1997; see also Kappas & Pecchinenda, 1999, for a detailed description of the paradigm). In these previous studies we could show, for example, that manipulations of relative speed of monsters and player symbol affected self-reports, such as ratings of coping potential, and physiological activation (see also Pecchinenda, 2001). During the game, there are specific events that are congruent with the goal defined by the game context (e.g., killing a monster) or goal incongruent (e.g., being killed by a monster). Our research interest here does not lie in the elicitation of specific "basic" emotions, but rather in the manipulation of emotion-antecedent appraisals to establish the relationship between specific patterns of appraisals with subjective experience, as well as expressive and physiological responses (see Kappas, 2001; Johnstone, van Reekum, & Scherer, 2001). Based on the results that we have accumulated so far, we are convinced that this paradigm does produce affective reactions at all levels and that participants are very engaged in playing the game. Individual voice samples taken from the stream of the voice-controlled game, when they occur in immediate proximity of relevant events (such as being bitten by a monster, or killing a monster) should be adequate objects of judgment of affective content. However, one problem that does arise with such an approach is that self-report cannot be used to validate the affective state of the encoder. Partici-

---

[1]Actually the words used were *haut* (up), *bas* (down), *gauche* (left), and *droite* (right), given that our participants in the encoding and in the decoding studies were native speakers of French.

pants cannot comment on-line, the game cannot be interrupted without affecting the flow of the game, and retrospective judgments are doubtful at best, if specific events are concerned. Thus, for the present judgment study, we chose to operationalize the criterion for selecting the stimuli as combinations of specific objective stimulus events that we considered having a specific meaning for all players. Specifically, we chose one group of vocalizations in a context in which an event occurred that was congruent with the goal of the game (biting the monster and gaining points) while coping potential was high (player symbol being faster than the monsters) and another group of vocalizations from a context in which an event occurred that was goal incongruent (being bitten by the monsters and losing points) while coping potential was low (player symbol being slower than the monsters). These events are arguably to be considered positive and negative with respect to the goals of the players, respectively.

To demonstrate that our notions of these two types of events as being positive and negative respectively would be shared by others simply based on a short account of the context, we presented a short description on a questionnaire that was distributed in an undergraduate class in psychology. Participants ($n = 87$) were to indicate their ratings on a 100 mm visual scale with the anchors labeled *very unpleasant* and *very pleasant*, respectively. The midpoint was indicated using a vertical bar. There were no numbers or gradations on the scale and participants were simply instructed to put an X on the scale corresponding to their judgment to what degree each event described would be pleasant or unpleasant for the player. The contexts themselves were defined as:

Negative context—A person plays a Pacman-type video game where the goal consists of making the highest number of points possible without getting bitten by the monsters. After some seconds of play, the player does not manage to save himself from the monsters and he gets bitten. Thus, the player loses 50 points. (The final score on average was in the range of −150 to 100 points.)

Positive context—A person plays a Pacman-type video game where the goal consists of making the highest number of points possible without getting bitten by the monsters. After having eaten a power pill, the player catches a monster and gains 50 points. (The final score on average was in the range of −150 to 100 points.)

The order of the two scenarios was counterbalanced but presented on one letter-size sheet. Responses were measured with a ruler and entered as mm deviation from the midpoint (i.e., values could be between −50 mm and +50 mm). Analyses indicated that both contexts were well discriminated, $t(84) = 15.482$, $p < .0001$, and the means were in the mid range of either side of the neutral point, $M_{pleasant} = 21.588$ mm, $sd = 16.359$, $M_{unpleasant} = -21.052$ mm, $sd = 15.714$.

Having validated that the two contexts would be evaluated as positive and negative, respectively, we planned two experiments. In the first experiment, a number of participants were to evaluate a series of spontaneous vocalizations coming from a positive or negative context and judge whether the encoder (player) was in a positive or negative state (operationalized as whether he was in a pleasant or unpleasant situation). However, participants would be unaware of the specific context from which the vocalizations were taken. They were simply told that these samples came from recordings taken while the encoders played a voice-controlled video game that resembles Pacman. In a second experiment, the same vocalizations would be given to participants together with an account explaining from which specific context these vocalizations were taken. We hypothesized that (a) affective judgments of vocalizations would be influenced by beliefs about the situational context, and (b) that the influence of context would depend on the source clarity and (c) the strength of the vocal stimuli. We defined source clarity, consistent with Ekman et al. (1982), as inter-rater agreement for a given stimulus in the first experiment in which no specific context was provided. We defined strength as the mean extent to which a stimulus deviated from the neutral point in the first experiment. Note that we did not include message complexity in our hypotheses or design, as Ekman et al.'s definition applies well to judgments regarding specific emotion categories, where "blends" could be considered as complex. We believe that complexity does not apply for our study where participants are simply asked to provide valence judgments.

Experiment 1

Method

Participants. Fifteen students at Université Laval (8 female, 7 male) aged between 18 and 49 years participated in the study. They replied to notes attached at the university's bulletin boards and did not receive any remuneration for their participation.

Materials. Based on the protocols of an experiment where 30 participants played the voice-controlled video game, four encoders (two male, two female) were chosen who pronounced the word *haut* (up) and the word *bas* (down) in either context/situation as defined above. The criterion was that the word must have been uttered within 1 s of the event. The selection of the stimuli was based exclusively on the paper record of events during the game without listening to them first so as not to be influenced by whether they were "good" portrayals or not. The vocalizations were recorded using a headset-type microphone (http://www.audio-technica.com) and had been taped at a sampling rate of 48.1 kHz on digital audio tape (http://www.fostex.com), and then were transferred to a PC compatible computer. Using Kay Elemetrics CSL software (http://www.kayelemetrics.com), the individual words chosen were edited and transferred to a Macintosh sound file. Stimuli were redigitized at 22 kHz on an Apple Power Macintosh 8500 (http://www.apple.com). All stimuli and instructions were presented using a program written in Macromedia Authorware, version 3.5 (http://www.macromedia.com). The audio samples were presented using the integrated speakers in the Macintosh's Apple Vision 1710 AV monitor.

Design and Procedure

Sixteen stimuli (two words in two contexts spoken by each of the four encoders) were presented twice in two blocks. The order of stimuli was randomized for each block for each participant. After participants signed an informed consent form they were placed in front of the computer, which presented all further instructions. Judgments were made using the mouse on a 100 mm visual scale with the extremes labeled *very unpleasant* and *very pleasant*, respectively. There was a vertical bar indicating the midpoint of the scale. Participants had four trials to familiarize themselves with the task. The warming up stimuli were different from the 16 stimuli used for the study and were taken from different encoders as well. After the judgment of the stimuli, participants also judged the two scenarios that had been presented in the pilot study. We did not analyze their ratings regarding their evaluation of the scenarios, but they were simply to confirm that participants had understood the mode of responding to the instructions by clicking on the left side of the scale for the negative scenario and on the right side of the scale for the positive scenario. All participants responded correctly and hence all judgment data on the 16 stimuli were included in the analysis. After the experiment the experimenter asked a series of questions concerning the experiment and then provided a full debriefing and encouraged participants to ask questions if they had any.

Results

Ratings did not differentiate between encoding conditions. Overall stimuli were rated as slightly negative ($M = -6.234$). Figure 8–1 shows the mean of each stimulus plotted against the standard deviation for that stimulus over all judges. Means and standard deviations are taken as indices of the *strength* and the *ambiguity* of the stimuli, respectively. A visual inspection of the data shows that there

are no stimuli that are strong and ambiguous. However, the correlation between means and standard deviations is low and not significant [$r(16) = .368$].

Discussion

There are several reasons that could account for judges' failure to distinguish between the two encoding conditions. Obviously, there is the possibility that there were no or few cues in the vocal samples that could allow distinguishing between encoding conditions. This in turn could be because the encoders' affective states did not differ between the two conditions. Alternatively, encoders' affective states differed in the positive and negative context respectively, but their expressions did not differ. We do know that in previous studies using the joystick controlled version of our game there were clear differences regarding the situations where the player symbol was faster than the monsters compared to the situation where the player symbol was slower, in self-report, and for several physiological measures. We did not try to evaluate the self-report data (or trial-based physiology data) for our four encoders. The goal of this study was not to see whether there were objective differences in the vocalizations of the encoders as a function of encoding condition and, in any case, looking only at four encoders would render such an enterprise futile.

The distribution of the judgment data suggests that stimulus strength and ambiguity are not evenly distributed. Because there do not seem to be strong and ambiguous stimuli in our set, further analyses of the impact of situational context on judgments will not be analyzed in an ANOVA design, but instead using a

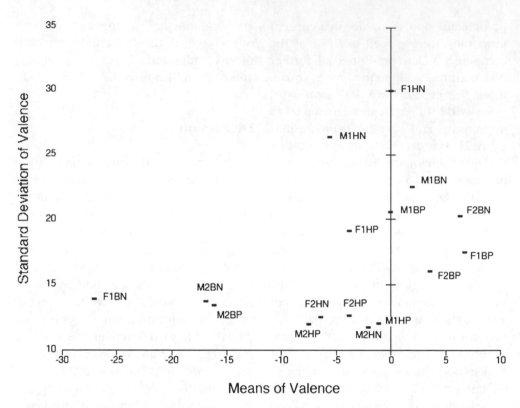

Figure 8–1. Means vs. standard deviations for the 16 stimuli judged in Experiment 1. Each stimulus is identified as a code specifying the gender and identity for each of the four encoders (M1, M2, F1, F2), the word pronounced (*haut*, *bas*), and whether the sample comes from a positive or a negative encoding situation (P, N). Thus M1HN is the encoder M1 pronouncing the word *haut* while being bitten by a monster in the video game (i.e., the negative encoding condition).

correlational approach, in which changes from the ratings obtained in the current experiment differ as a function of context are related to stimulus strength and ambiguity.

Experiment 2

Method

Participants. Twenty-five students at Université Laval (12 female, 13 male) aged between 19 and 40 years partici-

pated in the study. They replied to notes attached at the university's bulletin boards and did not receive any remuneration for their participation.

Materials. The same 16 stimuli used in Experiment 1 were presented to the participants. The description of the scenarios was the same used in the pilot study and is given verbatim above.

Design and Procedure

Sixteen stimuli (two words in two contexts spoken by each of the four encoders) were presented four times in four blocks. The order of stimuli was randomized for each block for each participant. In two of the four blocks participants were told that the next 16 stimuli would come from the positive context as defined above, while for the other two blocks the same stimuli were presented with the information that they were recorded in the negative context. The sequence of blocks was randomized for each participant in a way that a negative and a positive context would each be presented in the first two blocks and in the last two blocks, respectively. Otherwise the procedure was identical between the two experiments.

Results

Valence judgments were indeed strongly affected by the situational context (see Figure 8–2). When paired with the positive context, stimuli were judged as being more positive, $t(15) = -4.694, p < .0003$, and when paired with the negative context as being more negative, $t(15) = 4.070, p < .001$. Correlations were computed to evaluate whether the strength, operationalized as mean rating in the first experiment, or ambiguity, operationalized as mean standard deviation, affected the judgments in the second experiment. Here we looked at the mean ratings in the second experiment, as well

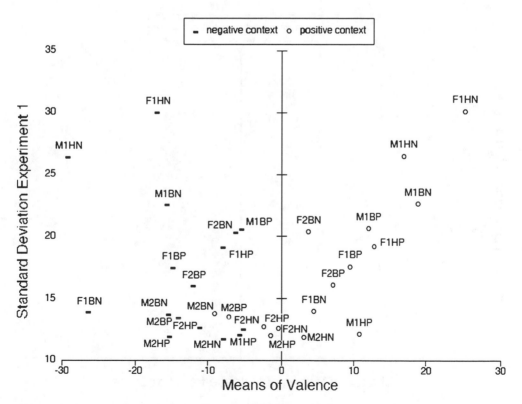

Figure 8–2. Means of valence ratings in Experiment 2 for each stimulus presented in a positive and in a negative context as a function of stimulus ambiguity, i.e., standard deviation of the valence ratings in Experiment 1.

as the difference between the ratings in the two experiments (see Figure 8–3). While the former represents the direct relationship between judgements and the stimulus clarity, the difference score indicates to what degree a stimulus was influenced by its context. The pattern of correlations observed differed for the positive and negative context. For the positive context there was a correlation of $r = .815, p < .0001$, between the SD of the first experiment and the mean ratings in Experiment 2 but not for the negative context. In contrast, for the negative context there was a correlation of $r = -.682$, $p < .0027$, between the SD of the first experiment and the difference of the

mean between the two experiments, but not for the positive context. This pattern is likely due to the fact that in general all stimuli were judged as being more negative than positive and the influence of specific stimuli, such as F1BN. This bias also complicates the interpretation of the correlations between strength of the stimuli and the impact of the situational context; there is a correlation of $r = -.670, p < .0035$, between the mean of the judgments in Experiment 1 and the impact of the negative context; i.e., stimuli that were already judged negative in the absence of a context were less affected than those which were weak or positive. As in the previous experiment,

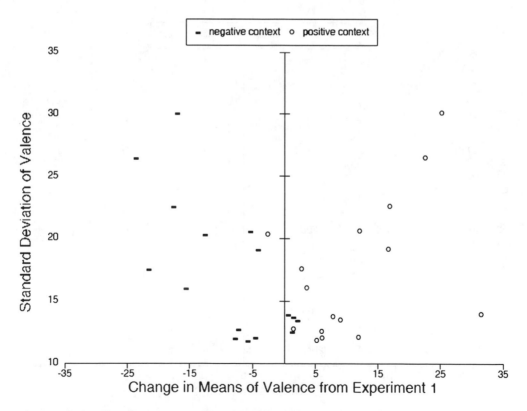

Figure 8–3. Change scores indicating the differences between the means of the valence ratings of Experiment 2 and Experiment 1 as a function of stimulus ambiguity, i.e., standard deviation of the valence ratings in Experiment 1.

there was no effect of the encoding situation on judgments or on the impact of the context.

Discussion

Our results clearly demonstrate that judgments of vocal stimuli were affected by decoders' beliefs about the situational context in which they were produced. This is the first time, to our knowledge, that such an effect has been demonstrated with spontaneous vocalizations and the first time that a context effect has been shown for adults' decoding of any type of affective vocalizations. We are not surprised by these findings and think it only logical that evaluations of affective vocalizations are influenced by the same type of information that has been shown to influence judgments of facial displays. Yet, this finding is far from trivial and underlines the necessity that models dealing with decoding processes in nonverbal communication are not specific to a particular channel of communication, but are general in nature.

It might be argued that we observed context effects because the vocal stimuli were not very clear. Indeed, the ratings of the stimuli in the first experiment were rather low and we would be surprised if the impact of context would have been less for stimuli that were evaluated as being very positive or very negative in the absence of contextual information or more general beliefs about context. Contrariwise, one might also argue that the fact that our stimuli were only mildly positive and negative made our manipulation more plausible. We had no reason to assume that the participants suspected that vocalizations were presented with a discordant context. As we stated in our introduction, we do not intend to make any claims as to the relative importance of voice vs. context. However, we do find it important to demonstrate that, at least under some circumstances, beliefs about the context clearly influence affective judgments.

We are also intrigued that we could show context influences despite the fact that we did not use categorical judgments, but a simple valence dimension. If our reading of Russell's model (e.g., 1997) of the interaction of dimensional judgments and attribution of emotion labels is correct, then we should not have been able to demonstrate an impact of context on the valence dimension itself. However, it is possible that the explicit situational context information we provided impacts the valence estimation via affective bias influences on nonverbal decoding. As Pell states:

> The past decade has seen burgeoning evidence of affective bias or priming in cognitive processing, where the encoding of a "target" event—typically, a written word, picture, or facial stimulus—is systematically influenced by shared affective evaluations of a spatially or temporally contiguous stimulus "prime" (Pell, 2005, p. 46).

In the present study the prime would be a mental activation of the game-event that supposedly led to the vocalization evaluated. Even if the evaluation of valence was automatic, as Russell (1997) argued for the context of facial expressions, an affective bias could moderate this automatic process. Clearly, more research is needed to test whether a vignette, as used in our study, can cause such priming effects.

We have also shown that the impact of beliefs regarding the situational context

is not independent of stimulus characteristics but interacts with them. Specifically, we could show that the ambiguity
of a stimulus clearly affected the impact
of the situational context—and to some
degree influenced the strength as well.
The particular pattern of influence is not
completely clear, as there are differences
in the results for the positive and the
negative context. However, our stimuli
are clearly not well distributed and some
of these differences represent this distribution or the negativity bias in our stimuli in general. We do not feel it necessary
to argue about the details of these patterns. It is clear that further studies must
follow that more carefully select the
material to be judged. For us it was more
important not to preselect stimuli as
good or bad to avoid fixing the outcome
of our study. We used a plausible selection method and objective criteria and
verified that our assumption regarding
whether the events that were the basis
for our selection would generally be
appraised as being positive or negative.
Thus, we believe that the current study
represents a fair test of the hypotheses
we have proposed and we feel reinforced
by our clear and positive findings. We
feel that the totality of our findings has
repercussions for the understanding of the
process of decoding all types of affective
displays. More generally, as has been
shown for faces before, it is true for voices
as well: decoding of affective expressions
is not simply based on the recognition of
specific features or configurations, but
instead an active construction based on
expectations, beliefs, and biases.

These findings have implications for
applied issues, such as the generation of
convincing portrayals of emotions in
computer-generated cartoons. Our results
suggest that vocalizations may be ambiguous on their own, but they are likely to
be perceived congruous with their context. Of course, further research needs to
be done to see whether these findings
hold true for larger segments of text. The
key to convincing artificial stimuli might
lie in ambiguity rather than adherence
to stereotypes.

Author Note. Part of the current data
was presented at the 10th Meeting of the
International Society for Research on
Emotions, in Würzburg, Germany, 1998.
We wish to thank Louise Binet for her
role in all stages of the decoding studies.
The encoding study was supported by
a grant from the Social Sciences and
Humanities Research Council of Canada
to Arvid Kappas. The decoding study was
supported by a grant from the Natural
Science and Engineering Research Coun-
cil of Canada to Arvid Kappas. Please
address correspondence to Arvid Kappas,
Jacobs University Bremen, School of
Humanities and Social Sciences, Campus
Ring 1, D-28759 Bremen, Germany;
(a.kappas@jacobs-university.de).

References

Bachorowski, J.-A., & Owren, M. J. (1995).
Vocal expression of emotion: Acoustic
properties of speech are associated with
emotional intensity and context. *Psychological Science, 6,* 219–224.
Carroll, J. M., & Russell, J. A. (1996). Do facial
expressions signal specific emotions?
Judging emotion from the face in context.
*Journal of Personality and Social Psy-
chology, 70,* 205–218.
de Gelder, B. (2000). Recognizing emotions
by ear and by eye. In R. D. Lane & L. Nadel

(Eds.), *Cognitive neuroscience of emotion* (pp. 84-105). New York: Oxford University Press.

Ekman, P., Friesen, W. V., & Ellsworth, P. (1982). What are the relative contributions of facial behavior and contextual information to the judgment of emotion? In P. Ekman (Ed.), *Emotion in the human face* (2nd ed., pp. 111-127). Cambridge, UK: Cambridge University Press.

Fernández-Dols, J.-M., & Carroll, J. M. (1997). Is the meaning perceived in facial expression independent of its context? In J. A. Russell & J. M. Fernández-Dols (Eds.), *The psychology of facial expression* (pp. 275-294). Cambridge, UK: Cambridge University Press.

Fernández-Dols, J.-M., Wallbott, H., & Sanchez, F. (1991). Emotion category accessibility and the decoding of emotion from facial expression and context. *Journal of Nonverbal Behavior, 15,* 107-123.

Goodenough, F. L., & Tinker, M. A. (1931). The relative potency of facial expression and verbal description of stimulus in the judgment of emotion. *Journal of Comparative Psychology, 12,* 365-370.

Hess, U., Kappas, A., & Scherer, K. R. (1988). Multichannel communication of emotion: Synthetic signal production. In K. R. Scherer (Ed.), *Facets of emotion: Recent research* (pp. 161-182). Hillsdale, NJ: Lawrence Erlbaum Associates.

Hortaçsu, N., & Ekinci, B. (1992). Children's reliance on situational and vocal expression of emotions: Consistent and conflicting cues. *Journal of Nonverbal Behavior, 16,* 231-247.

Johnstone, T., & Scherer, K. R. (2000). Vocal communication of emotion. In M. Lewis & J. M. Haviland-Jones (Eds.), *Handbook of emotions* (2nd ed., pp. 220-235). New York: Guilford.

Johnstone, T., van Reekum, C. M., & Scherer, K. R. (2001). Vocal expression correlates of appraisal processes. In K. R. Scherer, A. Schorr, & T. Johnstone (Eds.), *Appraisal processes in emotion: Theory, methods, research* (pp. 271-284). New York: Oxford University Press.

Jürgens, U. (1996). On the neurobiology of vocal communication. In H. Papousek, U. Jürgens, & M. Papousek (Eds.), *Nonverbal vocal communication* (pp. 31-42). New York: Cambridge University Press.

Kappas, A. (1995). Event-related facial activity: In pursuit of componential approaches to the expression of emotional reactions. *Psychophysiology, 32,* S6.

Kappas, A. (1997). His master's voice: Acoustic analysis of spontaneous vocalizations in an ongoing active coping task. *Psychophysiology, 34,* S5.

Kappas, A. (2001). A metaphor is a metaphor is a metaphor: Exorcising the homunculus from appraisal theory. In K. R. Scherer, A. Schorr, & T. Johnstone (Eds.), *Appraisal processes in emotion: Theory, methods, research* (pp. 157-172). New York: Oxford University Press.

Kappas, A. (2003). What facial expressions can and cannot tell us about emotions. In M. Katsikitis (Ed.), *The human face: Measurement and meaning* (pp. 215-234). Dordrecht, Netherlands: Kluwer Academic.

Kappas, A., & Hess, U. (1995). Nonverbal aspects of oral communication. In U. M. Quasthoff (Ed.), *Aspects of oral communication* (pp. 169-180). Berlin, Germany: DeGruyter.

Kappas, A., Hess, U., & Scherer, K. R. (1991). Voice and emotion. In R. S. Feldman & B. Rimé (Eds.), *Fundamentals of nonverbal behavior* (pp. 200-238). Cambridge, UK: Cambridge University Press.

Kappas, A., & Pecchinenda, A. (1996). The effect of sociality on event-related facial activity in the context of a video game. *Psychophysiology, 33,* S48.

Kappas, A., & Pecchinenda, A. (1999). Don't wait for the monsters to get you: A video game task to manipulate appraisals in real time. *Cognition and Emotion, 13,* 119-124.

Pecchinenda, A. (2001). The psychophysiology of appraisal. In K. R. Scherer, A. Schorr, & T. Johnstone (Eds.), *Appraisal processes in emotion: Theory, methods, research* (pp. 301–315). New York: Oxford University Press.

Pecchinenda, A., & Kappas, A. (1995). How do you deal with monsters? Relating appraisals to subjective, expressive, and ANS variations. *Psychophysiology, 32,* S59.

Pecchinenda, A., Kappas, A., & Smith, C. A. (1997). Effects of difficulty and ability in a dual-task video game paradigm on attention, physiological responses, performance, and emotion-related appraisal. *Psychophysiology, 34,* S70.

Pell, M. D. (2005). Nonverbal emotion priming: Evidence from the 'Facial Affect Decision Task.' *Journal of Nonverbal Behavior, 29,* 45–73.

Russell, J. A. (1997). Reading emotions from and into faces: Resurrecting a dimensional-contextual perspective. In J. A. Russell & J.

M. Fernández-Dols (Eds.), *The psychology of facial expression* (pp. 295–320). Cambridge, UK: Cambridge University Press.

Scherer, K. R. (1986). Vocal affect expression: A review and a model for future research. *Psychological Bulletin, 99,* 143–165.

van den Stock, J., Righart, R., & de Gelder, B. (2007). Body expressions influence recognition of emotions in the face and voice. *Emotion, 7,* 487–494.

Wallbott, H. G. (1988). In and out of context: Influences of facial expression and context information on emotion attributions. *British Journal of Social Psychology, 27,* 357–369.

Wallbott, H. G., & Scherer, K. R. (1986). Cues and channels in emotion recognition. *Journal of Personality & Social Psychology, 51,* 690–699.

CHAPTER 9

Modification of Emotional Speech and Voice Quality Based on Changes to the Vocal Tract Structure

Brad H. Story

Abstract

Speech production can be represented as the combination of a sound source and an acoustic filter. For vowels and vowel-like sounds, the sound source is the periodic airflow signal generated by the vibration of the vocal folds, whereas the filter is formed by the vocal tract airspace. Although the goal of speech production is to transmit a linguistic message to a listener, the structure and idiosyncratic use of the speech organs impose unique variations on both the source signal and filtering properties (formant frequencies) provided by the vocal tract. These variations create the acoustic characteristics that give rise to the "emotional quality" of the speech. In this chapter, a computational speech production model is used to demonstrate how structural modifications of the vocal tract can generate changes in the quality of the resultant speech. The results suggest that combining this type of modeling with psychoacoustic experiments could eventually provide a powerful means for learning about the emotional load carried in natural speech.

Introduction

The speech signal is a pattern of organized sounds that are transported by rapidly traveling waves to a willing listener. This pattern of sound carries within it the components of a (common) language, coded by the temporal variation of acoustic characteristics that provide cues for a listener's perception of a stream of vowels and consonants. Since speech is generated by both the mind and body of the speaker, information about the speaker's mental and physical state is inevitably transferred to the listener as well. Acoustic characteristics that signal gender, age, physique, dialect, health, and emotional state are often embedded in the speech sound and may unveil, at least in part, a speaker's identity, emotions, and intent. A listener effortlessly decodes the speech sound into a complex aural portrait of the speaker, which consists of the elements of language superimposed on a unique vocal "background" or "setting." Although speakers have precise control over the language component of the spoken message, they generally exercise little conscious control over those paralinguistic qualities that comprise their vocal background, unless conscious steps are taken to conceal or alter them.

The voiced sounds of speech are initiated by the vibration of the vocal folds. These vibrations create a source of oscillating airflow that acoustically encodes information relevant to the vibratory character of the vocal fold tissue. In turn, this flow generates a pressure wave that propagates through the vocal tract airspace formed by the relative positions of the tongue, jaw, lips, and velum, and effectively acquires information about the shape of the airspace that is eventually carried along to a listener's ear. Thus, the final output signal contains acoustic features that reveal information about the generation of the sound at its source as well as the vocal tract structure through which the source sound has traveled. During connected speech, the motor control commands executed by a speaker cause both the vocal folds and the vocal tract to undergo continuous (or nearly so) structural changes enacted by muscle contractions to produce a time-varying signal from which a listener can extract a message.

The human speech production system is similar enough across people that messages of common linguistic content can be easily produced. For a particular speaker, however, the sizes, shapes, and tissue properties of the speech articulators, as well as the speaker's idiosyncratic use of them, will determine the actual acoustic signal that is produced. It is these speaker-specific acoustic properties underlying the linguistic message that form the *quality* or *timbre* of the speech sound.

The aim of this article is to use a model of human speech production to demonstrate how some speech qualities that may be suggestive of emotional loading can be produced by changes to the underlying structure of the vocal tract. The model, which produces a speech signal, is based on a mathematical representation of the mechanics, aerodynamics, and acoustics of the sound source and vocal tract filter.

Model of Sound and Speech Production

Production of vowels and vowel-like sounds can be approximately represented as the combination of a sound *source* and a sound *filter* (e.g., Fant, 1960), where the source signal is the succession of airflow pulses generated by the periodic opening and closing of the space between the vocal folds (i.e., the glottis) as they vibrate. This signal is typically referred to as the *glottal flow*, and the temporal duration of each flow pulse determines the *fundamental frequency* (F_0) of a particular speech sound. In addition to the F_0, the source signal contains frequency components that are harmonically-related (integer multiples) to the F_0.

The primary filter is the airspace comprised of the pharyngeal and oral cavities, and is referred to as the *vocal tract*. Any particular shape of the vocal tract, resulting from the relative positions of the articulators, produces a pattern of acoustic resonances. As the source signal (wave) travels through the vocal tract, the resonances have the effect of enhancing the amplitude of some harmonics while suppressing others. Hence, the output sound results from the interaction of the source with the filter.

A quantitative, computational model of the source-filter representation of speech can be developed by mathematically describing the physical structure of, and the signals produced by, the vocal folds and the vocal tract. A simplified midsagittal picture of the vocal tract is shown in Figure 9-1a, where the articulatory organs and various parts of the airspace are indicated. Shown in Figure 9-1b is a vocal tract shape for a neutral vowel along a curve extending from larynx to lips based on measurements (e.g., Story, Titze, & Hoffman, 1996). For purposes of simplifying the mathematics, this curved airspace can be straightened into the tubular configuration shown in Figure 9-1c, where the horizontal axis indicates the distance (in cm) from the glottis

(vocal folds). Computational propagation of sound waves through this structure can be accomplished with a digital waveguide algorithm (e.g., Kelly & Lochbaum, 1962; Liljencrants, 1985; specifically for this study Story, 1995). Because the goal of this article is to demonstrate the effect of vocal tract modifications, the details of modeling the source will not be presented; however, source signals generated by such a model will be used and assumed to serve as a sufficient input to a given vocal tract shape.

The source-filter representation is illustrated graphically in Figure 9-2 with signals generated by the speech production model. Two flow pulses (cycles) of the glottal airflow signal are plotted in Figure 9-2a; for this example, they are repeated every 10 milliseconds, which is equivalent to a frequency of 100 Hz. This signal would effectively enter the tubular configuration of the vocal tract in Figure 9-2b at the point labeled "vocal folds." The flow pulses generate sound pressure waves that propagate through the tube, reflecting at each change in cross-sectional area. The pressure that is finally generated at the lip end of the vocal tract radiates outward, away from the speaker (to a listener). An output pressure waveform is shown in Figure 9-2c and is analogous to that produced by a microphone held near a speaker's lips.

The second row of plots in Figure 9-2 demonstrate the spectral (frequency and amplitude) characteristics of the source signal, the vocal tract, and the output sound pressure signal, respectively, from left to right. The fundamental frequency (F_0) of the glottal flow (source) is indicated by the first peak in the glottal flow spectrum (Figure 9-2c) and, as stated previously, is 100 Hz in this case. The peaks that occur successively, as frequency increases, are the "harmonics" of

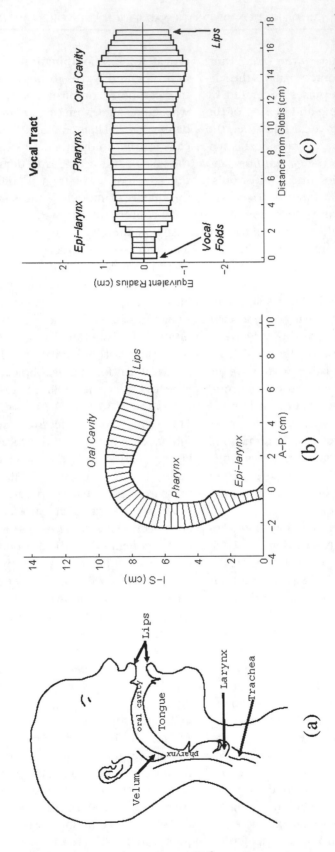

Figure 9–1. Transformation of the vocal tract from a midsagittal view to a tubular configuration. **(a)** Idealized midsagittal view of a neutral vowel, **(b)** vocal tract shape for a neutral vowel along a curve extending from larynx to lips based on measuements (e.g., Story, Titze, & Hoffman, 1996), and **(c)** tubular approximation of the neutral vowel.

126

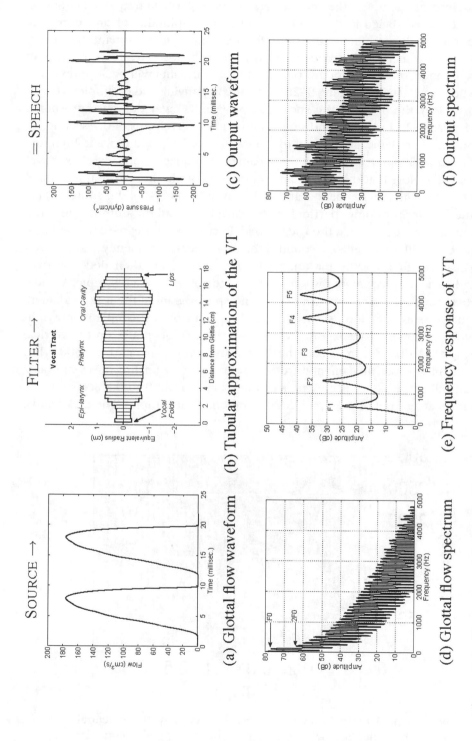

Figure 9–2. Illustration of the source-filter representation of speech. The upper row contains plots of the **(a)** glottal waveform, **(b)** tubular approximation to the vocal tract, and **(c)** the output waveform. The lower row shows the frequency-domain versions of each plot in the upper row: **(d)** glottal flow spectrum, **(e)** frequency response of the vocal tract, and **(f)** output spectrum.

127

the glottal flow signal and are related to the F_0 by integer multiples; the second harmonic ($2F_0$) is labeled in the figure. The amplitude of the harmonics tends to decrease with an increase in frequency.

The resonance frequencies of this particular vocal tract shape (Figure 9–2b) are indicated by the peaks in the spectrum of Figure 9–2e. In speech and singing, these peaks are typically referred to as the *formant frequencies*, hence the labels of F1–F5. Note that this spectrum does not represent the frequency and amplitude content of any particular sound, but rather the *effect* that the vocal tract shape would have on *any* sound that travels through it. For this reason, it is referred to as the *frequency response* of the vocal tract filter. The spectrum of the output pressure waveform shown in Figure 9–2e contains characteristics of both the glottal flow (source) and the vocal tract (filter). The fundamental frequency and all of the harmonics are present in this spectrum, but their amplitudes

have been modified by the vocal tract resonances (formant frequencies). Specifically, the amplitudes of any harmonic frequencies near a formant frequency will be enhanced, while those distant from the formants will be suppressed.

Accompanying audio samples s1.wav, s2.wav, and s3.wav demonstrate source and output waveforms of 0.7 seconds in duration, for low, medium, and high fundamental frequency source signals (male) combined with the vocal tract shape shown in Figure 9–2b; the source signal is played first and the output signal second. To create some degree of naturalness, the fundamental frequency was allowed to increase slightly then decrease over the time course of each sample. A wideband spectrogram of the low fundamental frequency output sample is shown in Figure 9–3. Frequency is on the vertical axis and ranges from 0 to 3000 Hz, whereas time is on the horizontal axis and extends from 0 to 0.7 seconds (the duration of the sample). The dark bands,

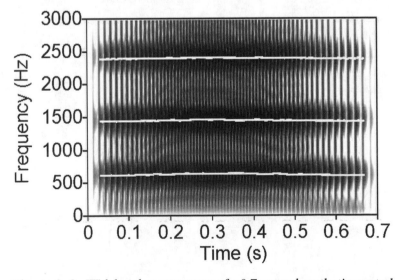

Figure 9–3. Wideband spectrogram of a 0.7 second synthetic neutral vowel. The white lines track the center of each formant frequency band.

whose centers are marked with white lines, indicate the formant frequencies and are the same as the F1, F2, and F3 peaks shown previously in Figure 9–2e. Because the vocal tract shape remained unchanged over the duration of this sample, the formant bands also remain unchanged.

Connected speech is produced by continuous variation of the voice source and the vocal tract shape, which is acousti-cally equivalent to a variation of the source spectrum and the frequency response (formant frequencies) of the vocal tract. As an example, a time-dependent variation of the vocal tract shape was generated by superimposing movement on the neutral vowel configuration (Story, 2005) shown in Figures 9–1 and 9–2, and used to create the audio samples discussed previously. The resulting time-varying vocal tract is depicted in Figure 9–4a.

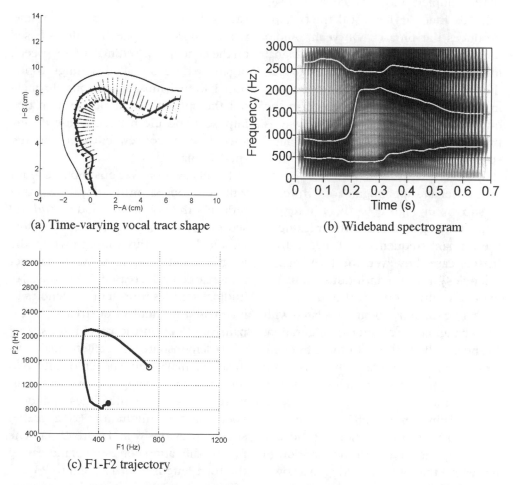

(a) Time-varying vocal tract shape

(b) Wideband spectrogram

(c) F1-F2 trajectory

Figure 9–4. Vocal tract and acoustic characteristics for the (synthesized) phrase "Oh yeah." **(a)** Time-dependent vocal tract shape changes; the solid and dashed lines are the starting and ending configurations, respectively, whereas the dotted lines are intermediate configurations. **(b)** Wideband spectrogram of the synthetic "Oh yeah" produced by the time-dependent vocal tract of (a). **(c)** F1-F2 vowel space trajectory for "Oh yeah."

To maintain continuity with anatomical landmarks it has been plotted in an idealized midsagittal form like that shown previously in Figure 9–1b. The outer profile of the tract is assumed to remain stationary, whereas the multiple inner profiles show the changing shape. The heavy solid line is the starting configuration, the heavy dashed line is the terminal configuration, and all of the light dotted lines represent configurations that exist during the time course of the utterance. When coupled with a voice source signal, this time-varying vocal tract shape produces the phrase, "Oh yeah." Audio sample s4.wav contains the source signal followed by the output signal; note that the source signal is identical to the one in s2.wav; hence, the difference in the output signals of s2.wav and s4.wav is produced entirely by the shape changes superimposed on the neutral vocal tract shape.

A wideband spectrogram of "Oh yeah" is shown in Figure 9–4b, where the white lines again indicate the tracking of the formant frequencies F1, F2, and F3. In this case, however, the formant frequencies almost continuously change over the duration of the utterance, reflecting the movement associated with the changing vocal tract configuration. In speech, the first two formant frequencies (F1 and F2) are usually considered to be of primary importance for vowel identification (e.g., Peterson & Barney, 1952). Thus, for vowel-like utterances, the acoustic representation can be simplified by plotting the time-variation of F2 against that of F1, resulting in a vowel space trajectory.

Such a trajectory is shown in Figure 9–4c for the "Oh yeah" phrase. The solid and open circles signify the F1 and F2 frequencies at the beginning and end of the phrase, respectively (i.e., at the left and right sides of the spectrogram in Figure 9–4b). The solid curved line connecting these points passes through the F1 and F2 frequencies that occur during the production of the phrase.

Modification of Quality

Laver (1980) outlined a convenient framework to describe speech qualities based on the concept of "settings" of the speech organs. These so-called settings represent habitual muscle tensions throughout the speech production system that impose a specific pattern of use during speech and consequently a specific speech quality.[1]

In this section, various modifications will be imposed on the vocal tract that reflect both *longitudinal* and *latitudinal* settings. According to Laver (1980), longitudinal settings are those in which the length of some, or all, of the vocal tract is increased or decreased. In contrast, latitudinal settings represent tendencies to maintain a particular constrictive or expansive effect on the vocal tract shape.

To demonstrate how longitudinal modifications may affect speech quality, two relatively large changes in overall length were imposed on the time-dependent vocal tract configuration ("Oh yeah") shown previously in Figure 9–4a. The first modification consisted of increasing the tract length from 17.5 cm to 23 cm, effectively simulating a very large person. The tract shape variation that will produce the phrase "Oh yeah" in the length-

---

[1]Laver (1980) referred to these as voice rather than speech qualities. But to avoid confusion with qualities attributed to the vocal folds and their vibratory characteristics, the term *speech quality* will be used here.

ened condition is shown in Figure 9–5a, whereas the corresponding F1-F2 trajectory is shown below this plot in Figure 9–5c. Note that increase in length causes the trajectory to be shifted downward and to the left, relative to that shown for the initial configuration in Figure 9–4c. The shape of the trajectory, however, is the same as in the initial case.

In the second modification, the overall vocal tract length was reduced from 17.5 cm to 11 cm. This length is roughly representative of a 5- to 8-year-old child (Fitch & Giedd, 1999). The tract variation and F1-F2 trajectories are shown in Figure 9–5b and Figure 9–5d, respectively. The effect of the length reduction is to increase both F1 and F2 over the course

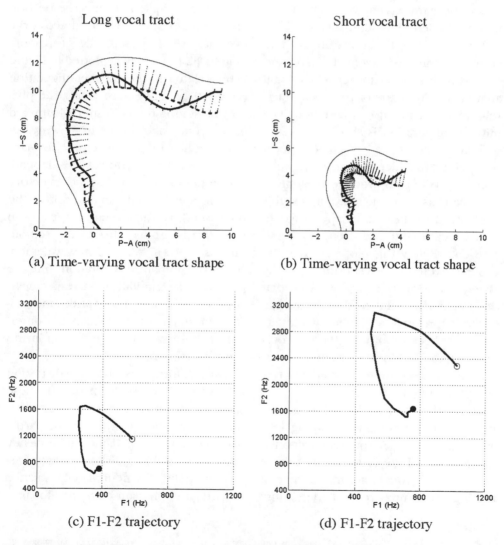

Long vocal tract   Short vocal tract

(a) Time-varying vocal tract shape   (b) Time-varying vocal tract shape

(c) F1-F2 trajectory   (d) F1-F2 trajectory

Figure 9–5. Effect of uniform vocal tract length changes on the F1-F2 trajectory of "Oh yeah." **(a)** Time-dependent vocal tract shape scaled to have a length of 23 cm. **(b)** Same as (a), but with vocal tract length scaled to 11 cm. **(c)** F1-F2 trajectory for lengthened tract. **(d)** F1-F2 trajectory for shortened tract.

of the entire trajectory; however, because the length change was uniformly distributed over the entire vocal tract, the shape of trajectory is essentially the same as in Figure 9–4c and Figure 9–5c. Audio samples s5.wav and s6.wav demonstrate the lengthened and shortened vocal tracts, respectively. The source signal in each of these samples is identical to that used to produce s4.wav (the initial configuration) so that all of the audible differences across these three samples can be attributed to the length modifications.

Latitudinal modifications are demonstrated by imposing constrictive and expansive biases on the cross-sectional area in specific parts of the vocal tract, relative to an initial configuration. The initial configuration is shown in Figure 9–6a and consists of a 19.8 cm long vocal tract with a time-dependent shape variation that will again produce the phrase "Oh yeah," as in previous examples (this is identical to the tract shape in Figure 9–4a except that the tract length is set to 19.8 cm). Below this plot is shown the F1-F2 trajectory corresponding to the change in vocal tract shape. Note that this trajectory is shifted downward and to the left, relative to that shown in Figure 9–4c, because of the 19.8 cm vocal tract length used for this example.

One of the settings described by Laver (1980) is a tendency to constrict the pharyngeal portion of the vocal tract relative to the other parts, resulting in a pharyngealized speech quality. As reported by Story and Titze (2002), this can be imposed on a vocal tract model by first altering the neutral tract shape (Figure 9–1b and Figure 9–1c, but with a length of 19.8 cm) such that the cross-sectional areas in the pharyngeal part were reduced slightly and those in the oral cavity increased. The same time-dependent shape changes used in the previous examples were then superimposed on the modified neutral shape, resulting in a modified version of the "Oh yeah" phrase. The time-dependent, and pharyngealized, vocal tract shape is shown in Figure 9–6b. The dotted ellipse indicates the portion of the vocal tract in which the constrictive bias was imposed. The corresponding F1-F2 trajectory is plotted in Figure 9–6e. Relative to the initial configuration (Figure 9–6a and Figure 9–6d), the pharyngeal setting tends to shift F1 upward in frequency and moves F2 downward. The amount by which either formant frequency is shifted, however, is dependent on the location within the trajectory (i.e., the specific point in time within the phrase). Thus, the overall shape of the trajectory is also modified by this setting. Audio samples s7.wav and s8.wav demonstrate the initial configuration and the pharyngealized modification, respectively. For no reason other than variety, the variation in fundamental frequency is different in these samples than it was in the previous examples.

Though formal psychoacoustic testing has not yet been performed with these samples, informal listening suggests that pharyngealization, along with the particular voice quality (fundamental frequency contour and glottal airflow characteristics), may shift the neutral vocal valance toward an unpleasant emotional load.[2]

---

[2]It is noted that Laver (1980) did not attach any emotional qualities to the pharyngealized or palatalized settings. Future psychoacoustic testing is necessary to formally determine whether such settings do carry an emotional load and what their valance might be. In addition, the emotional load and valance will undoubtedly be strongly related to the parameters of the voice (source) used to create the speech samples.

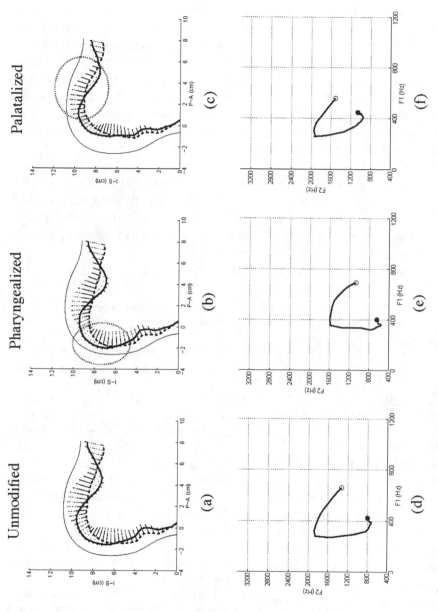

Figure 9–6. Effect of pharyngealization and palatalization on the vocal tract shape. **(a)** Same as the time-dependent vocal tract of Figure 9–4a, but with the length scaled to 19.8 cm. **(b)** Time-dependent vocal tract with pharyngeal constrictive bias (indicated with the dotted ellipse). **(c)** Time-dependent vocal tract with palatal constrictive bias (indicated with the dotted ellipse). **(d–e)** F1-F2 trajectories corresponding to the tract shape changes in (a–c).

133

A second latitudinal setting is a constrictive tendency in the palatal region of the vocal tract (Laver, 1980), and produces a *palatalized* quality. This type of setting was imposed on the model in the same manner as the pharyngealized setting, except that the cross-sectional areas within the oral cavity were slightly reduced while those in the pharynx were increased. The tract variations and F1-F2 trajectory are plotted in Figure 9–6c and Figure 9–6f, respectively. This setting has the effect of slightly decreasing F1 and increasing F2. But, as observed for the pharyngeal quality, the amount by which either formant is shifted depends on location within the trajectory, and results in a change in the shape of the F1-F2 trajectory. This quality is demonstrated in audio sample s9.wav. An informal listening evaluation of this particular palatalized quality suggests that it may be associated with a negative, if not sarcastic, vocal emotion.

Summary

Speech production can be represented as the combination of a sound source and an acoustic filter. For vowels and vowel-like sounds, the sound source is the periodic airflow signal generated by the vibration of the vocal folds, whereas the filter is formed by the vocal tract airspace. Although the goal of speech production is to transmit a linguistic message to a listener, the structure and idiosyncratic use of the speech organs impose unique variations on both the source signal and filtering properties (formant frequencies) provided by the vocal tract. These variations create the acoustic characteristics that give rise to the emotional quality of the speech, providing information about the speaker that may or may not be part of the intended message. A computational speech production model was used to demonstrate how structural modifications of the vocal tract can generate changes in the quality of the resultant speech. The results suggest that combining this type of modeling with psychoacoustic experiments could eventually provide a powerful means for learning about the emotional load carried in natural speech.

Acknowledgements. This work was supported in part by grant number R01 DC04789 from the National Institute on Deafness and Other Communication Disorders (NIDCD).

References

Fant, G. (1960). *The acoustic theory of speech production.* The Hague, Netherlands: Mouton.

Fitch, W. T., and Giedd, J. (1999). Morphology and development of the human vocal tract: A study using magnetic resonance imaging. *Journal of the Acoustical Society of America, 106,* 1511–1522.

Kelly, J., & Lochbaum, C. (1962). Speech synthesis. In (Ed.), *Proceedings of the 4th International Congress on Acoustics* (Vol. 1, pp. 1–4).

Laver, J. (1980). *The phonetic description of voice quality.* Cambridge, UK: Cambridge University Press.

Liljencrants, J. (1985). *Speech synthesis with a reflection-type line analog.* Unpublished doctoral dissertation, Royal Institute of Technology, Stockholm, Sweden.

Peterson, G. E., & Barney, H. L. (1952). Control methods used in a study of the vowels. *Journal of the Acoustical Society of America, 24*(2), 175–184.

Story, B. H. (1995) *Speech simulation with an enhanced wave-reflection model of the vocal tract*. Unpublished doctoral dissertation, University of Iowa, Iowa City.

Story, B. H. (2005). A parametric model of the vocal tract area function for vowel and consonant simulation. *Journal of the Acoustical Society of America*, *117*(5), 3231-3254.

Story, B. H., & Titze, I. R. (2002). A preliminary study of voice quality transformation based on modifications to the neutral vocal tract area function. *Journal of Phonetics*, *30*, 485-509.

Story, B. H., Titze, I. R., & Hoffman, E. A. (1996). Vocal tract area functions from magnetic resonance imaging. *Journal of the Acoustical Society of America*, *100*(1), 537-554.

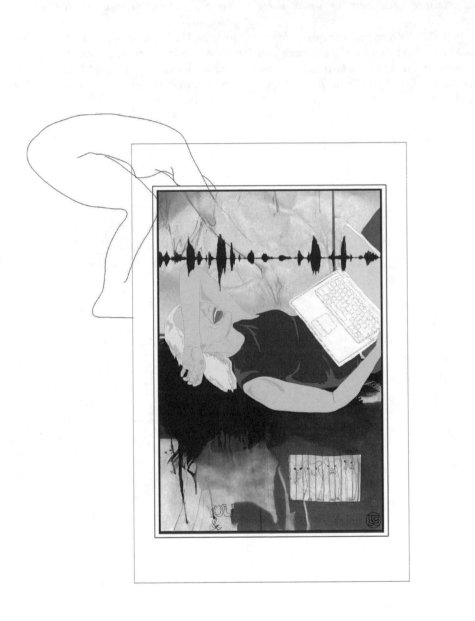

CHAPTER 10

Perception of Emotions Expressed via Speech and Nonlinguistic Vocalizations

Shirley Fecteau and Pascal Belin

Introduction

Vocal emotions have two main ways of expression, through nonlinguistic vocalizations and through speech prosody. Although emotional processing constitutes one of the most important research themes in neurosciences and psychology, only a few studies have explored the processing of emotional nonlinguistic vocalizations. The scientific community has shown greater interest in studying emotional processing through speech and facial expressions. However, much like speech, nonlinguistic vocalizations such as laughs or sighs represent an important source of information about the speaker, especially regarding his or her emotional state (for review, see Kreiman, 1997). The goal of this chapter is to sum-

marize the most relevant studies on perception of emotions expressed vocally. First a brief discussion on emotional prosody is presented, and then the main behavioral and neuroimaging studies on processing vocal emotions are summarized. We also discuss the differential contribution of the right and left hemispheres in vocal emotion processing, and we conclude with a short discussion of the importance of studying nonlinguistic vocalizations.

Emotional Prosody

Speech prosody is important for processing emotions (e.g., Monrad-Krohn, 1963; Joanette, Goulet, & Hannequin, 1990). However, prosodic stimuli carry emotional as well as linguistic informa-tion. Therefore, the language of speakers and decoders influences the production and the perception of emotions via prosodic stimuli. The effect of language on perception of emotional prosody is even observed in newborns before they talk. Indeed, newborns show differential responses, such as eye opening, to pres-entation of emotional prosody from maternal speech compared to a novel language (Mastropieri & Turkewitz, 1999). Syntactic structure is one of the linguis-tic components that may influence emo-tional processing of prosodic stimuli as direct interactions between prosodic and syntactic patterns have been shown (Steinhauer, Alter, & Friederici, 1999; Strelnikov, Vorobyev, Chernigovskaya, & Medvedev, 2005). Another influence stems from the fact that prosody is not the only source that can express emo-tions; the semantics can also carry an emotional load. The emotional informa-tion expressed by semantics can thus influence the emotion expressed by prosody and various methodological strategies have been developed in order to limit semantic influences. For instance, researchers have presented linguistic stimuli in which the semantics have no clear emotional load, such as numbers (Pfaff, 1954), weekdays (Osser, 1964), as well as letters of the alphabet (Dusen-bury & Knower, 1938; Wolf, Gorski, & Peters, 1972), produced with different emotional prosodic patterns. Another strategy is to manipulate stimuli acousti-cally to mask the intelligibility of the semantic content, such as using acoustic filters (Lakshminarayanan et al., 2003) and temporal inversion (Scott, Blank, Rosen, & Wise, 2000; Lakshminarayanan et al., 2003). However, most of these methods modify not only the semantics, but also the emotional prosodic patterns, result-ing in nonnatural vocal emotions.

The production of emotional prosodic patterns is also in part determined by cultural norms (Albas, McCluskey, & Albas, 1976; Mesquita, Frijda, & Scherer, 1997). Although recognition of vocal emotion is cross-culturally reliable, dif-ferences between cultures have been observed (Albas et al., 1976; Elfenbein & Ambady, 2002; Juslin & Laukka, 2003). In order to diminish the reference effect of language and culture, speechlike but semantically meaningless sentences have been developed by Scherer, Banse, and Wallbott (2001). These sentences have been built from several phonological and phonetic systems of Indo-European languages. However, a language/cultural effect was found when participants were performing a recognition task of emo-tional prosody. According to the authors, the segmental and suprasegmental infor-mation used by the decoders varies with the language and culture, even with these speechlike but semantically meaningless stimuli. Further studies are needed to better understand cultural influences on vocal emotion processing (prosody as well as nonlinguistic vocalizations); the influence of culture has been mainly studied using facial expressions (e.g., Elfenbein & Ambady, 2002).

Main Results on Perception of Vocal Emotion

Behavioral Studies

Our ability to perceive emotions expressed by prosody is good (see Russell, 2003 for a review; e.g., Scherer, 1981a,b; Banse & Scherer, 1996; Laukka, 2005), whether the stimuli are natural or acoustically manipulated (Johnson, Emde, Scherer, & Klinnert, 1986; Lakshminarayanan et al., 2003). Negative emotions seem to be better recognized than positive emotions during emotional categorization (Wallbott & Scherer, 1986) and judgment of emotional dimensions (Scherer et al., 2001). Age differences in processing emotional prosody have also been reported: older adults identified and discriminated emotions less accurately through prosodic information (Allen & Brosgole, 1993; Kiss & Ennis, 2001) and showed a decline in intensity ratings compared to younger adults (Thompson, Aidinejad, & Ponte, 2001). Sex differences in emotional prosody processing are discussed in Chapter 5 of the present volume by Annett Schirmer and Elizabeth Simpson. We do not know much about how we perceive emotional nonlinguistic vocalizations. Fecteau, Armony, Joanette, and Belin (2005a) found that judgment of emotional valence (i.e., whether the emotion expressed is positive, negative, or neutral) was consistent across participants. We also reported that younger adults rated vocalizations as more emotional than older individuals (higher valence for positive, lower for negative, and more intense for both positive and negative). These results are in line with age-related differences reported for emotional processing through prosody (e.g., Kiss & Ennis, 2001; Thompson et al., 2001) and facial expressions (e.g., Phillips, MacLean, & Allen, 2002). We also reported that the emotional load can influence episodic memory. Healthy participants showed a superior memory for emotional nonlinguistic vocalizations regardless of the valence (positive and negative emotions), compared to the neutral ones (Armony, Chochol, Fecteau, & Belin, in press).

Neuroimaging Studies

Vocal emotion processing elicits enhanced activity in several brain regions (see reviews by Adolphs, 2002; Phan, Wager, Taylor, & Liberzon, 2002; Russell, 2003; Schirmer & Kotz, 2005; see also a review on the neural substrates of voice perception by Belin, Fecteau, & Bédard, 2004). Among these regions, activations have been especially reported in the temporal and frontal cortices.

Temporal Regions

Enhanced activity in the superior temporal gyrus bilaterally has been observed during processing of emotional prosody (Kawashima et al., 1993; Buchanan et al., 2000; Wildgruber, Pihan, Ackermann, Erb, & Grodd, 2002; Mitchell, Elliott, Barry, Cruttenden, & Woodruff, 2003; Ethofer et al., 2005), as well as emotional nonlinguistic vocalizations (Phillips et al., 1998; Fecteau, Belin, Joanette, & Armony, 2007; Meyer, Zysset, von Cramon, & Alter, 2005). The superior temporal sulci also seem to be involved in emotional processing through prosody (Kotz et al., 2003; Grandjean et al., 2005) and vocalizations (Fecteau et al., 2007). This is consistent with a role of these regions in the analysis of the acoustic properties of the stimuli, which differs between emotionally loaded and neutral stimuli.

Frontal Regions

The frontal cortex has also been shown to be involved in emotional prosody processing, especially the inferior frontal cortex (Kawashima et al., 1993; Imaizumi et al., 1997; Buchanan et al., 2000; Mitchell et al., 2003; Wildgruber et al., 2004; 2005; Ethofer et al., 2005; see also a recent study using transcranial magnetic stimulation showing the involvement of the right fronto-parietal operculum in detection of emotional prosodic patterns by van Rijn et al., 2005). Emotional vocalizations elicited greater activity in the frontal cortex, such as the medial frontal cortex (Phillips et al., 1998), superior frontal gyrus (Morris, Scott, & Dolan, 1999) and the inferior frontal gyrus (Fecteau, Armony, Joanette, & Belin, 2005b; Meyer et al., 2005), when compared to various vocal sounds and silence.

Amygdala

The involvement of the amygdala in emotion processing is well documented (see review by Adolphs, 2002; Phelps & LeDoux, 2005). However, most studies of emotional prosody have failed to observe changes in amygdala activity (Imaizumi et al., 1997; Royet et al., 2000; Pourtois, de Gelder, Bol, & Crommelinck, 2005; see also the meta-analysis from Phan et al., 2002; but see Sander et al., 2005). With regards to emotional nonlinguistic vocalizations, conflicting results have been reported. Some studies found activations in the amygdala in response to emotional vocalizations (Phillips et al., 1998; Sander & Scheich, 2001; Fecteau et al., 2007 (see Figure 10-1), whereas others found no significant changes in activity (Morris et al., 1999; Meyer et al., 2005), and one study reported a decrease of activity for vocalizations of fear (Morris et al., 1999). The possible reasons of these conflicting results are discussed in Fecteau et al. (2007). Briefly, the lack of consistency of the amygdala responses to emotional vocalizations may be in part due to a neural saturation. The amygdala appears to be sensitive to habituation when the same emotional category is continuously

presented (Breiter et al., 1996) and most studies used block designs in which a given emotional category was presented for 30 to 60 s (Phillips et al., 1998; Morris et al., 1999; Sander & Scheich, 2001). Another important factor that presumably contributes to inconsistent results is that studies compared emotional vocalizations with various control stimuli, such as mildly happy vocalizations (Phillips et al., 1998), voiced nasal sounds (Morris et al., 1999), silence (Sander & Scheich, 2001), speech and nonvocal sounds (Meyer et al., 2005), and emotionally neutral vocalizations (Fecteau et al., 2007).

Differential Contribution of the Right and Left Hemisphere in Vocal Emotion Processing

Researchers have shown great interest in exploring the differential contribution of the right and left hemisphere in perception of emotional prosody and several hypotheses have been proposed (see review by Schirmer and Kotz, 2005).

The Right Hemisphere Dominance Hypothesis

Traditionally, processing emotional prosody has been attributed to activity in the right hemisphere, regardless of emotional valence (Joanette et al., 1990; Roland, 1993; Baum & Pell, 1999; Pihan, Altenmuller, Hertrich, & Ackermann, 2000). This hypothesis mainly came from studies in patients with unilateral brain damage to the right hemisphere (e.g., Heilman, Scholes, & Watson, 1975; Starkstein, Federoff, Price, Leiguarda, & Robinson, 1994; Ross, Thompson, & Yenkosky,

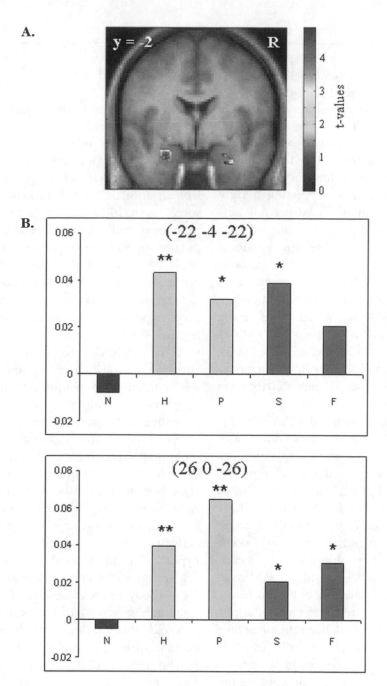

Figure 10–1. (**A**) Statistical parametric map, thresholded at p = 0.01 for visualization purposes, showing the bilateral amygdala activations for the contrast of emotional vs. neutral vocalizations. (**B**) Parameter estimates for each stimulus category are shown for the peaks in the left (*top*) and right (*bottom*) amygdala. Symbols indicate the level of significance associated with the paired t-test between each emotional category and the neutral vocalizations: **p <0.005 and *p <0.05. N: Neutral vocalizations; H: vocalizations of happiness; P: vocalizations of sexual pleasure; S: vocalizations of sadness; F: fearful screams. (Reproduced with permission from *Neuroimage*, *36*, Fecteau, S., Belin, P., Joanette, Y., & Armony, J. L., Bilateral amygdala activation for negative as well as positive emotional nonlinguistic vocalizations, 480–487, Copyright Elsevier [2007]).

1997; Schmitt, Hartje, & Willmes, 1997; Borod et al., 1998). In healthy subjects, behavioral studies of dichotic listening of prosodic stimuli (e.g., Schmitt et al., 1997) and nonlinguistic vocalizations (Carmon & Nachshon, 1973) have shown a left ear advantage for processing emotional stimuli, thus suggesting a right hemisphere dominance. Also, some neuroimaging studies in healthy subjects supported the right hemispheric dominance in processing emotional prosody (Kawashima et al., 1993; George et al., 1996; Buchanan et al., 2000; Kotz, Alter, Besson, Friederici, & Schirmer, 2000; Pihan et al., 2000; Rama et al., 2001; Wildgruber et al., 2002; Mitchell et al., 2003), as well as emotional nonlinguistic vocalizations (Sander & Scheich, 2001; Meyer et al., 2005).

However, some results did not support the right hemispheric dominance hypothesis in processing vocal emotions. Some studies reported bilateral responses to emotional prosody, and even stronger activations in the left hemisphere have been observed (e.g., Kotz et al., 2003). Moreover, the right hemispheric dominance hypothesis has not been clearly established in lesion studies. Although some patients with difficulties in identifying and discriminating emotional prosodic patterns predominantly presented lesions to the right hemisphere (Starkstein et al., 1994), deficits in perception of emotional prosody following lesions to the left hemisphere have also been reported (e.g., Cancelliere & Kertesz, 1990; van Lancker & Sidtis, 1992; Pell & Baum, 1997). Some studies with patients with left-hemisphere infarcts have even suggested a left hemispheric dominance in perception of emotional prosody (e.g., Pell, 1998).

Valence Hypothesis

The valence hypothesis suggests a left hemispheric dominance for processing positive emotions and a right hemispheric dominance for processing negative emotions (e.g., Sackeim et al., 1982; Ross, Homan, & Buck, 1994; Pell, 1998; Davidson & Irwin, 1999). However, some neuroimaging studies of emotional prosody did not support this hypothesis (George et al., 1996; Buchanan et al., 2000; Wildgruber et al., 2002; Kotz et al., 2003).

Some studies have supported both of these hypotheses according to the brain regions studied. For instance, findings from Sander, Roth, and Scheich (2003), studying neural substrates associated with perception of prosodic patterns of happiness and sadness, supported both hypotheses. Activations for emotional stimuli (versus vowel detection) in a temporo-parietal region of interest, although bilateral, were greater in the right hemisphere, thus supporting the right hemispheric dominance hypothesis. The authors also reported lateralized activations in support of the valence hypothesis in an occipital region of interest: stronger activations were observed for prosody expressing sadness in the right hemisphere than in the left one, whereas stimuli depicting happiness elicited greater responses in this region in the left hemisphere than in the right one.

Hypothesis of the Type of Emotion

Another hypothesis suggests that brain activations for primary emotions (e.g., happiness, sadness) are lateralized to the right hemisphere, whereas social emotions (e.g., culpability, shyness, envy) are lateralized to the left hemisphere (Ross et al., 1994). The study of social emotions is relatively recent and this hypothesis needs further investigation (for more details on social emotions, see Eisenberg, 2000).

Lateralization in Function of the Acoustic Parameters

Alternatively, it has been suggested that lateralization of prosody processing varies with the acoustic parameters. Most studies conceptualize emotional prosody as being a distinct entity instead of a manipulation of prosodic parameters to express an emotion. Processing a vocal emotion entails an acoustic analysis (Ethofer et al., 2005); and processing acoustic properties appears to involve lateralized brain areas (Zatorre & Belin, 2001; Boemio, Fromm, Braun, & Poeppel, 2005; Ethofer et al., 2005). According to a model proposed by van Lancker and Sidtis (1992), the left and right hemispheres are responsible for processing different aspects of emotional prosody. The right hemisphere is superior to the left one with regards to the extraction of fundamental frequency (F_0) information, whereas the left hemisphere is more involved in the extraction of temporal information. For instance, perception of the F_0 has been shown to involve the right hemisphere (e.g., Zatorre, Evans, Meyer, & Gjedde, 1992; Zatorre & Belin, 2001; Zatorre, Belin, & Penhune, 2002; but see Wildgruber et al., 2002), whereas the left hemisphere has been involved in temporal cues processing (e.g., Carmon & Nachshon, 1973; Zatorre et al., 1992;

Belin et al., 1998; Zatorre et al., 2002). Moreover, hemispheric differences have been reported according to the processed feature. For instance, in Ladd (1996) the lateral temporal lobe of the right hemisphere processed tonal direction, but not tonal range or height. Also, the right hemisphere has shown superiority in processing lower frequencies, such as the F_0, compared to higher frequencies (Ivry & Lebby, 1993, but see Wolf, 1977). However, in an elegant study from Wildgruber et al. (2002), superiority of the right hemisphere was observed during processing emotional prosody that was not explained by the acoustic structures of the F_0, nor the duration.

Some prosodic cues used to perceive emotional states are relatively specific and stable; for example, longer syllable length is strongly associated with prosody expressing sadness (e.g., Cosmides, 1983; Wallbott & Scherer, 1986; Banse & Scherer, 1996; Wildgruber et al., 2002). Moreover, relations between physiological changes underlying emotional states and changes in acoustic parameters have been reported (Scherer, 1986). Therefore, superiority of the right or the left hemisphere in emotional processing may be due in part to the fact that some acoustic cues play a greater role in the perception of a given emotion. This suggests that some cues and/or some aspects of these acoustic cues are processed in a lateralized fashion.

Several levels of processing are involved in the perception of vocal emotions and each of them modulates brain activity and can contribute to lateralized activity. For instance, attention modulates early acoustic processing (Rinne et al., 2005) as well as vocal emotional processing (Schirmer, Kotz, & Friederici,

2005; Sander et al., 2005), and attentional modulation seems to elicit greater activity in the right auditory cortex than the left one (e.g., Pugh et al., 1996). The type of task also presumably elicits differential patterns of brain activity. For instance, Peper and Irle (1997) showed that frontal regions are involved in decoding the emotional valence of prosodic stimuli, the dorsolateral, parietal, and temporal regions in categorization and matching tasks, whereas decoding arousal seems to involve all of these regions within the right hemisphere. Moreover, increases in cognitive demands when tasks require complex processes have been correlated with enhanced activity in the left hemisphere (frontal and temporal) in healthy subjects (e.g., Kotz et al., 2000; Pihan et al., 2000), as well as in patients with brain lesions (Tompkins & Flowers, 1985). Another important factor is that semantic information influences brain responses and greater activations have been observed in the left hemisphere (Vikingstad, George, Johnson, & Cao, 2000). Indeed, differential patterns of activation for prosodic stimuli with regards to availability of semantic content have been reported. Positive and negative emotions expressed through prosody when semantic information was not available (using acoustic filters) elicited enhanced activity in the inferior frontal gyrus, whereas activations in these regions when semantic content was available were observed only for positive emotions (Kotz et al., 2003). Neuroimaging techniques with better temporal resolution, such as event-related potentials, may describe differences between neural activity underlying emotional processing of prosodic and semantic information by distinguishing temporal patterns (e.g., Schirmer et al.,

2005). Linguistic prosody (i.e., modulation of acoustic parameters to communicate the phrasing and accentuation of words or sentences) is yet another candidate that influences neural activity associated with emotional prosody processing (as discussed by Ross et al., 1997; Pell, 1998; Baum & Pell, 1999). Weintraub, Mesulam, and Kramer (1981) and Brådvik et al. (1991) have even suggested that solely linguistic prosody is processed in the right hemisphere (studies from unilateral lesion to the right hemisphere). It is thus essential to carefully isolate these two types of prosody in order to study brain regions involved in processing emotional prosody.

Another important factor to consider in vocal emotion processing is that emotional stimuli can easily induce an emotional state, especially when a block design is used or when duration of the stimuli is long. In such cases, significant changes in gestures, facial expressions, and other physiological cues, such as arterial pressure and body temperature, are observed. Most studies of vocal emotions did not use electrophysiological measurements or questionnaires assessing the arousal of participants, and thus it is difficult to differentiate neural activity related to the perception of the stimuli from that related to mood induction effects. It may also be important to include different cognitive processes within a same study. For instance, it seems that the identification of the emotion and hedonic judgment are sometimes in *opposition*. In Wallbott and Scherer (1986), even if participants correctly identified sadness in prosodic stimuli, they judged these stimuli as being pleasant. These dichotomies remain to be explored by behavioral, electrophysiological, and neuroimaging studies.

Future studies need also to explore the distinction between emotion recognition and emotion understanding. It has been suggested that the mirror neuron system is one of the essential mechanisms involved in how humans understand emotions. According to this hypothesis, we understand emotions as we understand any other actions (e.g., Gallese, Keysers, & Rizzolatti, 2004). Specifically, it is hypothesized that we understand a given emotion expressed by a peer because part of the neural network that represents that given emotion is activated. For instance, the observation of a face expressing fear may engage part of the amygdala (Carr, Iacoboni, Dubeau, Mazziotta, & Lenzi, 2003), whereas observation of a face expressing disgust may recruit part of the insula (Wicker et al., 2003), in conjunction with the classical mirror neuron system neural networks, which include the rostral part of the inferior parietal lobe and the pars opercularis of the inferior frontal gyrus (Broca's area) (for more details see Rizzolatti, Fogassi, & Gallese, 2001). As far as we know, no studies have explored the mirror neuron system using vocal emotions; neuroimaging studies are needed to characterize the possible contribution of this mirror system in vocal emotion processing. (Editor: in agreement February 2006, but for a more popular discussion of valence, feelings, emotions and specific neuronal cells responses to selective visual (sic!) stimuli. See Scientific American: Mind, February/March 2006).

In summary, despite the distributed nature of the perceptual processing of vocal emotions, the right hemisphere, in particular the inferior frontal regions, seems to be a critical component of the system, which appears to work in collaboration with more posterior regions of the right hemisphere (such as the medial temporal gyrus), frontal regions of the left hemisphere, as well as subcortical structures. Ethofer et al. (2005) studied the connectivity of brain areas associated with emotional prosody and showed that processing emotional prosody first requires an acoustic analysis involving the right temporal cortex, after which the information is processed within the bilateral inferior frontal cortices.

Conclusion

Overall, the goal of this chapter was to discuss emotional processing through prosody and nonlinguistic vocalizations in an attempt to show that it is essential to further explore emotional nonlinguistic vocalizations. It is important to relate the literature on speech, facial expressions, and body gestures to the one on nonlinguistic vocalizations to have a complete view of how humans process emotions. The study of vocalizations will contribute to the understanding of other aspects of emotional processing that may not be possible (or different) using prosody. For instance, prosody and nonlinguistic vocalizations do not cover the same emotional spectrum. Indeed, the range of acoustic parameters used in prosodic patterns does not allow the expression of a set of emotions as large as that in vocalizations and limits the emotional intensity as well as spontaneity of expression (e.g., Scherer, 1981a; Barr, Hopkins, & Green, 2000). Moreover, language and culture represent confounding factors in emotional perception of prosodic stimuli. Cultural and language differences between speakers and decoders are at the center of emotional processing (Ekman, 1994; Russell, 1994; Mesquita et al., 1997; Scherer et al., 2001), as each individual uses his culture and language as references to identify emotions expressed through prosodic stimuli. These limits motivate the exploration of emotional nonlinguistic vocalizations, as these are less susceptible to be influenced by language and culture than emotional stimuli with linguistic or pseudolinguistic information. Laughs (Ruch & Ekman, 2001) and cries (Drummond, McBride, & Wiebe, 1993) produced by the human newborn constitute one of the earliest and most powerful means of communication, promoting a cascade of interactions between the infant and its parents (e.g., Cosmides, 1983; Barr et al., 2000). As such it must be stressed that processing emotions through vocalizations goes beyond linguistic codes.

Acknowledgments. This work was supported by the Fonds de la Recherche en Santé Québec and the Canadian Institutes of Health Research (SF), National Sciences and Engineering Research Council of Canada, Fonds Québecois de la Recherche sur la Nature et les Technologies, Canadian Institutes of Health Research, and Canadian Foundation for Innovation (PB).

References

Adolphs, R. (2002). Neural systems for recognizing emotion. *Current Opinion in Neurobiology*, *12*, 169–177.

Albas, D. C., McCluskey, K. W., & Albas, C. A. (1976). Perception of the emotional content of speech: A comparison of two Canadian groups. *Journal of Cross-Cultural Psychology*, 7, 481–489.

Allen, R., & Brosgole, L. (1993). Facial and auditory affect recognition in senile geriatrics, the normal elderly and young adults. *International Journal of Neuroscience*, *68*, 33–42.

Armony, J. L., Chochol, C,. Fecteau, S., & Belin, P. (in press). Laugh (or cry) and you will be remembered: Influence of emotional expression on memory for vocalizations. *Psychological Science*.

Banse, R., & Scherer, K. R. (1996). Acoustic profiles in vocal emotion expression. *Journal of Personality and Social Psychology*, *70*, 614–636.

Barr, R. G., Hopkins, B., & Green, J. A. (2000). *Crying as a sign, a symptom, & a signal*. New York: Cambridge University Press.

Baum, S. R., & Pell, M. D. (1999). The neural bases of prosody: Insights from lesion studies and neuroimaging. *Aphasiology*, *13*, 581–608.

Belin, P., Fecteau, S., & Bédard, C. (2004). Thinking the voice: Neural correlates of voice perception. *Trends in Cognitive Sciences*, *8*, 129–135.

Belin, P., McAdams, S., Smith, B., Savel, S., Thivard, L., Samson, S., et al. (1998). The functional anatomy of sound intensity discrimination. *Journal of Neuroscience*, *18*, 6388–6394.

Boemio, A., Fromm, S., Braun, A., & Poeppel, D. (2005). Hierarchical and asymmetric temporal sensitivity in human auditory cortices. *Nature Neuroscience*, *8*, 389–395.

Borod, J. C., Cicero, B. A., Obler, L. K., Welkowitz, J., Erhan, H. M., Santschi, C., et al. (1998). Right hemisphere emotional perception: Evidence across multiple channels. *Neuropsychology*, *12*, 446–458.

Brådvik, B., Dravins, C., Holtas, S., Rosen, I., Ryding, E., & Ingvar, D. H. (1991). Disturbances of speech prosody following right hemisphere infarcts. *Acta Neurologica Scandinavica*, *84*, 114–126.

Breiter, H. C., Etcoff, N. L., Whalen, P. J., Kennedy, W. A., Rauch, S. L., Buckner, R. L., et al. (1996). Response and habituation of the human amygdala during visual processing of facial expression. *Neuron, 17,* 875-887.

Buchanan, T. W., Lutz, K., Mirzazade, S., Specht, K., Shah, N. J., Zilles, K., et al. (2000). Recognition of emotional prosody and verbal components of spoken language: An fMRI study. *Cognitive Brain Research, 9,* 227-238.

Cancelliere, A. E., & Kertesz, A. (1990). Lesion localization in acquired deficits of emotional expression and comprehension. *Brain and Cognition, 13,* 133-147.

Carmon, A., & Nachshon, I. (1973). Ear asymmetry in perception of emotional nonverbal stimuli. *Acta Psychologica (Amsterdam), 37,* 351-357.

Carr, L., Iacoboni, M., Dubeau, M. C., Mazziotta, J. C., & Lenzi, G. L. (2003). Neural mechanisms of empathy in humans: A relay from neural systems for imitation to limbic areas. *Proceedings of the National Academy of Sciences USA, 100,* 5497-5502.

Cosmides, L. (1983). Invariances in the acoustic expression of emotion during speech. *Journal of Experimental Psychology and Human Perception Performance, 9,* 864-881.

Davidson, R. J., & Irwin, W. (1999). The functional neuroanatomy of emotion and affective style. *Trends in Cognitive Sciences, 3,* 11-21.

Drummond, J. E., McBride, M. L., & Wiebe, C. F. (1993). The development of mothers' understanding of infant crying. *Clinical Nursing Research, 2,* 396-413.

Dusenbury, D., & Knower, F. H. (1938). Experimental studies of the symbolism of action and voice (III): A study of the specificity of meaning in facial expression. *Quarterly Journal of Speech, 24,* 424-435.

Eisenberg, N. (2000). Emotion, regulation, and moral development. *Annual Review of Psychology, 51,* 665-697.

Ekman, P. (1994). Strong evidence for universals in facial expressions: A reply to Russell's mistaken critique. *Psychological Bulletin, 115,* 268-287.

Elfenbein, H. A., & Ambady, N. (2002). On the universality and cultural specificity of emotion recognition: A meta-analysis. *Psychological Bulletin, 128,* 203-235.

Ethofer, T., Anders, S., Erb, M., Herbert, C., Wiethoff, S., Kissler, J., et al. (2006). Cerebral pathways in processing of affective prosody: A dynamic causal modeling study. *Neuroimage, 30,* 580-587.

Fecteau, S., Armony, J. L., Joanette, Y., & Belin, P. (2005). Judgment of emotional nonlinguistic vocalizations: Age-related differences. *Applied Neuropsychology, 12,* 40-48.

Fecteau, S., Armony, J. L., Joanette, Y., & Belin, P. (2005). A response in the human prefrontal cortex for human voice. *Journal of Neurophysiology, 94,* 2251-2254.

Fecteau, S., Belin, P., Joanette, Y., & Armony, J. L. (2007). Bilateral amygdala activation for negative as well as positive emotional nonlinguistic vocalizations. *Neuroimage, 36,* 480-487.

Gallese, V., Keysers, C., & Rizzolatti, G. (2004). A unifying view of the basis of social cognition. *Trends in Cognitive Sciences, 8,* 396-403.

George, M. S., Parekh, P. I., Rosinsky, N., Ketter, T. A., Kimbrell, T. A., Heilman, K. M., et al. (1996). Understanding emotional prosody activates right hemisphere regions. *Archives of Neurology, 53,* 665-670.

Grandjean, D., Sander, D., Pourtois, G., Schwartz, S., Seghier, M. L., Scherer, K. L., et al. (2005). The voices of wrath: Brain responses to angry prosody in meaningless speech. *Nature Neuroscience, 8,* 145-146.

Heilman, K. M., Scholes, R., & Watson, R. T. (1975). Auditory affective agnosia. Disturbed comprehension of affective speech. *Journal of Neurology, Neurosurgery & Psychiatry, 38,* 69-72.

Imaizumi, S., Mori, K., Kiritani, S., Kawashima, R., Sugiura, M., Fukuda, H., et al. (1997). Vocal identification of speaker and emotion activates different brain regions. *Neuroreport, 8,* 2809-2812.

Ivry, R. B., & Lebby, P. C. (1993). Hemispheric differences in auditory perception are similar to those found in visual perception. *Psychological Science, 4,* 41-45.

Joanette, Y., Goulet, P., & Hannequin, D. (1990). *Right hemisphere and verbal communication*. New York: Springer Verlag.

Johnson, W. F., Emde, R. N., Scherer, K. R., & Klinnert, M. D. (1986). Recognition of emotion from vocal cues. *Archives of General Psychiatry, 43*, 280–283.

Juslin, P. N., & Laukka, P. (2003). Communication of emotions in vocal expression and music performance: Different channels, same code? *Psychological Bulletin, 129*, 770–814.

Kawashima, R., Itoh, M., Hatazawa, J., Miyazawa, H., Yamada, K., Matsuzawa, T., et al. (1993). Changes of regional cerebral blood flow during listening to an unfamiliar spoken language. *Neuroscience Letters, 161*, 69–72.

Kiss, I., & Ennis, T. (2001). Age-related decline in perception of prosodic affect. *Applied Neuropsychology, 8*, 251–254.

Kotz, S. A., Alter, K., Besson, M., Friederici, A. D., & Schirmer, A. (2000). The interface between prosodic and semantic processes: An ERP study. 7th Annual Meeting of the Cognitive Neuroscience Society, San Francisco, April 2000. *Journal of Cognitive Neuroscience, Supplement 123*.

Kotz, S. A., Meyer, M., Alter, K., Besson, M., von Cramon, D. Y., & Friederici, A. D. (2003). On the lateralization of emotional prosody: An event-related functional MR investigation. *Brain and Language, 86*, 366–376.

Kreiman, J. (1997). Listening to voices: Theory and practice in voice perception research. In K. Johnson & J. Mullenix (Eds.), *Talker variability in speech research* (pp. 85–108). New York: Academic Press.

Ladd, D. R. (1996). *Intonational phonology*. Cambridge, UK: Cambridge University Press.

Lakshminarayanan, K., Ben Shalom, D., van Wassenhove, V., Orbelo, D., Houde, J., & Poeppel, D. (2003). The effect of spectral manipulations on the identification of affective and linguistic prosody. *Brain and Language, 84*, 250–263.

Laukka, P. (2005). Categorical perception of vocal emotion expressions. *Emotion, 5*, 277–295.

Mastropieri, D., & Turkewitz, G. (1999). Prenatal experience and neonatal responsiveness to vocal expressions of emotion. *Developmental Psychobiology, 35*, 204–214.

Mesquita, B., Frijda, N. H., & Scherer, K. R. (1997). Culture and emotion. In P. B. Berry & T. S. Saraswathi (Eds.), *Handbook of cross-cultural psychology* (pp. 255–297). Boston: Allyn & Bacon.

Meyer, M., Zysset, S., von Cramon, D. Y., & Alter, K. (2005). Distinct fMRI responses to laughter, speech, and sounds along the human peri-sylvian cortex. *Cognitive Brain Research, 24*, 291–306.

Mitchell, R. L., Elliott, R., Barry, M., Cruttenden, A., & Woodruff, P. W. (2003). The neural response to emotional prosody, as revealed by functional magnetic resonance imaging. *Neuropsychologia, 41*, 1410–1421.

Monrad-Krohn, G. H. (1963). The third element of speech: Prosody and its disorders. In L. Halpern (Ed.), *Problems of dynamic neurology* (pp. 101–117). Jerusalem, Israel: Hebrew University Press.

Morris, J. S., Scott, S. K., & Dolan, R. J. (1999). Saying it with feeling: Neural responses to emotional vocalizations. *Neuropsychologia, 37*, 1155–1163.

Osser, H. (1964). A distinctive feature analysis of the vocal communication of emotion. *Dissertation Abstracts, 25*, 3708.

Pell, M. D. (1998). Recognition of prosody following unilateral brain lesion: Influence of functional and structural attributes of prosodic contours. *Neuropsychologia, 36*, 701–715.

Pell, M. D., & Baum, S. R. (1997). Unilateral brain damage, prosodic comprehension deficits, and the acoustic cues to prosody. *Brain and Language, 57*, 195–214.

Peper, M., & Irle, E. (1997). Categorical and dimensional deciding of emotional intonations in patients with focal brain lesions. *Brain and Language, 58*, 233–264.

Pfaff, P. L. (1954). An experimental study of the communication of feeling without contextual material. *Speech Monographs*, *21*, 155-156.

Phan, K. L., Wager, T., Taylor, S. F., & Liberzon, I. (2002). Functional neuroanatomy of emotion: A meta-analysis of emotion activation studies in PET and fMRI. *Neuroimage*, *16*, 331-348.

Phelps, E. A., & LeDoux, J. E. (2005). Contributions of the amygdala to emotion processing: From animal models to human behavior. *Neuron*, *48*, 175-187.

Phillips, L. H., MacLean, R. D., & Allen, R. (2002). Age and the understanding of emotions: Neuropsychological and sociocognitive perspectives. *Journal of Gerontology B: Psychological Sciences and Social Sciences*, *57*, P526-P530.

Phillips, M. L., Young, A. W., Scott, S. K., Calder, A. J., Andrew, C., Giampietro, V., et al. (1998). Neural responses to facial and vocal expressions of fear and disgust. *Proceedings of the Royal Society of London B Biological Science*, *265*, 1809-1817.

Pihan, H., Altenmuller, E., Hertrich, I., & Ackermann, H. (2000). Cortical activation patterns of affective speech processing depend on concurrent demands on the subvocal rehearsal system. A DC-potential study. *Brain*, *123*, 2338-2349.

Pourtois, G., de Gelder, B., Bol, A., & Crommelinck, M. (2005). Perception of facial expressions and voices and of their combination in the human brain. *Cortex*, *41*, 49-59.

Pugh, K. R., Offywitz, B. A., Shaywitz, S. E., Fullbright, R. K., Byrd, D., Skudlarski, P., et al. (1996). Auditory selective attention: An fMRI investigation. *Neuroimage*, *4*, 159-173.

Rama, P., Martinkauppi, S., Linnankoski, I., Koivisto, J., Aronen, H. J., & Carlson, S. (2001). Working memory of identification of emotional vocal expressions: An fMRI study. *Neuroimage*, *13*, 1090-1101.

Rinne, T., Pekkola, J., Degerman, A., Autti, T., Jaaskelainen, I. P., Sams, M., et al. (2005). Modulation of auditory cortex activation by sound presentation rate and attention. *Human Brain Mapping*, *26*, 94-99.

Rizzolatti, G., Fogassi, L., & Gallese, V. (2001). Neurophysiological mechanisms underlying the understanding and imitation of action. *Nature Reviews Neuroscience*, *2*, 661-670.

Roland, P. E. (1993). *Brain activation*. New York: John Wiley.

Ross, E. D., Homan, R. W., & Buck, R. (1994). Differential hemispheric lateralization of primary and social emotions: Implications for developing a comprehensive neurology for emotions, repression, and the subconscious. *Neuropsychiatry, Neuropsychology, and Behavioral Neurology*, *7*, 1-19.

Ross, E. D., Thompson, R. D., & Yenkosky, J. (1997). Lateralization of affective prosody in brain and the callosal integration of hemispheric language functions. *Brain and Language*, *56*, 27-54.

Royet, J. P., Zald, D., Versace, R., Costes, N., Lavenne, F., Koenig, O., et al. (2000). Emotional responses to pleasant and unpleasant olfactory, visual, and auditory stimuli: A positron emission tomography study. *The Journal of Neuroscience*, *20*, 7752-7759.

Ruch, W., & Ekman, P. (2001). The expressive pattern of laughter. In A. Kaszniak (Ed.), *Emotion, qualia, and consciousness* (pp. 426-443). Tokyo: World Scientific.

Russell, J. A. (1994). Is there universal recognition of emotion from facial expression? A review of the cross-cultural studies. *Psychological Bulletin*, *115*, 102-141.

Russell, J. A. (2003). Core affect and the psychological construction of emotion. *Psychological Review*, *110*, 145-172.

Sackeim, H. A., Greenberg, M. S., Weiman, A. L., Gur, R. C., Hungerbuhler, J. P., & Geschwind, N. (1982). Hemispheric asymmetry in the expression of positive and negative emotions: Neurologic evidence. *Archives of Neurology*, *39*, 210-218.

Sander, D., Grandjean, D., Pourtois, G., Schwartz, S., Seighier, M. L., Scherer, K. R., et al. (2005). Emotion and attention interactions in social cognition: Brain regions involved in processing anger prosody. *Neuroimage, 28*, 848-858.

Sander, K., Roth, P., & Scheich, H. (2003). Left-lateralized fMRI in the temporal lobe of high repressive women during the identification of sad prosodies. *Cognitive Brain Research, 16*, 441-456.

Sander, K., & Scheich, H. (2001). Auditory perception of laughing and crying activates human amygdala regardless of attentional state. *Cognitive Brain Research, 12*, 181-198.

Scherer, K. R. (1981). Speech and emotional states. In J. Darby (Ed.), *Speech evaluation in psychiatry* (pp. 189-220). New York: Grune & Stralton.

Scherer, K. R. (1981). Vocal indicators of stress. In J. Darby (Ed.), *Speech evaluation in psychiatry* (pp. 171-187). New York: Grune & Stralton.

Scherer, K. R. (1986). Vocal affect expression: A review and a model for future research. *Psychological Bulletin, 99*, 143-165.

Scherer, K. R., Banse, R., & Wallbott, H. G. (2001). Emotion inferences from vocal expression correlate across languages and cultures. *Journal of Cross-Cultural Psychology, 32*, 76-92.

Schirmer, A., & Kotz, S. A. (2006). Beyond the right hemisphere: Brain mechanisms mediating vocal emotional processing. *Trends in Cognitive Sciences, 10*, 24-30.

Schirmer, A., Kotz, S. A., & Friederici, A. D. (2005). On the role of attention for the processing of emotions in speech: Sex differences revisited. *Cognitive Brain Research, 24*, 442-452.

Schmitt, J. J., Hartje, W., & Willmes, K. (1997). Hemispheric asymmetry in the recognition of emotional attitude conveyed by facial expression, prosody and propositional speech. *Cortex, 33*, 65-81.

Scott, S. K., Blank, C. C., Rosen, S., & Wise, R. J. (2000). Identification of a pathway for intelligible speech in the left temporal lobe. *Brain, 123*, 2400-2406.

Starkstein, S. E., Federoff, J. P., Price, T. R., Leiguarda, R. C., & Robinson, R. G. (1994). Neuropsychological and neuroradiological correlates of emotional prosody comprehension. *Neurology, 44*, 515-522.

Steinhauer, K., Alter, K., & Friederici, A. D. (1999). Brain potentials indicate immediate use of prosodic cues in natural speech processing. *Nature Neuroscience, 2*, 191-196.

Strelnikov, K. N., Vorobyev, V. A., Chernigovskaya, T. V., & Medvedev, S. V. (2006). Prosodic clues to syntactic processing—A PET and ERP study. *Neuroimage, 29*, 1127-1134.

Thompson, L. A., Aidinejad, M. R., & Ponte, J. (2001). Aging and the effects of facial and prosodic cues on emotional intensity ratings and memory reconstructions. *Journal of Nonverbal Behavior, 25*, 101-125.

Tompkins, C. A., & Flowers, C. R. (1985). Perception of emotional intonation by brain damaged adults: The influence of task processing levels. *Journal of Speech and Hearing Research, 28*, 527-583.

van Lancker, D., & Sidtis, J. J. (1992). The identification of affective prosodic stimuli by left and right hemisphere damaged subjects: All errors are not created equal. *Journal of Speech and Hearing Research, 35*, 963-970.

van Rijn, S., Aleman, A., van Diessen, E., Berckmoes, C., Vingerhoets, G., & Kahn, R. S. (2005). What is said or how it is said makes a difference: Role of the right fronto-parietal operculum in emotional prosody as revealed by repetitive TMS. *European Journal of Neuroscience, 21*, 3195-3200.

Vikingstad, E. M., George, K. P., Johnson, A. F., & Cao, Y. (2000). Cortical language lateralization in right handed normal subjects using functional magnetic resonance imaging. *Journal of the Neurological Sciences, 175*, 17-27.

Wallbott, H. G., & Scherer, K. R. (1986). Cues and channels in emotion recognition. *Journal of Abnormal and Social Psychology, 51*, 690-699.

Weintraub, S., Mesulam, M. M., & Kramer, L. (1981). Disturbances in prosody: A right-hemisphere contribution to language. *Archives of Neurology*, *38*, 742–744.

Wicker, B., Keysers, C., Plailly, J., Royet, J. P., Gallses, V., & Rizzolatti, G. (2003). Both of us disgusted in my insula: The common neural basis of seeing and feeling disgust. *Neuron*, *40*, 655–664.

Wildgruber, D., Hertrich, I., Riecker, A., Erb, M., Anders, S., Grodd, W., et al. (2004). Distinct frontal regions subserve evaluation of linguistic and emotional aspects of speech intonation. *Cerebral Cortex*, *14*, 1384–1389.

Wildgruber, D., Pihan, H., Ackermann, H., Erb, M., & Grodd, W. (2002). Dynamic brain activation during processing of emotional intonation: Influence of acoustic parameters, emotional valence, and sex. *Neuroimage*, *15*, 856–869.

Wildgruber, D., Riecker, A., Hertrich, I., Erb, M., Grodd, W., Ethofer, T., et al. (2005). Identification of emotional intonation evaluated by fMRI. *Neuroimage*, *24*, 1233–1241.

Wolf, C. G. (1977). The processing of fundamental frequency in a dichotic matching task. *Brain and Language*, *4*, 70–77.

Wolf, G., Gorski, R., & Peters, S. (1972). Acquaintance and accuracy of vocal emotions. *Journal of Communication*, *22*, 300–305.

Zatorre, R. J., & Belin, P. (2001). Spectral and temporal processing in human auditory cortex. *Cerebral Cortex*, *11*, 946–953.

Zatorre, R. J., Belin, P., & Penhune, V. B. (2002). Structure and function of auditory cortex: Music and speech. *Trends in Cognitive Sciences*, *6*, 37–46.

Zatorre, R. J., Evans, A. C., Meyer, E., & Gjedde, A. (1992). Lateralization of phonetic and pitch discrimination in speech processing. *Science*, *256*, 846–849.

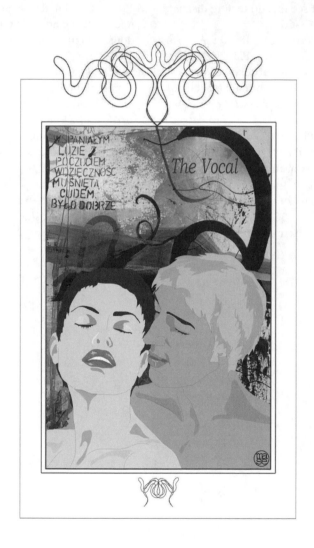

CHAPTER 11

Research on Vocal Expression of Emotion: State of the Art and Future Directions

Petri Laukka

Abstract

The current state of the art on the vocal expression of emotions is presented. The data on decoding accuracy show that vocal expressions of discrete emotions can be accurately communicated, also cross-culturally. Further, the data presently available suggest the presence of emotion-specific patterns of acoustic voice cues that can be used to communicate discrete emotions. Acoustic correlates of emotion dimensions are also reviewed. The patterns of voice cues for discrete emotions are largely consistent with Scherer's (1986) theoretical predictions for anger, fear, happiness, and sadness implying that the particular shapes of vocal expressions have their origin in the physiological effects of emotional reactions. Problems with current research are discussed and research directions are outlined.

Introduction

Among the nonverbal cues people use to infer the emotions of others in everyday life, voice cues (e.g., pitch, loudness, and speech rate) are among the most frequently reported (e.g., Planalp, DeFrancisco, & Rutherford, 1996). Scientific interest in vocal expression (i.e., how emotions are expressed nonverbally through the voice) has a long history, but progress has been slower than originally expected. This state of affairs may now be changing, however, as a result of growing interest in the affective sciences coupled with progress in speech science (see Cowie et al., 2001; Scherer, Johnstone, & Klasmeyer, 2003). This book is a good example of the increasing attention being paid to vocal expression of emotion at the moment. Thus, now is a good time to summarize what is currently known about voice and emotions. In this chapter I will give a brief review on the literature on vocal expression and outline some important concerns for future research. Throughout the chapter I will take a psychological perspective on voice and emotion, and will begin by considering what emotions are from the viewpoint of psychology.

What Is an Emotion?

From an evolutionary perspective, the key to understanding emotions is to look at what *functions* they serve (Keltner & Gross, 1999). From this perspective, emotions have evolved to deal with goal-relevant changes in our environment and may be described as relatively brief and intense reactions to these changes. Most researchers would agree that emotions consist of several components: cognitive appraisal, subjective feeling, physiological arousal, expression, action tendency, and regulation (Oatley & Jenkins, 1996).

The two research traditions that have most strongly influenced research on vocal expression are discrete and dimensional emotion theories. According to discrete emotion theories, each emotion represents a unique person-environment interaction with its own adaptation significance for the individual. Each discrete emotion is also thought to have its own unique pattern of cognitive appraisal, physiological activity, action tendency, and expression (Darwin, 1872/1998; Ekman, 1992). According to several discrete emotion theories there exist a limited number of "basic" emotions that have evolved to deal with particularly pertinent life problems such as competition (anger), danger (fear), cooperation (happiness), or loss (sadness; see Power & Dalgleish, 1997, pp. 86–99). It is also often assumed that environmental demands on behavior are reflected in distinct physiological patterns (Levenson, 1994). The strongest support for discrete emotions has traditionally come from studies of communication of emotions, which suggest that facial expressions are universally expressed and recognized (Ekman, 1992).

The dimensional approach to emotion has largely concentrated on one component of emotion, the subjective feeling state, and focuses on identifying emotions based on their placement on a small number of underlying dimensions. Wundt (1912/1924) suggested that three dimensions (pleasure-displeasure, strain-relaxation, excitement-calmness) could account for all differences among emotional states. Schlosberg (1941) proposed that the underlying structure of emotional experience can be characterized as an ordering of emotional states on the circumference of a circle. This model, now commonly referred to as the *circumplex* model of emotion, has proved highly influential. Today, most proponents of the circumplex model agree that two orthogonal dimensions underlie the circular ordering. Many authors have postulated an *activation* dimension and an evaluation, or *valence*, dimension (Larsen & Diener, 1992; Russell, 1980). The valence dimension relates to how well one is doing at the level of subjective experience, and ranges from displeasure to pleasure. The activation dimension, in turn, relates to a subjective sense of mobilization or energy, and ranges from sleep to frenetic excitement (Russell & Feldman Barrett, 1999).

The use of only two dimensions has been criticized on the grounds that this does not allow discrimination of certain emotional states (Larsen & Diener, 1992; Lazarus, 1991). Fear and anger, for example, are both unpleasant and highly active. In order to be able to capture qualitative differences among different emotional states, more dimensions are needed. A third dimension that is frequently mentioned in the literature is *potency* (Osgood, Suci, & Tannenbaum, 1957). Potency may be seen as a dimension that involves cognitive appraisal of an individual's coping potential, or power, in a particular situation; and it has been variably referred to as potency, dominance, power, or control. It has been suggested that this is an important dimension for the differentiation of negative emotions (Smith & Ellsworth, 1985). Another dimension that is generally recognized but poorly understood is *emotion intensity*. Emotions vary not only in quality but also in quantity; a person can be just a little

angry or very angry. The relative intensity of emotions is of great importance for the behavioral and physiological responses of an emotion (e.g., Brehm, 1999; Sonnemans & Frijda, 1994).

The communication of emotions is often viewed as crucial to social relationships and survival (Buck, 1984). Emotion expressions can serve as incentives of social behavior through two interrelated mechanisms (Keltner & Kring, 1998). First, by expressing emotions we can communicate important information to others, thereby influencing their behaviors, and the recognition of others' expressions allows us to make quick inferences about their probable behaviors (Darwin, 1872/1998; Plutchik, 1994). Second, expressions can regulate social behavior by evoking emotional responses in the decoder (e.g., Russell, Bachorowski, & Fernández-Dols, 2003).

Several researchers have proposed that the production and perception of emotion expressions are organized by innate mechanisms (e.g., Buck, 1984; Ekman, 1992; Lazarus, 1991, Tomkins, 1962). Support for this notion comes from, for instance, more or less intact facial and vocal expressions of emotion in children born deaf and blind (Eibl-Eibesfeldt, 1973), and universality of emotion expressions (Elfenbein & Ambady, 2002; Juslin & Laukka, 2003). However, as also noted by several researchers, expressions are shaped to a certain degree by salient cultural display rules and contextual factors, such as the immediate social environment (Ekman, 1972; Izard, 1977). A useful distinction can here be made between so-called *push* and *pull* effects in the determinants of emotion expressions (Scherer, 1989). Push effects involve various internal processes of the organism that are influenced by the emotional response. Pull effects, on the other hand, involve external conditions such as social norms. In any given case of emotion expression, both push and pull effects can be present and affect the resulting expression.

A consequence of the coexistence of push and pull effects is that there is no one-to-one relationship between expression and other components of emotion (e.g., subjective feeling). Individuals are most likely to report an emotion, and theorists are most likely to claim that an emotion has occurred, to the extent that many components of emotion co-occur (such as cognitive appraisal, subjective feeling, physiological arousal, expression; see Ekman, 1993).

Studies on Vocal Expression

Most studies have considered vocal expression as a means to communication. Hence, fundamental issues include (a) the *content* (What is communicated?), (b) the *accuracy* (How accurately is it communicated?), and (c) the *code* (How is it communicated?). The following sections first review the methods that have been used to address these questions, and then review the literature on decoding and encoding of emotions, respectively.

Methods of Collecting Vocal Expressions

A majority of studies on vocal expression have used some variant of the *standard content paradigm*. That is, someone (e.g., an actor) is instructed to read some verbal material aloud, while simultaneously portraying particular emotions chosen by the investigator. The emotion portrayals are first recorded and then evaluated in listening experiments to see whether listeners are able to decode the intended emotions. The same verbal material is used in portrayals of different emotions, and most typically has consisted of single words or short phrases. The assumption is that because the verbal material remains the same in the different portrayals, whatever effects appear in listeners' judgments should mainly be the result of the voice cues produced by the speaker. Other common methods include the use of emotional speech from real conversations (Eldred & Price, 1958; Greasley, Sherrard, & Waterman, 2000; Huttar, 1968), induction of moods in the speaker using various methods (Bachorowski & Owren, 1995; Bonner, 1943; Millot & Brand, 2001), and the use of speech synthesis to create emotional speech stimuli (Burkhardt, 2001; Cahn, 1990; Murray & Arnott, 1995).

Listeners' responses have most often been collected through forced-choice procedures, where the listener is asked to select one among several emotion labels. Another fixed-alternative method is to ask listeners to rate the stimuli on scales representing either emotion labels or emotion dimensions (Scherer, Banse, Wallbott, & Goldbeck, 1991). Free descriptions have also been used, though more sparsely.

The use of forced-choice methodology produces an ecologically valid task, but the fixed number of alternatives may produce artifacts. Some of the problems with the forced-choice method are alleviated by the use of rating scales, but the listeners' responses are still being influenced by the alternatives present. There have been several suggestions as to how one can improve the validity of the fixed-choice methodology, for instance by correcting for guessing (Wagner, 1993), or including "other emotion" as a response alternative (Frank & Stennet, 2001). The use of free descriptions is the least biasing task, but free descriptions are difficult to classify. It has been reported that free descriptions and the forced-choice task yield similar results, though free descriptions give more detailed information (Greasley et al., 2000).

Decoding of Vocal Expressions

It was early agreed that emotions can be communicated accurately through vocal expressions, a finding that is supported by common, everyday experience (Kramer, 1963). In the most comprehensive review to date, Juslin and Laukka (2003) conducted a meta-analysis of the literature on decoding accuracy of discrete emotions in both within-cultural and cross-cultural communication. Included in the analysis were studies that presented forced-choice decoding data relative to some independent criterion of encoding intention. To be able to compare accuracy scores from different studies with different numbers of response alternatives in the decoding task, the accuracy scores were transformed to Rosenthal and Rubin's (1989) effect size index for one-sample, multiple-choice-type data, pi. This index transforms accuracy scores involving any number of response alternatives to a standard scale of dichotomous choice, on which .50 is the null value and 1.00 corresponds to 100% correct decoding. The results of the meta-analysis, in terms of the pi index, are shown in Table 11-1. Also shown in the table are additional data regarding surprise and disgust taken from Laukka and Juslin (2002).

The means and confidence intervals presented in Table 11-1 suggest that the decoding accuracy is typically significantly higher than what would be expected by chance alone for both within-cultural and cross-cultural vocal expression. However, the accuracy was significantly higher (t-test, $p < .01$) for within-cultural expression (pi = .90) than for cross-cultural expression (pi = .85). Among the individual emotions, anger and sadness were best decoded, followed by fear, happiness, and surprise. Disgust and tenderness received the lowest accuracy although it must be noted that the estimates for these emotions were based on fewer data points. The pattern of results visible in Table 11-1 is consistent with previous reviews of vocal expression featuring fewer studies, but differs from the pattern found in studies of facial expression, in which happiness is usually better decoded than other emotions (Elfenbein & Ambady, 2002).

Conclusions (decoding): (a) The communication of emotions may reach an accuracy well above chance level, at least for broad emotion categories corresponding to basic emotions (that is, anger, disgust, fear, happiness, sadness, surprise, tenderness). (b) Vocal expressions of emotion are accurately decoded cross-culturally, although the accuracy is somewhat lower than for within-cultural vocal expression.

Encoding Studies of Vocal Expression

Almost from the beginning of empirical research on vocal expressions, researchers started to acoustically analyze the emotional speech, hoping to find acoustic voice cues that signal various emotional states

Table 11–1. Summary of results from meta-analysis of decoding accuracy for discrete emotions

	Anger	Disgust	Fear	Happiness	Sadness	Surprise	Tenderness	Overall
Within-Cultural Expression								
Mean accuracy (PI)	.93	.83	.88	.87	.93	.90	.82	.90
95% CI	.021	.089	.037	.040	.020	.061	.083	.020
Number of studies	32	11	26	30	31	14	6	42
Number of speakers	278	138	273	253	225	170	49	488
Cross-Cultural Expression								
Mean accuracy (PI)	.91	.76	.82	.74	.91	.80	.71	.85
95% CI	.017	—	.062	.040	.018	.265	—	.025
Number of studies	6	1	5	6	7	3	1	9
Number of speakers	69	16	66	68	71	20	3	75

Note. Adapted from "Communication of Emotions in Vocal Expression and Music Performance: Different Channels, Same Code?" by P. N. Juslin and P. Laukka, 2003, *Psychological Bulletin, 129,* pp. 770–814. Reprinted with permission from the American Psychological Association.

(see Fairbanks & Provonost, 1939; Scripture, 1921; Skinner, 1935). Soon enough it was discovered that it was difficult to find specific voice cues that could be used as reliable indicators of vocal expressions. As a consequence of the difficulties in finding specific patterns of voice cues for discrete emotions, some authors have concluded that voice cues only reflect the activation dimension of emotions (Davitz, 1964; Pakosz, 1983).

Voice cues that can be measured from an acoustic speech signal can be broadly divided into those related to (a) *fundamental frequency (F$_0$)*, (b) *voice intensity*, (c) *voice quality*, and (d) *temporal aspects* of speech. The respiratory process of the lungs builds up subglottal pressure. This pressure, in combination with vocal fold adduction and tension, leads to vibration of the vocal folds. The frequency with which the vocal folds open and close across the glottis during phonation is termed F_0. This is subjectively heard as the pitch of the voice, and mainly reflects the differential innervation of the laryngeal musculature and the extent of subglottal pressure. Voice intensity is subjectively heard as the loudness of the voice, and is determined by respiratory and phonatory action. It reflects the effort required to produce the speech. Voice quality is subjectively heard as the timbre of the voice, and is largely determined by the settings of the supralaryngeal vocal tract and the phonatory mechanisms of the larynx. Temporal aspects of speech, finally, concern the temporal sequence of the production of sounds and silence (such as speech rate, pausing).

In the most extensive review to date, Juslin and Laukka (2003) investigated whether there are distinct patterns of voice cues that correspond to discrete emotions. The main results from their review of the code usage literature are shown in Table 11-2. In this table, patterns of voice cues used to express different emotions, as reported in 77 studies of vocal expression, are displayed. Also included in the table are results from a review on the acoustical correlates of emotion dimensions including 15 studies (see Laukka, Juslin, & Bresin, 2005).

The results in Table 11-2 strongly suggest that there are emotion-specific patterns of voice cues that convey discrete emotions. This general pattern of the results is also supported by research published after the Juslin and Laukka (2003) review (e.g., Airas & Alku, 2006; Audibert, Aubergé, & Rilliard, 2005; Bänziger, 2004; Barrett & Paus, 2002; Cook, Fujisawa, & Takami, 2006; Gendrot, 2003; Hozjan & Kacic, 2003; Lakshminarayanan et al., 2003; Lee & Narayanan, 2005; Linnankoski, Leinonen, Vihla, Laakso, & Carlson, 2005; Oudeyer, 2003; Toivanen, Väyrynen, & Seppänen, 2004; Viscovich et al., 2003).

As shown in Table 11-2, the same voice cues are often used in a similar way for conveying more than one emotion. For instance, F_0 rises and speech rate increases for both anger and fear. Therefore F_0 and speech rate are not perfect indicators of respective emotion. This inconsistency in code usage has been explained in terms of the coding of the communicative process (Juslin & Laukka, 2003). Any voice cue taken alone is not sufficient for communicating emotion expressions, but what are needed are combinations of several cues. The acoustic voice cues that are involved in expression of emotions thus seem to be partly redundant, and the relevant cues are coded probabilistically (the cues are not

Table 11–2. Patterns of acoustic voice cues used to express discrete emotions and emotion dimensions in studies of vocal expression

Voice Cue	Category	Number of Studies for Each Emotion Label							
		Anger	Fear	Happiness	Sadness	Tenderness	Activation	Valence	Potency
F_0 mean	High	33	28	34	4	1	8	—	1
	Medium	5	8	2	1	—	—	—	4
	Low	5	3	2	40	4	—	2	4
F_0 variability	High	27	9	33	2	—	7	4	4
	Medium	4	6	2	1	5	—	—	—
	Low	4	17	1	31	5	—	2	—
F_0 contour	Up	6	6	7	—	1	—	1	1
	Down	2	—	—	11	3	—	—	—
Jitter (F_0 perturbation)	High	6	4	5	1	—	—	—	6
	Low	1	4	3	5	—	—	—	—
Voice intensity mean	High	30	11	20	1	—	5	—	6
	Medium	1	3	6	2	—	—	—	—
	Low	1	8	—	29	4	—	2	—
Voice intensity variability	High	9	7	8	2	—	1	—	2
	Medium	1	4	3	1	—	—	—	—
	Low	2	1	2	8	—	—	1	—
Voice onsets (attack)	Fast	1	1	2	1	1	1	1	—
	Slow	1	1	—	1	—	1	—	1
High-frequency energy[a]	High	22	8	13	—	—	4	—	2
	Medium	—	2	3	—	—	—	—	—
	Low	—	6	1	19	3	—	2	—
F1 mean	High	6	1	5	1	—	1	—	1
	Medium	—	—	1	—	—	—	—	—
	Low	—	3	—	5	—	—	1	—

Number of Studies for Each Emotion Label

Voice Cue	Category	Anger	Fear	Happiness	Sadness	Tenderness	Activation	Valence	Potency
F1 bandwidth	Narrow	4	—	2	—	—	1	—	1
	Wide	—	2	1	3	—	—	—	—
Precision of articulation	High	7	2	3	—	—	1	—	1
	Medium	—	2	2	—	—	—	—	—
	Low	—	2	—	6	1	—	1	—
Glottal waveform[b]	Steep	6	2	2	—	—	1	—	—
	Rounded	—	4	—	4	—	—	—	—
Speech rate	Fast	28	24	22	1	—	5	2	2
	Medium	3	3	5	5	1	—	—	—
	Slow	4	2	6	30	3	1	—	3
Proportion of pauses	Large	—	2	1	11	1	—	—	—
	Medium	—	3	2	—	—	—	—	—
	Small	8	4	3	1	—	2	1	—
Micro-structural regularity[c]	Regular	—	—	2	—	1	—	—	—
	Irregular	3	2	—	4	—	—	—	—

Note. Results are shown in terms of the number of studies that have reported a particular finding for each emotion label and voice cue. Text in bold typeface indicates the most frequent finding for each voice cue. For a detailed description of the included studies and voice cues, the reader is referred to Juslin and Laukka (2003). Data regarding emotion dimensions is taken from Laukka et al. (2005).

[a]High-frequency energy refers to the relative proportion of acoustic energy above versus below a certain cut-off frequency (e.g., 500 Hz or 1000 Hz). As the proportion of high-frequency energy in the acoustic spectrum increases, the voice sounds more "sharp" and less "soft" (von Bismarck, 1974).

[b]The glottal waveform has mainly been studied by means of inverse filtering (e.g., Laukkanen, Vilkman, Alku, & Oksanen, 1996).

[c]Microstructural regularity refers to the regularity/irregularity of F_0, voice intensity, and/or duration (see Davitz, 1964).

Adapted from "Communication of Emotions in Vocal Expression and Music Performance: Different Channels, Same Code?" by P. N. Juslin & P. Laukka, 2003, *Psychological Bulletin, 129*, pp. 770–814. Reprinted with permission from the American Psychological Association.

perfectly reliable indicators of the expressed emotion; see Juslin & Scherer, 2005). The redundancy between the cues largely reflects the sound production mechanisms of the voice. For instance, an increase in subglottal pressure increases not only the intensity of the voice, but also F_0 to some degree (Borden, Harris, & Raphael, 1994). The probabilistic nature of the cues reflects individual differences among encoders and structural constraints of the verbal material, as well as the fact that the same cue can be used in the same way in more than one expression. The redundancy and probabilistic nature of the voice cues entail that decoders have to combine many cues for successful communication to occur. This is not simply a matter of pattern matching, however, because the cues contribute in an additive fashion to listeners' judgments (see Ladd, Silverman, Tolkmitt, Bergmann, & Scherer, 1985). Each cue is neither necessary nor sufficient, but the larger the number of cues used, the more reliable the communication becomes (Juslin, 2000). Obviously, this emphasizes the importance of considering a large number of voice cues in studies of vocal expression.

The nature of the coding described above has more important implications. Because the voice cues are intercorrelated to some degree, more than one way of using the cues might lead to a similarly high level of decoding accuracy (Juslin, 2000). This might explain why accurate communication is regularly found in studies of vocal expression, despite considerable inconsistency in code usage. Multiple cues that are partly redundant yield a robust communicative system that is forgiving of deviations from optimal code usage. However, this robustness comes with a price. The redundancy of the

cues means that the same information is conveyed by many cues, which limits the complexity of the information that can be conveyed (Shannon & Weaver, 1949).

There are few theories of vocal expression of emotion. The one stringent attempt to formulate a theory of vocal expression was made by Scherer (1986). The general principle that underlies this theory is that physiological variables to a large extent determine the nature of phonation and resonance in vocal expression. For instance, anger yields increased tension in the laryngeal musculature coupled with increased subglottal air pressure. This will change the production of sound at the glottis and hence change the timbre of the voice. In other words, depending on the specific physiological state, we may expect to find specific acoustic features in the voice. Based on his component process theory of emotion, Scherer (1986) made detailed predictions about the patterns of vocal cues associated with different emotions. The predictions were based on the idea that emotions involve sequential cognitive appraisals, or *stimulus evaluation checks* (SEC), of stimulus features like novelty, intrinsic pleasantness, goal significance, coping potential, and norm/self compatibility (for further elaboration of appraisal dimensions, see Scherer, 2001). The outcome of each SEC is assumed to have a specific effect on the somatic nervous system, which, in turn, affects the musculature associated with voice production. In addition, each SEC outcome is assumed to affect various aspects of the autonomous nervous system (e.g., mucus and saliva production) in ways that strongly influence voice production. Scherer (1986) offered detailed predictions for acoustic cues associated with anger, disgust, fear, happiness, and sadness. The results shown in Table 11–2 are generally consistent with Scherer's (1986) predictions. In a direct test, 82% of 32 comparisons of the predictions matched the results of the review, while some predictions may have to be revised (Juslin & Laukka, 2003).

Finally, as evident from Table 11–2, the results regarding acoustical correlates of emotion dimensions are weaker than the evidence regarding discrete emotions, but at least activation and potency do have clear acoustical correlates. The results also show that voice cues allow a more fine-grained differentiation of emotional states than merely activation and valence. However, a dimensional approach to vocal expression may still be a viable alternative if one wishes to study milder affective states (e.g., moods, attitudes, or stress) that do not correspond to full-blown emotions (Laukka et al., 2005). It has been suggested that such affective states can be usefully described in terms of broad emotion dimensions (Russell & Feldman Barrett, 1999), and that such affective states play an important role in everyday vocal expression (Cowie & Cornelius, 2003). Thus, a dimensional approach can contribute to the understanding of how the voice offers subtle cues to affective states in everyday life.

Conclusions (encoding): (a) The results strongly suggest that there are emotion-specific patterns of acoustic voice cues that can be used to communicate discrete emotions in vocal expression. (b) The patterns of voice cues for discrete emotions are largely consistent with Scherer's (1986) theoretical predictions for anger, fear, happiness, and sadness, which implies that the particular shapes of vocal expressions have their origin in the physiological effects of emotional reactions.

Future Directions

In the light of the results presented above, it may now be time to start looking beyond the simple, though admittedly important, question about whether discrete emotions can or cannot be conveyed by vocal expressions. To find evidence of emotion-specific patterns of voice cues is only a first step toward the understanding of vocal emotion expression. In order for further progress to be made, research on vocal expression now needs to start asking more subtle questions. In the following, I will outline some areas that will be of crucial importance for future research.

A crucial issue is what emotional states should be investigated in studies on vocal expression. Many studies have not used well-defined emotion labels, but instead have chosen the labels to be investigated on an ad hoc basis. Most studies have used labels that more or less correspond to basic emotions. However, it seems to be the case that such labels do not capture the full amount of differentiation that may be possible in vocal expression. For example, different variants of anger (like irritation and rage) may differ with respect to their acoustic patterns, even though they do belong to the same emotion family (anger). Banse & Scherer (1996) used such more fine-grained descriptions of emotions and showed that these differences did have an impact on the patterning of voice cues. Also, Juslin and Laukka (2001) showed that emotion intensity had a large effect on voice cues. Sometimes the differences between different intensities of the same emotion were larger than differences between different emotions with the same intensity. Thus it is very important to control for emotion intensity when designing studies on vocal expression. Another promising route is to study the appraisal processes of emotions directly to see how they relate to the listener's perception and voice cues (Johnstone, Van Reekum, Hird, Kirsner, & Scherer, 2005; Johnstone, Van Reekum, & Scherer, 2001). Finally, if one aims at capturing the essence of expression in spontaneous conversational speech, it may be better to look for less prototypical expressions because everyday expressions often are masked, or strategically posed, and thus may convey quite complex affective states (e.g., Cowie & Cornelius, 2003; Devillers, Vidrascu, & Lamel, 2005). Thus if one is interested in studying everyday conversations for applied purposes like improving the naturalness of speech synthesis or enhancing automatic speech recognition, it may be a good strategy to concentrate efforts on weaker affective states involving the effects of stress, attitudes, and positive versus negative moods.

Another crucial issue is which methodology should be employed for studying vocal expression. So far, a large majority of empirical studies (as reviewed in Table 11–2) has been conducted on posed vocal expressions. It is generally assumed that emotion portrayals need to be similar to naturally occurring expressions in order to be effective. Nevertheless, posed expressions may be influenced by conventionalized stereotypes of vocal expression and may also yield expressions that are more intense and prototypical than naturally occurring expressions (Scherer, 1986). Unfortunately, the actual extent to which posed expressions are similar to natural expression is an empirical question that requires further research, and more studies need to be con-

ducted in naturalistic settings in order to increase the ecological validity of the findings. It can be argued that the choice of methodology should be informed by the research questions that one wishes to address. For instance, if one wishes to study effects of weaker affective states on voice production, mood-induction methods or recordings of real conversations combined with dimensional listening tests could be a successful combination. If, on the other hand, one wishes to study discrete emotions of a fairly strong intensity, one may be forced to rely on emotion portrayals to a large extent. Induction methods are effective in inducing moods (Westermann, Spies, Stahl, & Hesse, 1996), but it is harder to induce intense emotional states in controlled laboratory settings. However, to conduct vocal expression studies where relatively intense discrete emotions are induced in controlled laboratory settings is an important undertaking for future research. Finally, the use of speech synthesis enables one to conduct controlled experiments where different voice cues can be manipulated separately or in combination, in order to investigate diverse hypotheses about cue utilization in vocal expression. All hypotheses derived from empirical studies should be verified experimentally using speech synthesis techniques where cues are manipulated in a systematic fashion.

Besides providing evidence of distinct patterns of voice cues that correspond to discrete emotions, Table 11–2 also revealed many gaps in the literature that can be used to guide further research (Juslin & Laukka, 2003). Many voice cues have not been systematically investigated, and thus the results for many cues are preliminary at best. To date, acoustic measures that are averaged over time are most commonly utilized. However, to be able to capture the dynamic nature of speech, more detailed analyses of local features must be conducted. This could be done, for instance, by using continuous measurements of listener responses that can then be coupled with time-linked measurements of voice cues. In addition, more research needs to be directed to the spectral parameters of speech to clarify the relationships between voice quality, voice production, and acoustic measurements.

It has been reported that expression of emotions can be mediated by personality characteristics (Feldman Barrett & Niedenthal, 2004; Gross, John, & Richards, 2000). This entails that some people are more expressive than others and may be more emotional than others, something that has been often reported in studies of vocal expression. Future studies should take the issue of individual differences seriously and, besides using large numbers of encoders and decoders, also systematically study the reasons for these differences.

Various other issues also deserve attention. First, there is a need for more cross-cultural research, especially on the possible universality of code usage. It would be worthwhile to make more fine-grained comparisons of encoding and decoding of vocal expressions, taking into account the relations between the particular cultures (Elfenbein & Ambady, 2003). Second, the organization of the production and perception of vocal expression has not received much attention, though it is an issue of great relevance for how to conceptualize vocal emotions. Laukka (2003; 2005) found categorical effects in the perception of vocal expressions, which tentatively supports a discrete-emotions view on per-

ception of vocal expression. Third, the face and the voice together constitute the most effective means of communication of emotions (de Gelder, 2000), but more research is needed on the interaction of these two modalities. Interesting future topics thus include the bimodal expression of emotion in the face and voice (Massaro & Egan, 1996) and the influence of facial expressions on the acoustics of vocal expression (Tartter, 1980). Finally, studies on the neural bases of production and perception of emotional speech are an important way forward in this area (Adolphs, Damasio, & Tranel, 2002; Gandour et al., 2003; George et al., 1996). Work on the production of vocal expressions is especially missing today. Knowledge about the underlying brain mechanisms responsible for perception and production of vocal expressions will be crucial for a deeper understanding of how vocal expression works. To conclude, much progress has been made in research on vocal expression. However, much work also remains to be done, which promises vocal expression will be a dynamic area of research for years to come.

References

Adolphs, R., Damasio, H., & Tranel, D. (2002). Neural systems for recognition of emotional prosody: A 3-D lesion study. *Emotion, 2*, 23–51.

Airas, M., & Alku, P. (2006). Emotions in vowel segments of continuous speech: Analysis of the glottal flow using the normalized amplitude quotient. *Phonetica, 63*, 26–46.

Audibert, N., Aubergé, V., & Rilliard, A. (2005). The prosodic dimensions of emotions in speech: The relative weights of parameters.

In *Proceedings of the 9th European Conference on Speech Communication and Technology* (pp. 525-528). Lisbon, Portugal: International Speech Communication Association.

Bachorowski, J.-A., & Owren, M. J. (1995). Vocal expression of emotion: Acoustical properties of speech are associated with emotional intensity and context. *Psychological Science, 6*, 219-224.

Banse, R., & Scherer, K. R. (1996). Acoustic profiles in vocal emotion expression. *Journal of Personality and Social Psychology, 70*, 614-636.

Bänziger, T. (2004). *Communication vocale des émotions: Perception de l'expression vocale et attributions émotionnelles.* Unpublished doctoral dissertation, Université de Genève, Geneva, Switzerland.

Barrett, J., & Paus, T. (2002). Affect-induced changes in speech production. *Experimental Brain Research, 146*, 531-537.

Bonner, M. R. (1943). Changes in the speech pattern under emotional tension. *American Journal of Psychology, 56*, 262-273.

Borden, G. J., Harris, K. S., & Raphael, L. J. (1994). *Speech science primer: Physiology, acoustics and perception of speech* (3rd ed.). Baltimore: Williams & Wilkins.

Brehm, J. W. (1999). The intensity of emotion. *Personality and Social Psychology Review, 3*, 2-22.

Buck, R. (1984). *The communication of emotion.* New York: Guilford Press.

Burkhardt, F. (2001). *Simulation emotionaler Sprechweise mit Sprachsyntheseverfahren* [Simulation of emotional speech by means of speech synthesis]. Unpublished doctoral dissertation, Technische Universität Berlin, Berlin, Germany.

Cahn, J. E. (1990). The generation of affect in synthesized speech. *Journal of the American Voice I/O Society, 8*, 1-19.

Cook, N. D., Fujisawa, T. X., & Takami, K. (2006). Evaluation of the affective valence of speech using pitch substructure. *IEEE Transactions on Audio, Speech, and Language Processing, 14*, 142-151.

Cowie, R., & Cornelius, R. R. (2003). Describing the emotional states that are expressed in speech. *Speech Communication, 40*, 5-32.

Cowie, R., Douglas-Cowie, E., Tsapatsoulis, N., Votsis, G., Kollias, S., Fellenz, W., et al. (2001). Emotion recognition in human-computer interaction. *IEEE Signal Processing Magazine, 18*(1), 32-80.

Darwin, C. (with introduction, afterword, and commentaries by P. Ekman). (1998). *The expression of the emotions in man and animals.* New York: Oxford University Press. (Original work published 1872)

Davitz, J. R. (1964). Auditory correlates of vocal expressions of emotional meanings. In J. R. Davitz (Ed.), *The communication of emotional meaning* (pp. 101-112). New York: McGraw-Hill.

de Gelder, B. (2000). Recognizing emotions by ear and by eye. In R. D. Lane & L. Nadel (Eds.), *Cognitive neuroscience of emotion* (pp. 84-105). New York: Oxford University Press.

Devillers, L., Vidrascu, L., & Lamel, L. (2005). Challenges in real-life emotion annotation and machine learning based detection. *Neural Networks, 18*, 407-422.

Eibl-Eibesfeldt, I. (1973). The expressive behavior of the deaf-and-blind born. In M. von Cranach & I. Vine (Eds.), *Social communication and movement: Studies of interaction and expression in man and chimpanzee* (pp. 163-193). New York: Academic Press.

Ekman, P. (1972). Universals and cultural differences in facial expression of emotion. In J. Cole (Ed.), *Nebraska symposium on motivation* (vol. 19, pp. 207-283). Lincoln, NE: University of Nebraska Press.

Ekman, P. (1992). An argument for basic emotions. *Cognition and Emotion, 6*, 169-200.

Ekman, P. (1993). Facial expressions and emotion. *American Psychologist, 48*, 384-392.

Eldred, S. H., & Price, D. B. (1958). A linguistic evaluation of feeling states in psychotherapy. *Psychiatry, 21*, 115-121.

Elfenbein, H. A., & Ambady, N. (2002). On the universality and cultural specificity of emotion recognition: A meta-analysis. *Psychological Bulletin, 128,* 203-235.

Elfenbein, H. A., & Ambady, N. (2003). Cultural similarity's consequences. A distance perspective on cross-cultural differences in emotion recognition. *Journal of Cross-Cultural Psychology, 34,* 92-110.

Fairbanks, G., & Provonost, W. (1939). An experimental study of the pitch characteristics of the voice during the expression of emotion. *Speech Monographs, 6,* 87-104.

Feldman Barrett, L., & Niedenthal, P. M. (2004). Valence focus and the perception of facial affect. *Emotion, 4,* 266-274.

Frank, M. G., & Stennet, J. (2001). The forced-choice paradigm and the perception of facial expressions of emotion. *Journal of Personality and Social Psychology, 80,* 75-85.

Gandour, J., Wong, D., Dzemidzic, M., Lowe, M., Tong, Y., & Li, X. (2003). A cross-linguistic fMRI study of perception of intonation and emotion in Chinese. *Human Brain Mapping, 18,* 149-157.

Gendrot, C. (2003). Rôle de la qualité de la voix dans la simulation des émotions: Une étude perceptive et physiologique [The role of voice quality in the simulation of emotions: A study of perception and physiology]. *Revue PArole, 27,* 137-158.

George, M. S., Parekh, P. I., Rosinsky, N., Ketter, T. A., Kimbrell, T. A., Heilman, K. M., et al. (1996). Understanding emotional prosody activates right hemisphere regions. *Archives of Neurology, 53,* 665-670.

Greasley, P., Sherrard, C., & Waterman, M. (2000). Emotion in language and speech: Methodological issues in naturalistic settings. *Language and Speech, 43,* 355-375.

Gross, J. J., John, O. P., & Richards, J. M. (2000). The dissociation of emotion expression from emotion experience: A personality perspective. *Personality and Social Psychology Bulletin, 26,* 712-726.

Hozjan, V., & Kacic, Z. (2003). Context-independent multilingual emotion recognition from speech signals. *International Journal of Speech Technology, 6,* 311-320.

Huttar, G. L. (1968). Relations between prosodic variables and emotions in normal American English utterances. *Journal of Speech and Hearing Research, 11,* 481-487.

Izard, C. E. (1977). *Human emotions.* New York: Plenum.

Johnstone, T., Van Reekum, C. M., Hird, K., Kirsner, K., & Scherer, K. R. (2005). Affective speech elicited with a computer game. *Emotion, 5,* 513-518.

Johnstone, T., Van Reekum, C. M., & Scherer, K. R. (2001). Vocal expression correlates of appraisal processes. In K. R. Scherer, A. Schorr, & T. Johnstone (Eds.), *Appraisal processes in emotion: Theory, methods, research* (pp. 271-284). New York: Oxford University Press.

Juslin, P. N. (2000). Cue utilization in communication of emotion in music performance: Relating performance to perception. *Journal of Experimental Psychology: Human Perception and Performance, 26,* 1797-1813.

Juslin, P. N., & Laukka, P. (2001). Impact of intended emotion intensity on cue utilization and decoding accuracy in vocal expression of emotion. *Emotion, 1,* 381-412.

Juslin, P. N., & Laukka, P. (2003). Communication of emotions in vocal expression and music performance: Different channels, same code? *Psychological Bulletin, 129,* 770-814.

Juslin, P. N., & Scherer, K. R. (2005). Vocal expression of affect. In J. Harrigan, R. Rosenthal, & K. R. Scherer (Eds.), *The new handbook of methods in nonverbal behavior research* (pp. 65-135). New York: Oxford University Press.

Keltner, D., & Gross, J. J. (1999). Functional accounts of emotions. *Cognition and Emotion, 13,* 467-480.

Keltner, D., & Kring, A. M. (1998). Emotion, social function, and psychopathology. *Review of General Psychology, 2,* 320-342.

Kramer, E. (1963). Judgment of personality characteristics and emotions from nonverbal properties of speech. *Psychological Bulletin, 60,* 408-420.

Ladd, D. R., Silverman, K. E. A., Tolkmitt, F., Bergmann, G., & Scherer, K. R. (1985). Evidence of independent function of intonation contour type, voice quality, and F_0 range in signaling speaker affect. *Journal of the Acoustical Society of America, 78,* 435–444.

Lakshminarayanan, K., Shalom, D. B., van Wassenhove, V., Orbelo, D., Houde, J., & Poeppel, D. (2003). The effect of spectral manipulations on the identification of affective and linguistic prosody. *Brain and Language, 84,* 250–263.

Larsen, R. J., & Diener, E. (1992). Promises and problems with the circumplex model of emotion. In M. S. Clark (Ed.), *Review of personality and social psychology* (Vol. 13, pp. 25–59). Newbury Park, CA: Sage.

Laukka, P. (2003). Categorical perception of emotion in vocal expression. *Annals of the New York Academy of Sciences, 1000,* 283–287.

Laukka, P. (2005). Categorical perception of vocal emotion expressions. *Emotion, 5,* 277–295.

Laukka, P., & Juslin, P. N. (2002, July). *Accuracy of communication of emotions in speech and music performance: A quantitative review.* Paper presented at the 7th International Conference on Music Perception and Cognition, Sydney, Australia.

Laukka, P., Juslin, P. N., & Bresin, R. (2005). A dimensional approach to vocal expression of emotion. *Cognition and Emotion, 19,* 633–653.

Laukkanen, A.-M., Vilkman, E., Alku, P., & Oksanen, H. (1996). Physical variations related to stress and emotional state: A preliminary study. *Journal of Phonetics, 24,* 313–335.

Lazarus, R. S. (1991). *Emotion and adaptation.* New York: Oxford University Press.

Lee, C. M., & Narayanan, S. (2005). Towards detecting emotions in spoken dialogs. *IEEE Transactions on Speech and Audio Processing, 13,* 293–303.

Levenson, R. W. (1994). Human emotion: A functional view. In P. Ekman & R. J. Davidson (Eds.), *The nature of emotion: Fun-*

damental questions (pp. 123–126). New York: Oxford University Press.

Linnankoski, I., Leinonen, L., Vihla, M., Laakso, M.-L., & Carlson, S. (2005). Conveyance of emotional connotations by a single word in English. *Speech Communication, 45,* 27–39.

Massaro, D. W., & Egan, P. B. (1996). Perceiving affect from the voice and the face. *Psychonomic Bulletin & Review, 3,* 215–221.

Millot, J.-L., & Brand, G. (2001). Effects of pleasant and unpleasant ambient odors on human voice pitch. *Neuroscience Letters, 297,* 61–63.

Murray, I. R., & Arnott, J. L. (1995). Implementation and testing of a system for producing emotion-by-rule in synthetic speech. *Speech Communication, 16,* 369–390.

Oatley, K., & Jenkins, J. M. (1996). *Understanding emotions.* Oxford, UK: Blackwell.

Osgood, C. E., Suci, G. J., & Tannenbaum, P. H. (1957). *The measurement of meaning.* Urbana, IL: University of Illinois Press.

Oudeyer, P.-Y. (2003). The production and recognition of emotions in speech: Features and algorithms. *International Journal of Human-Computer Studies, 59,* 157–183.

Pakosz, M. (1983). Attitudinal judgments in intonation: Some evidence for a theory. *Journal of Psycholinguistic Research, 12,* 311–326.

Planalp, S., DeFrancisco, V. L., & Rutherford, D. (1996). Varieties of cues to emotion in naturally occurring situations. *Cognition and Emotion, 10,* 137–153.

Plutchik, R. (1994). *The psychology and biology of emotion.* New York: Harper-Collins.

Power, M., & Dalgleish, T. (1997). *Cognition and emotion: From order to disorder.* Hove, UK: Psychology Press.

Rosenthal, R., & Rubin, D. B. (1989). Effect size estimation for one-sample multiple-choice-type data: Design, analysis, and meta-analysis. *Psychological Bulletin, 106,* 332–337.

Russell, J. A. (1980). A circumplex model of affect. *Journal of Personality and Social Psychology, 39,* 1161–1178.

Russell, J. A., Bachorowski, J.-A., & Fernández-Dols, J.-M. (2003). Facial and vocal expressions of emotion. *Annual Review of Psychology, 54*, 329-349.

Russell, J. A., & Feldman Barrett, L. (1999). Core affect, prototypical emotional episodes, and other things called emotion: Dissecting the elephant. *Journal of Personality and Social Psychology, 76*, 805-819.

Scherer, K. R. (1986). Vocal affect expression: A review and a model for future research. *Psychological Bulletin, 99*, 143-165.

Scherer, K. R. (1989). Vocal correlates of emotional arousal and affective disturbance. In H. Wagner & A. Manstead (Eds.), *Handbook of social psychophysiology* (pp. 165-197). New York: Wiley.

Scherer, K. R. (2001). Appraisal considered as a process of multi-level sequential checking. In K. R. Scherer, A. Schorr, & T. Johnstone (Eds.), *Appraisal processes in emotion: Theory, methods, research* (pp. 92-120). New York: Oxford University Press.

Scherer, K. R., Banse, R., Wallbott, H. G., & Goldbeck, T. (1991). Vocal cues in emotion encoding and decoding. *Motivation and Emotion, 15*, 123-148.

Scherer, K. R., Johnstone, T., & Klasmeyer, G. (2003). Vocal expression of emotion. In R. J. Davidson, K. R. Scherer, & H. H. Goldsmith (Eds.), *Handbook of affective sciences* (pp. 433-456). New York: Oxford University Press.

Schlosberg, H. (1941). A scale for the judgment of facial expressions. *Journal of Experimental Psychology, 29*, 497-510.

Scripture, E. W. (1921). A study of emotions by speech transcription. *Vox, 31*, 179-183.

Shannon, C. E., & Weaver, W. (1949). *The mathematical theory of communication.* Urbana, IL: University of Illinois Press.

Skinner, E. R. (1935). A calibrated recording and analysis of the pitch, force and quality of vocal tones expressing happiness and sadness. *Speech Monographs, 2*, 81-137.

Smith, C. A., & Ellsworth, P. C. (1985). Patterns of cognitive appraisal in emotion. *Journal of Personality and Social Psychology, 48*, 813-838.

Sonnemans, J., & Frijda, N. H. (1994). The structure of subjective emotional intensity. *Cognition and Emotion, 8*, 329-350.

Tartter, V. C. (1980). Happy talk: Perceptual and acoustic effects of smiling on speech. *Perception & Psychophysics, 27*, 24-27.

Toivanen, J., Väyrynen, E., & Seppänen, T. (2004). Automatic discrimination of emotion from spoken Finnish. *Language and Speech, 47*, 383-412.

Tomkins, S. (1962). *Affect, imagery, and consciousness: Vol. 1. The positive affects.* New York: Springer.

Viscovich, N., Borod, J., Pihan, H., Peery, S., Brickman, A. M., Tabert, M., et al. (2003). Acoustical analysis of posed prosodic expressions: Effects of emotion and sex. *Perceptual and Motor Skills, 96*, 759-771.

von Bismarck, G. (1974). Sharpness as an attribute of the timbre of steady state sounds. *Acustica, 30*, 146-159.

Wagner, H. L. (1993). On measuring performance in category judgment studies of nonverbal behavior. *Journal of Nonverbal Behavior, 17*, 3-28.

Westermann, R., Spies, K., Stahl, G., & Hesse, F. W. (1996). Relative effectiveness and validity of mood induction procedures: A meta analysis. *European Journal of Social Psychology, 26*, 557-580.

Wundt, W. (1924). *An introduction to psychology* (R. Pintner, Trans.). London: Allen & Unwin. (Original work published in 1912).

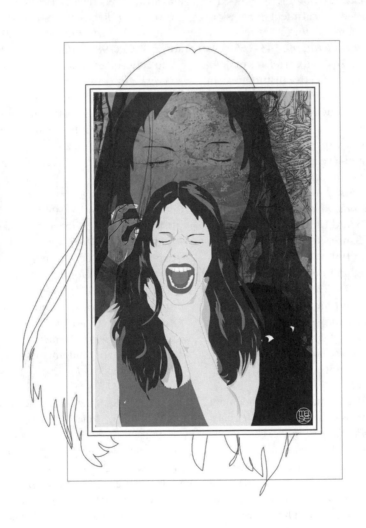

CHAPTER 12

The Role of Voice in the Expression and Perception of Emotions

Anne-Maria Laukkanen, Paavo Alku, Matti Airas, and Teija Waaramaa

Abstract

In this chapter we summarize the results of our series of investigations on the emotional expressivity of voice, mainly studied in terms of source characteristics, formant frequencies, and spectral slope of the speech sound. Perception of various simulated emotional samples was classified according to psychophysiological activation and valence inherent in the expressions. Voice source was parameterized among other parameters using a time-domain quantity, the normalized amplitude quotient (NAQ). Voice source varied significantly between the emotions expressed, and the variation was independent of F_0 and SPL variation.

NAQ was shown to reflect the activation dimension of the activation-evaluation space. The order of emotions in which the NAQ mean value changed from the smallest to the largest was anger, neutral, joy, sadness, and tenderness. This order was the same for both genders but the variation in NAQ values among all emotions was greater in females than in males.

Voice source parameters seem to be used for coding the activity level related to various emotional states, while higher formant frequencies, F2–F4, seem to be used for coding the valence of the emotion, being stereotypically higher in positive emotions. The type of glottal source also appears to affect the valence dimension of emotional expression, either reflecting knowledge of stereotypic voice production patterns in various emotions or through affecting the spectral slope and, thus, the prominence of formants. Gender differences are discussed.

Introduction

Voice characteristics can be studied on at least at three levels: physiological, acoustic, and perceptual. The number of vocal fold vibrations per second at the physiological level corresponds to the fundamental frequency (F_0) of the sound, which in turn corresponds (more or less directly) to the perceived pitch. Similarly, the amplitude of vocal fold vibrations varies in relation to sound pressure level (SPL) and to the perception of vocal loudness. The perceptual concept of *voice color* or *timbre* refers to the distribution of sound energy along the frequency scale at the physiological level. Physiologically, then, the voice colour is the combined result of the vibratory characteristics of the vocal folds and the articulatory setting of the vocal tract. The amplitude of vibration of the vocal folds correlates to the amplitude of the spectrum fundamental, and glottal closing time affects the spectral slope—that is, the relative strength of the overtones as compared to the amplitude of the fundamental (Fant, 1979; Gauffin & Sundberg, 1989). The positioning of the articulators together with the physiological properties

of the vocal tract determines the vocal tract resonances, the so-called formants. In addition, the closeness in frequency of sound components to each other contributes to the perceptual quality along the smooth/rough axis (see Sundberg, 1977).

Vibratory characteristics of the vocal folds are related both to F_0 and SPL and to phonation type as well as to the so-called register (Hanson, Gerratt, & Berke, 1990; Holmberg, Hillman, & Perkell, 1988; 1989; Kempster, Preston, Mack, & Larson, 1986; Kitzing & Sonesson, 1974; Sonesson, 1960; Timcke, von Leden, & Moore, 1958). Thus also, the energy distribution of the sound varies along these dimensions. The relative open time of the glottis tends to increase with F_0 and decrease as SPL rises. Furthermore, the relative open time is higher in falsetto register compared to modal ("chest") register. The relative closing time of the glottis is shorter and the closed time longer in modal register than in falsetto. The closing time typically decreases and closed time increases with SPL (Hanson et al., 1990; Holmberg et al., 1988; Holmberg, Hillman, Perkell, & Gress, 1994; Sonesson, 1960; Sundberg, Fahlstedt, & Morell, 2005; Sundberg, Scherer, & Titze, 1990).

The degree of adduction of the vocal folds in relation to subglottal pressure characterizes different phonation types along the axis of breathy phonation (low adduction), flow phonation (somewhat firmer adduction, better than normal voice quality, like an operatic singer's or a trained speaker's voice), normal phonation (still firmer adduction), and pressed or overpressed phonation in pathological cases (excessively high adduction) (Izdebski, 1984). The relative open and closing time of the glottis decreases when adduction rises. The spectral slope becomes steeper when closing time increases, and therefore the speech spectrum in falsetto declines faster than that in modal or pressed phonation. Increased glottal open time is related to prominence of the voice fundamental (e.g., Fant, 1993). Thus, in falsetto and breathy phonation, a more prominent fundamental is expected than in modal register or in normal or pressed phonation. (Gauffin & Sundberg, 1989; Izdebski, 1984). Moreover, the vocal tract impedance may modify the shape of the glottal flow pulse, and if the supralaryngeal impedance is sufficiently high compared to the laryngeal impedance, it may even enhance or impair the vibratory characteristics of the vocal folds (Müller, 1939; Titze, 1988). Vocal tract impedance is related to resonance frequencies, and it is highest at formant frequencies, especially at that of the first formant, F1. Changing the length or diameter of the vocal tract (for example, by raising or lowering the larynx, spreading or protruding the lips, or narrowing or widening the pharynx) modifies the vocal tract formants and the impedance.

In addition to the sound energy distribution along the frequency range, the voice quality may be defined to include such characteristics as the degree of aperiodicity in the signal (period-to-period changes in period length = jitter, or changes in amplitude = shimmer), which corresponds to the perception of clarity or harshness/roughness of the voice—or the degree of turbulent noise, which when excessively high adds a whispery component to the sound. Sufficiently wide and slow (over several periods) changes in F_0 or amplitude are perceived as trembling quality.

Acoustic Expression of Emotions

F_0, SPL, and temporal aspects of speech have been of primary interest in studying the expression of emotions (Murray & Arnott, 1993). Voice quality, in turn, has been so far studied to a lesser extent in relation to emotions even though its relevance to the field has been acknowledged already for a long time (Scherer, 1981; 1986). Some extensive studies (such as Banse & Scherer, 1996) also have included spectral parameters, which may be considered to portray some voice quality features. Laukkanen, Vilkman, Alku, and Oksanen (1995; 1997) studied the role of voice quality in conveyance of emotions in terms of glottal flow and formant frequencies. Some recent studies also address vocal expression of emotions from the point of view of voice quality and glottal flow characteristics (Airas & Alku, 2006; Gobl & Ní Chasaide, 2003; Waaramaa, Alku, & Laukkanen, 2006; Waaramaa, Laukkanen, Alku, Björkner, & Leino, 2007). Since studying voice quality typically involves inverse filtering, we will now discuss some of our inverse filtering studies on vocal emotions.

Inverse Filtering in the Study of Voice

Most studies on vocal fold vibration and glottal volume velocity waveform (referred to as glottal waveform from here on) have been performed using vowel phonations where either the F_0 or SPL has been kept constant. In contrast, only a few studies have investigated vocal fold vibration and glottal waveform during the production of normal speech and in the vocal communication of emotions, where F_0, SPL, and voice quality change simultaneously (Airas & Alku, in press; Childers & Lee, 1991; Cummings & Clements, 1990; Gobl & Ní Chasaide, 2003; Monsen, Engebretson, & Vemula, 1978; Pierrehumbert, 1989).

Laukkanen, Vilkman, Alku, and Oksanen (1996) addressed vocal parameters during production of sentence stress, simulating different emotional states. One male and two female subjects produced a nonsense utterance, [pa:p:a *pa*:p:a pa:p:a], simulating neutrality, surprise, sadness, enthusiasm, and anger, with the main stress placed on the italicized syllable. These emotional states were chosen because they may represent both high and low psychophysiological activity levels and positive and negative valences (surprise—low activity, positive valence, sadness—low activity, negative valence, enthusiasm—high activity, positive valence, anger—high activity, negative valence; see Murray & Arnott, 1993). Oral pressure during [p] was used as an estimate of subglottal pressure.

The utterances were 64–100% correctly identified in a listening test. Glottal waveform was estimated from the acoustic speech signal using the IAIF method (Alku, 1992). The time-based parameters speed quotient (SQ) and quasi-open quotient (QOQ), which characterize the glottal waveform, were measured from the inverse filtered signal (Timcke et al., 1958; Hacki, 1989, respectively).

Results showed that SQ and QOQ varied significantly between the emotions expressed. There was a significant emotional state-related glottal waveform variation also independently of F_0 level and SPL. Additionally, changes in subglottal (oral) pressure were not explicable in terms of changes in F_0 and SPL alone (Laukkanen et al., 1996). These findings suggest that the type of the glottal source was also used independently to express emotional states.

Based on these data a separate research project, focusing in particular on the role of the glottal flow in production of emotional speech, was conducted in the Helsinki University of Technology between 2003 and 2005 as a part of a larger consortium (for details, see Airas & Alku, in press; 2006). Speech data of this study were produced by nine professional stage actors (four females; aged between 26 and 45 years; all native speakers of Finnish) using five different emotions: neutral, sadness, joy, anger, and tenderness. These emotions were selected because they differ in the activation-evaluation space: sadness and tenderness have low activation, while joy and anger have high activation. Both sadness and anger have a negative valence, while the valence of joy and tenderness is positive. The category neutral stands for weak emotional expression and was assumed to have neutral valence and middle level of activation.

The actors read a text passage of Finnish prose (83 words) whose contents could be expressed easily using different emotions. The subjects were allowed to select freely the vocal means to express the emotion. Each emotion was simulated 10 times, in a random order given by the prompter. The recordings of the speech data, conducted in a radio anechoic chamber, were done with a condenser microphone (Brüel & Kjær 4188) placed at a distance of 50 cm from the speaker. Data were saved onto digital tapes with a DAT recorder (Sony DTC-690). Because estimation of the glottal flow with inverse filtering is most reliable for nonnasalized vowels with high first formant, three segments of vowel [a:] were cut from each recorded speech sample for further analyses. These selected segments were located in predefined positions at the beginning, middle, and end of each sample, and they were always surrounded by an unvoiced plosive or fricative.

Normalized Amplitude Quotient (NAQ) and Emotions

The estimation of the glottal flow was computed from the vowel segments using an inverse filtering method described in Alku (1992). The glottal flow waveforms obtained were expressed in numerical forms using the NAQ (Alku, Bäckström, & Vilkman, 2002). NAQ is a parameter that measures the characteristics of a glottal flow pulse during its most important phase, the closing phase of the cycle. NAQ quantifies the time-domain behavior of the glottal flow by using two amplitude domain values, the level of the maximum flow and the level of the negative peak amplitude of the flow derivative, which makes the parameter

straightforward to be extracted and robust against noise present in glottal flows estimated from natural speech. Similar to the widely used Closing Quotient (Holmberg et al., 1988; Alku & Vilkman, 1996), NAQ is a relative time-domain parameter where the time-length of the glottal closing phase is normalized with respect to the length of the fundamental period. NAQ has been shown to reflect time-domain features of the glottal flow both in different phonation types (Alku et al., 2002) and in different singing styles (Sundberg, Thalen, Alku, & Vilkman, 2004). In general, a large NAQ value corresponds to a smooth glottal flow pulse, which, for example, is used in production of soft voices or in breathy phonation. A small NAQ value, in turn, reflects shortening of the glottal closing phase, which typically corresponds to the use of a pressed phonation type or production of loud voices.

The behavior of the glottal flow in the analyzed five emotions is expressed with NAQ in Figure 12–1 for all the subjects as well as separately for females and males. Statistical analyses were computed with ANOVA and Tukey's honestly significant difference test. In general, ANOVA indicated that both emotion and gender had a statistically significant effect on NAQ ($p < 0.001$). When both of the genders were combined, the neutral emotion differed significantly from tenderness and sadness. For male subjects, however, the neutral emotion differed significantly only from tenderness. Likewise, joy differed significantly from anger, sadness, and tenderness when both genders were combined, but among males only from tenderness. Interestingly, joy exhibited the smallest minimum NAQ value, although it was the most centered emotion according to mean and median.

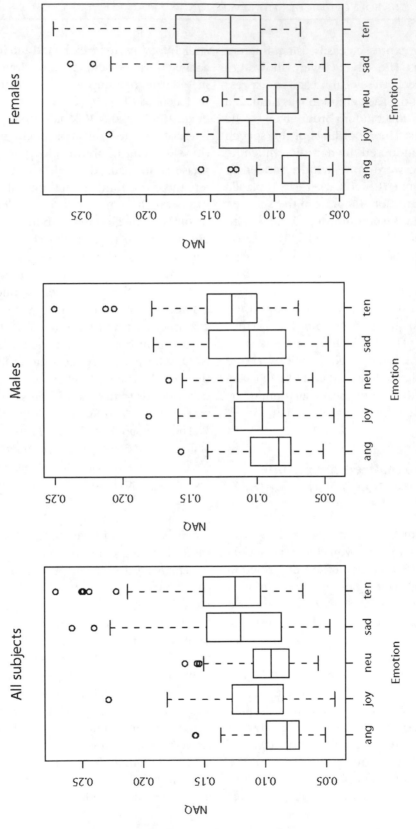

Figure 12–1. Box plots of NAQ values with regard to different genders and emotions.

Among all the emotions analyzed, NAQ values of sadness showed the highest standard deviation. Tenderness scored the highest NAQ value mean, and the standard deviation was nearly as large as in sadness. Tenderness alone differed significantly from anger, joy, and neutral emotions among both males and females.

The order of emotions in which the NAQ mean value changed from the smallest to the largest was anger, neutral, joy, sadness, and tenderness. This order was the same for both genders. Importantly, when comparing males and females, it could be noted that the variation in NAQ values among all emotions was greater in females than in males. In other words, the study indicates that females used larger glottal flow dynamics in production of different emotions than males. This gender difference is consistent with the findings that have been reported on the sending accuracy of the facial expression of emotions (Manstead, 1992).

The focus of the study by Airas and Alku (in press) was to assess whether NAQ varies with regard to different emotions. The results were promising in showing that estimation of the glottal flow from continuous speech can be used for analysis of emotional content of speech. Moreover, the selected glottal flow parameter, NAQ, was shown to reflect the activation dimension of the activation-evaluation space. While it appears that NAQ correlates well with emotional and voice quality changes, it has to be noted that it is only a single parameter and therefore cannot alone represent all the rich features embedded in vocal emotions. Further work is required to assess the relative importance of NAQ (and other similar glottal flow parameters) together with more traditional features such as F_0 and SPL.

Perceptual Evaluation of Emotional Sounds

Earlier results suggest that glottal waveform may be highly significant perceptually (Rosenberg, 1971; Childers, Yea, & Boccheri, 1985; Colton, 1982). Laukkanen et al. (1995) focused on the role of voice quality in the perception of emotions in speech in their earlier study. The first 200 ms of the main stress-carrying syllable of a nonsense utterance produced expressing neutral state, surprise, sadness, enthusiasm, and anger were played at equal sound volume to listeners. Surprise, sadness, and anger were best identified. When the differences in F_0 level were artificially eliminated, neutrality, surprise, and anger were still recognized. This seemed to be due to differences in intrasyllabic F_0 change and glottal waveform.

In a further study (Laukkanen et al., 1997), the differences in both F_0 level and the intrasyllabic F_0 changes were artificially eliminated and only the first 200 ms of the primarily stressed syllable replayed at equal sound volume to 10 listeners. Glottal waveform was estimated using the IAIF inverse filtering method (Alku, 1992). The listeners seemed to categorize the samples to represent emotions with either high or low psycholphysiological activity level. This seemed to be based on signs of vocal effort level in the signal. Significant correlations were found between perception of vocal effort and the glottal source characterizing parameters SQ and QOQ as well as F1. Valence of the perceived emotion was in this material significantly related to F1 and F4. The type of glottal source, however, also seemed to contribute to the perception of valence. Samples with moderate effort tended to be perceived as positive.

The Recent Tampere Studies

A series of studies of the role of various acoustic voice parameters on the perception of emotions was carried out in the University of Tampere during 2003–2005, partly related to the consortium mentioned in the previous section. The material consisted of vowel [a:] extracted from the prose samples recorded by nine professional actors simulating neutrality, joy, anger, sadness, and tenderness as well as [a: o: e:] produced on a single pitch by 14 student actors expressing love, anger, and sadness. Samples were analyzed for duration, F_0, SPL, jitter and shimmer, signal-to-noise (S/N) ratio, alpha ratio [SPL (1–5 kHz)—SPL (50 Hz–1 kHz)], formant frequencies F1–F4, and their relations to each other. The [a:] samples were inverse filtered and NAQ was calculated.

When the role of F_0 was excluded by using monopitch samples, F2 and F3 seemed to be of importance in the perception of valence (Waaramaa-Mäki-Kulmala, Laukkanen, & Leino, 2003; Waaramaa et al., 2007). According to the results by Waaramaa et al.(2006), semisynthetic [a:] samples with artificially 30% raised F3 were perceived more often as positive than the samples with original, artificially 30% lowered or removed F3. However, the results suggest that the role of F3 alone is not crucial in determining the perceived valence, and that also energy distribution in the spectra may have some importance in valence perception. This may reflect the fact that the type of glottal source determines the spectrum slope of the signal and therefore also the perceptual relevance of various formants. Figure 12–2 shows sound energy distribution in two vowel samples expressing

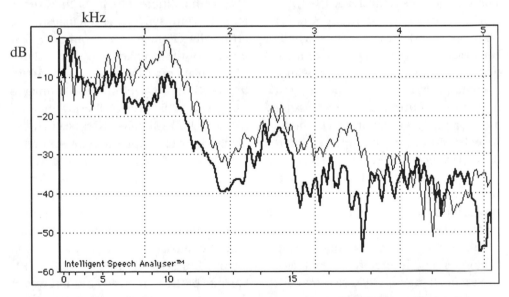

Figure 12–2. Long-term-average spectra of the vowel [a:] in tenderness (*thin line*) and in sadness (*thick line*) produced by a male actor. Horizontal lower axis: bark scale, upper axis: frequency in kHz. Vertical axis: relative amplitude in dB. Figure made with ISA (Intelligent Speech Analyser), a signal analysis system developed by Raimo Toivonen (M. Sc. Eng.).

sadness and tenderness. F4 is slightly higher in the sample of tenderness and the overall spectral slope is less steep, which is prone to make the voice quality brighter in general.

Discussion

On the basis of the studies reviewed here (Laukkanen et al. 1995; 1996; 1997; Airas & Alku, 2006; Waaramaa et al., 2006, Waaramaa et al., 2007), the glottal waveform seems to play a remarkable role in conveying emotional content of speech. After elimination of differences in F_0, SPL, and duration, samples were still perceived to signal some emotional states based on the characteristics of the glottal waveform and formant frequencies. Samples with low SQ and high QOQ reflecting low vocal effort level tended to be perceived as expressions of emotional states with low psychophysiological activity level, such as sadness, tenderness, or surprise (Laukkanen et al., 1997). Samples with high SQ and low QOQ, on the other hand, tended to be perceived as expressions of enthusiasm or anger.

These results of the expressive role of voice source are in accordance with the theory on *glottal mimicry* presented by Fónagy (1962). The basic dualism was not perfect, though. The subjects of the study by Laukkanen et al., 1997 perceived joy, fear, and sadness in samples with opposite glottal waveform characteristics. This is not likely to be just a sign of the listeners' insecurity in their judgments. Instead, it may illustrate the fact that emotional states and their expressions may take different forms depending on the vocalizer's evaluation of the situation.

For example, the subject may be depressive and acquiescent in sadness and fear and therefore use low activity level, or he or she may be full of grief and desire to change the negative situation, thus exploiting a high activity level.

Strength and activity level related to an emotion has been suggested to be mainly expressed by pitch, loudness, and duration, while valence of an emotion is assumed to be communicated by rhythm and voice quality (Murray & Arnott, 1993). In the study by Laukkanen et al., 1997, there was reasonable consistency between the intended and the perceived valence, suggesting that perception of valence has still been possible regardless of the elimination of F_0, SPL, and temporal differences between the samples, and the regression analysis suggested that only F1 and F4 (in vowel [a:]) had significant effect on the perception of valence. In further work by Waaramaa et al. (2007), F3 was found to have relevance in valence coding for specific vocalic back open unrounded to semiclosed rounded segments [a:, o:], while F2 seemed to play a role in open back-to-front semiopen unrounded [a:, e:] vocalic segments.

The experiments with semisynthetic material (Waaramaa et al., 2006) also suggested that F3 and spectral slope have some role in coding the valence. Similarly, Laukkanen et al., 1997 concluded that the voice source type seemed to affect the perception of valence. This is naturally to be expected because the voice source type, in turn, relates to the spectral slope. The findings of for instance Gobl and Ní Chasaide (2003) and Alku and Airas (in press) suggest that the pressed vocal quality (and thus also the steepness of the spectral slope) correlates with the emotion activation rather than valence.

Of interest to these findings is the evidence from Trojan (1952), who demonstrated an emotion/attitude-related covariation in the size of the pupil and the pharynx and the voice quality. Unpleasant experiences and resistance awakened by them related to a narrowing of the pupil and the pharynx and to the use of a tense voice (*Kraftstimme*; with increased adduction/pressure). Pleasant experiences, in turn, led to opposite physiological changes and a lax, tender voice quality (*Schonstimme*). This dualistic theory of *automatic rhythm* by Trojan can be challenged because it does not take into account that both tenderness and sorrow may obviously be expressed with low laryngeal effort and thus with little adduction and most likely with an open pharynx. On the other hand, it is tempting to postulate (on the basis of Laukkanen et al., 1997) a deeper relation between perceived effort and valence, based on estimation of vitality.

Low effort may be seen to reflect low vitality, which in turn may be a sign of a poor condition and therefore inherently judged as negative, while sufficiently high effort is related to good vitality, and therefore judged as positive. Too high an effort, in turn, may be already judged as a possible threat, and therefore it is given a negative valence. The results by Gobl and Ní Chasaide (2003) and Airas and Alku (2006), however, seem to be in conflict with this suggestion. NAQ may be low in neutral samples and high in positive.

In the experimental setup used by Waaramaa et al. (2007) the role of F_0 was eliminated by asking the subjects to produce pure monopitch voice samples. It is likely that when F_0 was preset the subjects (student actors) used other means of expression to compensate for the role of F_0. The results obtained for the mono-pitch samples were in line with those obtained by Laukkanen et al., 1997. SPL, alpha ratio, and NAQ seemed to be used to code the psychophysiological activity and formants F2– F4 to code valence.

According to Laukkanen et al., 1997, very low or very high F1 tended to be related to perceived negative valence, and contrastively high F3 and F4 seemed to be related to positive valence. The reason why high F1 would be related to negative valence is most likely the fact that in anger a high F1 (wide mouth opening) is used to raise SPL. Based on the fact that smiling increases all formant frequencies it can be expected that higher formant frequencies are related to positive valence of emotional states. This agrees with Sychra and Sedlacek (1970), who showed a correlation between brightness of the voice timbre (implying higher formant frequencies and possibly also a less tilting spectral slope) and joy, whereas grief correlated with darkness.

According to the theory of a frequency code (Ohala, 1983; 1984), which applies both to apes and humans, higher F_0 and formant frequencies are used to express positive, surrendering attitudes, whereas lower F_0 and formant frequencies signal threat and dominance. The rationale behind this behavior is the fact that bigger and thus more powerful creatures usually have lower F_0 and lower formant frequencies, while the opposite is true for smaller and less powerful creatures.

The artificial pitch-manipulation in Laukkanen et al. (1997) led to some samples with unintentionally crackling sound quality. Such samples were perceived more often as negative in valence. The presence of this crackling noise in the signal fits the findings of Sychra and Sedlacek (1970) and those of Blood, Mahan, and Hyman (1979). Sychra and Sedlacek (1970) showed a correlation between perceived joy and purity of voice, while grief, in turn, correlated with hoarseness and the emotion of anger with harshness. (More on the correlations of the pathologic voice quality and the perception of unintended emotions is discussed in Volume 2, Chapter 8.)

Blood et al. (1979) reported that voice disorders evoked more negative judgments of personality and appearance of the speaker than normal voices. It is possible that hoarse and harsh voice quality tend to elicit negative perception because strong emotions, especially negative ones like fear or anger, may result in a hoarse voice quality, as they may impair the laryngeal control. This has profound implications on vocal interaction in social settings of patients with various types of dysphonias (Izdebski, 2006).

The perception of emotional states of vocal expressions is obviously a complex task implying an unconscious multifactor analysis of various characteristics. Because communication of emotions is of great importance for survival and for daily social life, expression of emotions must contain much redundancy. Consequently, many vocal cues can be eliminated and still perception of some emotional states or at least the valence of the emotion, if not the emotion itself, is possible. The results of, for example, Lieberman and Michaels (1962) already suggested this. The results obtained by Laukkanen et al. (1995 and 1997) and Waaramaa et al. (2007) confirm the suggestion.

Conclusions

Voice source parameters seem to be used for coding the activity level related to various emotional states, while higher formant frequencies, F2–F4, seem to be used for coding the valence of the emotion. The type of glottal source also appears to affect the valence dimension of emotional expression, either reflecting knowledge of stereotypic voice production patterns of various emotions or affecting the spectral slope and, thus, the prominence of formants.

References

Airas M, Alku P. (2006). Emotions in vowel segments of continuous speech: Analysis of the glottal flow using the normalised amplitude quotient. *Phonetica, 63*, 26–46.

Alku, P. (1992). Glottal wave analysis with Pitch Synchronous Iterative Adaptive Inverse Filtering. *Speech Communication, 11*, 109–118.

Alku, P., Bäckström, T., & Vilkman, E. (2002). Normalized amplitude quotient for parameterization of the glottal flow. *Journal of the Acoustical Society of America, 112*, 701–710.

Alku, P., & Vilkman, E. (1996). A comparison of glottal voice source quantification parameters in breathy, normal, and pressed phonation of female and male speakers. *Folia Phoniatrica et Logopaedica, 48*, 240–254.

Banse, R., & Scherer, K. R. (1996). Acoustic profiles in vocal emotion expression. *Journal of Personality and Social Psychology, 70*, 614–636.

Blood, G. W., Mahan, B. W., & Hyman, M. (1979). Judging personality and appearance from voice disorders. *Journal of Communication Disorders, 12*, 63–68.

Childers, D. G., & Lee, C. K. (1991). Vocal quality factors: Analysis, synthesis and perception. *Journal of the Acoustical Society of America, 90*, 2394–2410.

Childers, D. G., Yea, J. J., & Boccheri, E. L. (1985, July). *Source/vocal-tract interaction in speech and singing synthesis*. Paper presented at the Stockholm Music Acoustic Conference, Sweden.

Colton, R. H. (1982). Discrimination of glottal waveform variations. In V. L. Lawrence (Ed.), *Transcripts of the 11th Symposium Care of Professional Voice, Part 1: Scientific Papers* (pp. 61–68). New York: The Voice Foundation.

Cummings, K. E., & Clements, M. A. (1990, April). *Analysis of glottal waveforms across stress styles*. Paper presented at the International Conference on Acoustics, Speech and Signal Processing, Albuquerque, New Mexico.

Fant, G. (1979). Glottal source and excitation analysis. *Speech Transmission Laboratory, Quarterly Progress and Status Report, 1*, 85–107.

Fant, G. (1993). Some problems in voice source analysis. *Speech Communication, 13*, 7–22.

Fónagy, I. (1962). Mimik auf glottaler Ebene. *Phonetica, 8*, 209–219.

Gauffin, J., & Sundberg, J. (1989). Spectral correlates of glottal voice sourcewaveform characteristics. *Journal of Speech and Hearing Research, 32*, 556–565.

Gobl, C., & Ní Chasaide, A. (2003). The role of voice quality in communicating emotion, mood and attitude. *Speech Communication, 40*, 189–212.

Hacki, T. (1989). Klassifizierung von Glottisdysfunktionen mit Hilfe der Elektroglottographie. *Folia Phoniatrica et Logopaedica, 41*, 43–48.

Hanson, D. G., Gerratt, B. R., & Berke, G. S. (1990). Frequency, intensity and target matching effects on photoglottographic measures of open quotient and speed quotient. *Journal of Speech and Hearing Research, 33*, 45–50.

Holmberg, E. B., Hillman, R. E., & Perkell, J. S. (1988). Glottal airflow and transglottal air pressure measurements for male and female speakers in soft, normal and loud voice. *Journal of the Acoustical Society of America, 84*, 511–529.

Holmberg, E. B., Hillman, R. E., & Perkell, J. S. (1989). Glottal airflow and transglottal air pressure measurements for male and female speakers in low, normal and high pitch. *Journal of Voice, 3*, 294–305.

Holmberg, E. B., Hillman, R. E., Perkell, J. S., & Gress, C. (1994). Relationships between intra-speaker variation in aerodynamic measures of voice production and variation in SPL across repeated recordings. *Journal of Speech and Hearing Research, 37*, 484–495.

Izdebski, K. (1984). Overpressure and breathiness in spastic dysphonia. An acoustic (LTAS) and perceptual study. *Acta Otolaryngolica Scandinavia, 97*, 122–129.

Izdebski, K. (2007). Pathologic phonation connotes and evokes wrong emotive reactions in listeners. Chapter 8, Volume 2, in K. Izdebski. *The emotions of the human voice* . San Diego, CA: Plural Publishing.

Kempster, G., Preston, J., Mack, R., & Larson, C. (1986). A preliminary investigation relating laryngeal muscle activity to changes in EGG waveform. In T. Baer, C. Sasaki, & K. S. Harris (Eds.), *Vocal fold physiology: Laryngeal function in phonation and respiration* (pp. 339–348). San Diego, CA: College-Hill Press.

Kitzing, P., & Sonesson, B. (1974). A photoglottographical study of the female vocal folds during phonation. *Folia Phoniatrica et Logopaedica, 26*, 138–149.

Laukkanen, A.-M., Vilkman, E., Alku, P., & Oksanen, H. (1995, August). On the perception of emotional content in speech. In K. Elenius & P. Branderud (Eds.), *Proceedings of the XIIIth International Congress of Phonetic Sciences* (Vol. 1, pp. 246–249). Stockholm, Sweden: Stockholm University.

Laukkanen, A.-M., Vilkman, E., Alku, P., & Oksanen, H. (1996). Physical variations related to stress and emotional state: A preliminary study. *Journal of Phonetics. 24*, 313–335.

Laukkanen, A.-M., Vilkman, E., Alku, P., & Oksanen, H. (1997). On the perception of emotions in speech: The role of voice quality. *Logopedics Phoniatrics Vocology, 22*, 157–168.

Lieberman, P., & Michaels, S. B. (1962). Some aspects of fundamental frequency and envelope amplitude as related to the emotional content of speech. *Journal of the Acoustical Society of America*, 7, 922-927.

Manstead, A. S. R. (1992). *Handbook of individual differences: Biological perspectives.* Chichester, UK: Wiley.

Monsen, R. B., Engebretson, A. M., & Vemula, N. R. (1978). Indirect assessment of the contribution of subglottal air pressure and vocal-fold tension to changes of fundamental frequency in English. *Journal of the Acoustical Society of America*, 64, 65-80.

Müller, E. (1939). Über den Einfluss von Ansatz- und Windrohr auf die Stimmlippenbewegung eines Kehlkopfmodelles. *Archiv für Sprach- und Stimmphysiologie*, 3, 1-28.

Murray, I. R., & Arnott, J. L. (1993). Toward the simulation of emotion in synthetic speech: A review of the literature on human vocal emotion. *Journal of the Acoustical Society of America*, 93, 1097-1108.

Ohala, J. J. (1983). Cross-language use of pitch: An ethological view. *Phonetica*, 40, 1-18.

Ohala, J. J. (1984). An ethological perspective on cross-language utilization of F_0 in the voice. *Phonetica*, 41, 1-16.

Pierrehumbert, J. B. (1989). A preliminary study of the consequences of intonation for the voice source. *Speech Transmission Laboratory, Quarterly Progress and Status Report*, 4, 23-36.

Rosenberg, A. E. (1971). Effect of glottal pulse shape on the quality of natural vowels. *Journal of the Acoustical Society of America*, 49, 583-590.

Scherer, K. R. (1981). Speech and emotional states. In J. Darby (Ed.), *Speech evaluation in psychiatry* (pp. 189-203). New York: Grune & Stratton.

Scherer, K. R. (1986). Vocal affect expression: A review and a model for future research. *Psychological Bulletin*, 99, 143-165.

Sonesson, B. (1960). On the anatomy and vibratory pattern of the human vocal folds. With special reference to a photoelectrical method for studying the vibratory movements. *Acta Otolaryngologica* (Suppl. 156),.

Sundberg, J. (1987). The science of he singing voice. Illinois: ,Northern University Press.

Sundberg, J., Fahlstedt, E., & Morell, A. (2005). Effects on the glottal voice source of vocal loudness variation in untrained female and male voices. *Journal of the Acoustical Society of America*, 117, 879-885.

Sundberg, J., Scherer, R., & Titze, I. (1990). Phonatory control in male singing. A study of the effects of subglottal pressure, fundamental frequency and mode of phonation on the voice source. *Speech Transmission Laboratory, Quarterly Progress and Status Report*, 4, 59-79.

Sundberg, J., Thalen, M., Alku, P., & Vilkman, E. (2004). Measuring perceived phonatory pressedness in singing from flow glottograms. *Journal of Voice*, 18, 56-62.

Sychra, A., & Sedlacek, K. (1970). *Relations between the acoustic, articulatory and psychological parameters of the emotional expressions in speech*. Paper presented at the 6th International Congress of Phonetic Sciences, Prague, Czechoslovakia.

Timcke, R., von Leden, H., & Moore, P. (1958). Laryngeal vibrations: Measurements of the glottic wave. *AMA Archives of Otolaryngology*, 68, 1-19.

Titze, I. R. (1988). A framework for the study of vocal registers. *Journal of Voice*, 3, 183-194.

Trojan, F. (1952). Experimentelle Untersuchungen uber den Zusammenhang zwischen dem Ausdruck der Sprechstimme und dem vegetativen Nervensystem. *Folia Phoniatrica et Logopaedica*, 4, 65-92.

Waaramaa, T., Alku, P., & Laukkanen, A.-M. (2006). The role of F3 in the vocal expression of emotions. *Logopedics, Phoniatrics, Vocology, 31*(4), 153-156.

Waaramaa, T., Laukkanen, A.-M, Alku, P., Björkner, E., & Leino, T. (2007). Perception of emotions in mono-pitched vowels. In L. Rantala (Ed.), *Kuormittumista, koulutusta, kuntoutusta. Kirjoituksia vokologiasta ja logopediasta.* [Vocal loading, training, rehabilitation. Studies in vocology and logopedics.] Puheopin laitoksen raportteja 5/2007. Tampereen yliopisto, pp. 74–99. [Reports of the Department of Speech Communication and Voice Research, University of Tampere, Tampere, Finland.]

CHAPTER 13

Universality and Diversity in the Vocalization of Emotions

Jörg Zinken, Monja Knoll, and Jaak Panksepp

Introduction

There is no doubt that prosodic channels play an important part in emotional communication (Bachorowski & Owren, 1995; Frick, 1985; Viscovich et al., 2003). A relationship between emotional experiences and acoustic properties of vocalization was already suggested by Darwin (1872), and it finds support from primate research (Jürgens, 2006).

The aim of this paper is to discuss universals in the vocal expression of emotion. In particular, we will share perspectives on the theoretical modeling of *universality* and *diversity* underlying research in this field. Our analysis will be based on diverse lines of evidence emerging from an increasingly substantial body of empirical research. Results from this research show an ambiguous picture, but they are most frequently

interpreted as confirmation for the existence of universal mechanisms in the vocal communication of emotions. This research, briefly summarized in the first section, provides the background for discussions in the remainder of the chapter. In the second section, we scrutinize the notions of universality and diversity framing much of the current debate. In particular, we argue that misleading juxtapositions of universality versus diversity still seem to underlie the design and interpretation of empirical studies. Proposals for an alternative framing of universality and diversity are provided in the third section. In particular, we argue that universals of different types of affect vocalization need to be studied within their respective semiotic systems. The *symptomatic* communication of raw affect can be studied to discover evolved acoustic action patterns. Such patterns are continuous across species, and universal

185

across human communities. However, research into the cross-cultural recognizability of emotion from the voice has used speech stimuli obtained by asking speakers (mostly professional actors) to *pose* various emotions. Such *iconic* communication of affect can be studied as an aspect of advanced sign use in humans. Such sign use is diverse across cultures, but becomes universal in histories of engagement. In the fourth section, we discuss new questions that such a perspective brings into view, and we close with a set of conclusions in the fifth section.

Universality and Diversity in the Vocalization of Emotions: An Overview of Empirical Research

Results from Cross-Cultural Recognition Studies

The vocal expression of emotions has not received nearly as much attention as the facial expression of emotions. This is all the more true for analysis of universality and diversity in the vocal expression of emotions. Nevertheless, there is now a growing body of empirical research addressing these questions, including meta-analyses (Elfenbein & Ambady, 2002; Juslin & Laukka, 2003).[1]

Empirical research on the universality of vocal expression of emotions has largely focused on the ability of raters to recognize emotions expressed in speech samples produced by a member of a different culture (e.g., Albas, McCluskey, & Albas, 1976; Bezooijen, Otto, & Heenan, 1983; Scherer, Banse, & Wallbott, 2001).[2,3] Recognition studies consistently show an ambiguous picture. Virtually all studies report that emotions are recognized from voice with above-chance accuracy across cultures (Elfenbein & Ambady, 2002). At the same time, all studies show that the accuracy of recognition decreases with the cultural distance between the speaker and the rater (Elfenbein & Ambady, 2002; Scherer et al., 2001).

These results have received widely differing interpretations, depending on whether the authors were interested in universality or in diversity. For example, Scherer and his colleagues (Scherer, 1999a; 1999b; Scherer et al., 2001) tend to interpret the literature as providing support for the existence of a universal core of mechanisms for inferring emotions from the voice. Beside the fact that emotions are recognized with above-chance accuracy across cultures, they have found a similarity in confusion patterns. For example, the vocal expression of fear by a German-speaking actor was most frequently mistaken for sadness rather than any other emotion by both

---

[1]In most cases, cross-cultural studies of emotion recognition identify language with culture, so that the contrasted "cultural" groups are defined by the native languages. However, this is not always the case. In some studies, *culture* has been defined ethnically or geographically (Elfenbein & Ambady, 2002). The results have been similar to those where cross-linguistic diversity was studied. For example, Australian speakers of English were worse than American speakers of English at recognizing emotions from the voice of an American speaker.

[2]These studies aim to investigate people's ability to *recognize* emotion from voice. However, given the design of these studies, which require participants to choose an emotion from a list of alternatives, it seems more appropriate to interpret the results as indicating an ability to *discriminate* between emotions (Frick, 1985).

[3]The study of recognition of emotions bears parallels with the extensive literature on basic color terms using Munsell color chips: participants are asked to apply a local label to an array of foreign stimuli. It has been argued that this methodology produces rather than uncovers conceptual universals (Saunders, 1995).

German and Indonesian raters (Scherer et al., 2001).

However, the same results also indicate a systematic relation between cultural proximity and accuracy of emotion recognition. Notably, vocal expression of emotion by German-speaking actors in the study by Scherer and colleagues (2000) was recognized most accurately by speakers of German, less accurately by speakers of other Germanic languages (Dutch, English), less accurately still by speakers of other Indo-European languages (French, Italian), and least accurately by speakers of the only non-Indo-European language included, Bahasa Indonesia.[4] Although Indonesian raters still achieved above-chance accuracy, their accuracy rates were significantly lower than those of the German-speaking participants. Some evidence also suggests that the similarity in confusion patterns decreases with linguistic-cultural distance between speakers and raters. In a study on emotion recognition from the voice of English speakers by English, Spanish, and Japanese raters, the confusions in the judgments by Spanish speakers were similar to those of English raters, whereas those of Japanese raters were more dissimilar (Graham, Hamblin, & Feldstein, 2001).

The diversity evident from these studies becomes even more interesting when we take into account that the languages and cultures studied so far are not actually very diverse. For example, the most extensive cross-linguistic study in this area seems to be Scherer et al. (2001), who asked speakers of seven languages from nine countries to rate the emotions expressed in voice samples produced by German-speaking actors. However, of the seven languages included, six were Indo-European languages. With approximately 6000 languages currently spoken around the globe, this is hardly a representation of actual linguistic diversity, and it is unclear what conclusions about universality can be drawn from such a narrow and relatively homogeneous sample of languages.

Furthermore, only a few specific emotions have been studied systematically, and these usually relate to the different extant proposals regarding "basic" emotions. If universal mechanisms exist that guide the recognition of emotion from voice, or the vocal expression of emotion, these should surely exist for basic emotions. Given this restriction to a few basic emotions, the ambiguity of the results from recognition studies seems quite surprising. We would not expect such a result if the vocal expression of these emotions was itself grounded in universal mechanisms.[5]

An interpretation de-emphasising universal mechanisms might suggest that what these results show is the degree of familiarity of raters with the speaker's

---

[4]The only exception from this genetic trend was French-speaking Swiss, who achieved better recognition rates than speakers of Germanic languages (Dutch, English). The authors suggest that this is because of the fact that most Swiss speakers of French have some knowledge of German. More specifically, we would argue that it is the communication histories between French-speaking and German-speaking Swiss that leads to this result; cf. section The Relation between Universality and Diversity: A Systems Model.

[5]Indeed, when humans are asked to express a single word, such as *mom* or any other single-syllable word in four basic emotional intonations (happy, sad, angry, and scared), the forced choice emotional detection rate approaches 100% in American students (greater than 90% in four separate studies, Panksepp, 1985–1991, unpublished data). However, such emotional sounds could not be distinguished from EEG recordings from the cortical surface processed with sophisticated Event Related Desynchronization signal-detection algorithms, probably because the recording sites were far from the source generators (Panksepp, 2000).

culture. This notion is also supported by a much earlier study that was concerned with the effects of familiarity on the enhancement of emotion recognition within the same culture (Hornstein, 1967). It was found that the prosodic emotional communication between compatible college roommates improved during the first 3 months of living together. In contrast, incompatible roommates' emotional communication did not improve. In the remainder of the article, we will argue that recognition studies utilizing posed emotions can address such "developing universals," but not evolved universal "mechanisms."

Results from Cross-Cultural Studies on Infant-Directed Speech

Another area that has sought to combine research into prosody and emotional responsivity is that of speech directed to infants (e.g., Burnham, Kitamura, & Vollmer-Conna, 2002; Fernald, 1989; Fernald & Simon, 1984; Kuhl, 1994). The prosody of infant-directed speech (IDS) has been extensively analyzed and is characterized by higher pitch, exaggerated pitch contours, hyperarticulation of vowels, shorter utterances, and longer pauses (Burnham et al., 2002; Fernald & Simon, 1984; Stern, Spieker, Barnett, & MacKain, 1983; Trainor, Austin, & Desjardins, 2000). Independent raters of such speech perceived high positive emotional affect (Burnham et al., 2002; Kitamura & Burnham, 2003). These prosodic modifications are generally assumed to be universal, and several cross-cultural studies have found support for this (e.g., Fernald al, 1989; Kuhl, 2000; Scherer et al., 2001).

As a large proportion of research into IDS deals with the analysis of natural interactions, specific emotions (e.g., happiness, sadness) have rarely been addressed; instead content-filtered speech samples are normally rated for generalized emotional affect (such as positive, negative). What makes IDS an extremely relevant case study for the discussion of the expression of vocal emotion is the prelinguistic stage of the infant. This vocal expression of emotion toward infants is only possible through the modification of prosodic channels, as the lexical content of IDS is presumably not understood at this developmental stage. A second reason why we have decided to include IDS in this discussion is the fundamental assumption of universality in this area.

This viewpoint of universality is often maintained regardless of the fact that differences are apparent across cultures. For instance, differences were found in the way mothers express vocal affect between Australian English and Thai (Kitamura, Thanavishuth, Burnham, & Luksaneeyanawin, 2002). Thai is a tonal language, in which pitch is used to convey lexical meaning. Kitamura et al. (2002) found that Thai mothers compared to Australian English mothers restricted their pitch excursions in order to not disrupt tonal information. The authors concluded that instead of using heightened pitch to convey emotional affect as found in the English speaking mothers, Thai mothers may use different vocal characteristics (final particles to express mood and status) and maybe increased affective linguistic content.

Similarly, pitch contours in Mandarin Chinese (another tonal language) IDS are less exaggerated than in American

English IDS and are more similar to adult-directed speech (ADS) in Mandarin Chinese (Papousek & Hwang, 1991). This study also compared both IDS and ADS to foreign-directed speech (FDS), and interestingly found that Mandarin Chinese FDS had more exaggerated pitch contours than both IDS and ADS. In contrast to this, British English mothers' FDS does not show the same exaggerated pitch contours, and was found to be more similar to ADS, while IDS exhibited exaggerated pitch contours (Knoll, Walsh, MacLeod, O'Neill, & Uther, 2007). This shows that exaggerated pitch contours in tonal languages might have a different, more linguistic function compared to the nontonal languages, and we can therefore not assume that these acoustic features per se are indices of certain emotional states across all cultures. Many more examples of these slight but important differences in prosodic modifications across cultures in IDS exist. Japanese IDS has lower, less exaggerated pitch values than American IDS, but this is obviated by a higher affective linguistic content (Toda, Fogel, & Kawai, 1990; Viscovich et al., 2003). Another language that also exhibits lower pitch values in IDS but higher pitch values in ADS is Quiche (Mayan language, Bernstein Ratner & Pye, 1984). The authors explained their findings in terms of the utilization of pitch as an indication of status rather than affect.

The important aspect here is first that IDS shows slight differences in prosodic modifications across cultures, and that universality of the vocal expression of emotions per se can therefore not be completely maintained. We also suggest that prosodic modifications, regardless of how they are perceived by independent raters, might have a variety of different functions. For instance, in the case of the British English FDS, raters perceived low-pass filtered speech samples of FDS as more negative than ADS despite similar pitch contours and pitch values. The only difference that was found between those two speech conditions was the aforementioned hyperarticulation of vowels, which should have a linguistic but not an emotional function (Knoll & Uther, 2004). The research into IDS shows that regardless of features held in common in IDS across cultures, there are also differences that cannot be discounted and which would require an alternative, less simplistic explanation than the common universality versus diversity debate can offer.

The Relation between Universality and Diversity: Linear Models

Similarities and differences are both evident in the recognition of vocal expressions of emotion across cultures. This has been interpreted as showing that the vocal expression of emotions itself has both cross-culturally universal and diverse facets. Similarly, the acoustic properties of IDS show both similarities and differences across cultures. It seems then that instead of asking whether emotional expression is universal or diverse we should ask questions about the relationship between universality and diversity in emotional expression. This statement seems to be uncontentious and is endorsed so commonly in the introduction sections of research articles (e.g., Scherer et al., 2001) that it might even seem like a "shallow platitude" (Ellsworth, 1994).

However, explicit metatheoretical discussions of what we imagine the relation between universality and diversity to be are comparatively sparse (Manstead & Fischer, 2002).

We will argue in this section that the relation between universality and diversity has been modeled, more implicitly than explicitly, as the two poles of a single continuum.[6] This model is evident in the conviction underlying much of the empirical literature that if we find similarities in behavior across raters, then this will diminish the existence or at least the relevance of diversity. It is evident, conversely, in the argument that if we can illustrate diversity across cultures, then this decreases the convincingness, or relevance, of theories assuming the existence of universals. These *if-then* arguments are only valid if we can think of the truth about the expression of emotions as a point moving between the two poles on a continuum, or between two scales, so that an increase in universality necessarily decreases diversity and vice versa. A continuum model is also evident in some interpretations of differences in the recognizability of different emotions. For example, van Bezooijen and colleagues found that some emotions, such as sadness, were fairly well recognized from the voice across cultures, whereas others, such as joy, were relatively poorly recognized (Bezooijen et al., 1983). They concluded that some emotions are expressed in culturally specific ways, whereas others are universally expressed in the same way; in other words, emotions can fall on different places along a universality-diversity continuum.

A continuum model is evident also in the way universality and diversity may come together in the *process* of the vocal expression of emotions. This process is sometimes imagined as a sequential motion along the continuum, as represented in Figure 13-1.

The basic opposition between a universal and a diverse pole is here supplemented with a vertical metaphor: the evaluation of diverse practices being a surface behavior that is initiated by universal underlying mechanisms. The vocal expression of emotion is imagined to be initiated by universal evolved mecha-

---

[6]The figures discussed in this section are not intended as reconstructions of anybody's explicit theoretical views. Rather, they are meant as reconstructions of the nontechnical models and assumptions that underlie explicit scientific thinking (Black, 1962).

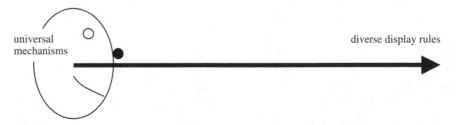

Figure 13–1. The expression of emotions as a sequence from universal to local steps.

nisms. In a second step, this expression is adapted to local, potentially diverse, display rules. This sequential model is evident, for example, in Scherer's metaphors of *push* and *pull* effects. Physiological changes in the organism constitute the push effects that initiate a vocal expression of emotion. Pull effects subsequently work on this expression to "suppress," "amplify," or "modify" it according to local display rules (Scherer, 1999b).

This model is also evident in the historical development of a division of labor between academic disciplines in the study of the expression of emotions. Much of the psychological literature treats the interest in diversity of emotional expression as belonging to the realm of anthropology and ethnology, which study local practices of showing emotions. Psychologists, on the other hand, have identified their subject as the universal mechanisms of emotion expression, which are thought of as an evolved potential that is itself universally shared across cultures, and possibly across species.

Accordingly, the interest in universality and the interest in diversity are effectively conceptualized as two distinct enterprises concerned with the different ends of the continuum. Interest in universality goes with a focus on evolved mechanisms, and interest in diversity goes with a focus on local practice. These views can be brought together by considering universality and diversity on different levels of generality. For example, the intrinsic capacities for infant musicality can lead to a host of culture specific learning principles that help weave a child into its local social ecology (Trevarthen, 2000).

Nevertheless, many authors still frame the debate as concerning universality *versus* diversity (e.g., Elfenbein & Ambady,

2002; Scherer, 2000), even when they explicitly acknowledge the importance of accommodating *both* universality and diversity. It seems that the research traditions of being either interested primarily in universals or in diversity are so strong that they still frame the current debate.

The continuum model can account for the empirical findings in the sense that it is able to incorporate both universality and diversity. However, this does not make it an appropriate model, and we will now consider that there are some problems associated with it. The model suggests that we can uncover universally evolved mechanisms of vocal emotion expression by identifying areas of overlap in the behavior (mostly recognition behavior) of members of different cultures. Those emotions for which we can find satisfying degrees of overlap (whatever these are) are emotions for which universal mechanisms of vocal expression exist. We have stripped away the diversity and identified the universal core.

We believe that this research strategy is not justified as long as intentional emotion portrayals are used. The reason is that intentional vocal communication and vocal affect bursts belong to two different semiotic systems (Borod, 2000). Affective vocalizations shared across species, which can be described as evolved universal mechanisms, belong to a symptomatic system. Posed emotion portrayals, on the other hand, require advanced abilities of sign use and belong to an iconic system. Both systems have their universals, but the relation between overlap in behavior in one system, and the structure and functions of the other system, is not as straightforward as the continuum model suggests. We will elaborate on this contention in the next section.

The Relation between Universality and Diversity: A Systems Model

In this section, we want to spell out an alternative model of the relation between universal and diverse factors in the vocal expression of emotions, represented in Figure 13–2. Again, this figure is not intended as a technical model, but as a figurative handle for the following discussion. In particular, we do not suggest, as it might seem from the figure: (a) that affect bursts occur independently of context; (b) that evolved universals are independent of evolving universals.

The gist of this model is that it separates affect burst behavior (the affective system) from intentional communicative behavior (the communicative system). Evolved mechanisms implicated in vocal bursts of emotion are part of the ancient affective systems that humans share with other primates and possibly other mammals (Panksepp & Bernatzky, 2002). There is presently little doubt that there are intrinsic emotional-vocal control mechanisms in the mammalian brain, with a great deal of cross-species coherence (Hauser, 1996; Jürgens, 1998). Vocal communication of emotions builds on the acoustics of affect bursts, but universality of such communication cannot be attributed to, and should not be sought in, just evolved mechanisms. In what follows we present this argument in more detail, discussing universality first in the affective system, and then in the communicative system.

Affect Vocalizations as Evolved Action Systems: Figure 13–2(a)

Emotional vocalizations occurring in all mammals can be described as evolved action systems (Panksepp, 1982; 2005). It would seem that such vocalizations, indicative of affective states experienced by other mammals, should also be a natural part of the vocal repertoire of the human species. These action systems would be part of what Scherer calls push effects.

Affective vocalizations might not so much relate to cognitive aspects of emo-

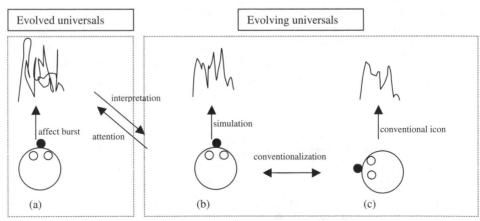

Figure 13–2. Systems model of the vocal expression of emotion.

tions such as anger or happiness, but rather to fundamental affective states that are part and parcel of motivational arousals shared by many species, states that we can refer to in English with words such as being enraged, joyous, cold, lustful, etc. (Panksepp, 2005). Of course, the terms of a particular language might be associated with various evaluations, expectations, or action "scripts" (Wierzbicka, 1991) that might be quite specific to that language. Nevertheless, we believe that many of the raw feelings that exist beyond words are shared across human cultures and across species. It is the symptomatic vocal expression of fundamental affective states, rather than the iconic vocal communication of emotions, that we would expect to exhibit similarities in acoustic properties across cultures (Juslin & Laukka, 2003; Panksepp & Bernatzky, 2002).

The recognizability of such raw emotional sounds is also reasonable from the point of view that certain emotional (or affective) states are associated with distinct physiological changes such as increased muscle tension and sympathetic arousal. For instance, tension in both the respiratory and laryngeal muscles can lead to louder and higher pitched speech (Frick, 1985). These physiological changes would presumably occur cross-culturally during the expression of certain affective states if these were accompanied by increased muscle tension and subsequent sympathetic arousal.

The existence of intrinsic brains circuits for a variety of basic emotions, which can yield vocal outputs (Jürgens, 1998), from essentially the same subcortical brain regions in all mammalian species that have been studied (Newman, 1988) provides powerful testimony for the existence of intrinsic emotional vocal control in all mammals. Perhaps the most compelling example is the squeal of pain. However, one critical question is whether these sounds are communicatory or merely by-products of emotional expressions.

There is increasing animal data that many of these sounds do contribute to communication and infection of emotional states among interacting animals. For instance, happy laughter type 50 kHz chirps in rats facilitate social and sexual choices (Burgdorf & Panksepp, 2006), and 22 kHz distress calls reduce the likelihood that colony members will leave burrows to explore and forage. The infantile separation-distress vocalizations in many species motivate maternal retrieval and attention, and hence have clear survival value (Panksepp, 2003). It is not hard to imagine that such emotional sounds, even after enculturation, will still have distinct kinds of emotional impact even in highly encephalized species where learned display rules tend to override instinctual ones. Indeed, it does remain possible that the roots of cultural practices such as musical expressions of emotions still rely on our capacities for making and appreciating intrinsic emotional sounds (Panksepp & Bernatzky, 2002) as our capacity to mold such raw materials into complex communications through the engines of culture.

Symptomatic vocalizations might be difficult to study in humans. One reason for this is the methodological difficulty of using words relating to complex categories such as *joy* or *sadness* in an attempt to study nonlinguistic affective states. Another reason is that human societies seem to impose constraints on the expression of affective states, so that humans, at least adults, have a tendency to cover up these states to make their vocal expressions socially acceptable (cf. Scherer's notion of pull effects). The final usage or contribution of these acoustic cues to the communication of emotions would differ depending on cultural conventionalization processes, which could be very diverse, depending on how different cultures viewed the propriety and usefulness of emotional frankness.

Societal restrictions in the form of display rules are therefore one factor in the development of diversity. However, such social expectations are not the only, and probably not the fundamental, factor that leads to a diversity of vocal expression of emotions across cultures. The influence of society on human behavior is not a purely negative, constraining one. Rather, the motive for communication itself leads people to modify their voice, as we will argue in the following sections. Thus, as soon as intentionality becomes part of communication, diversity begins to impose new levels of complexity upon universality.

Attention to and Interpretation of Natural Signs (Symptoms): Figure 13–2(b) and (c)

Whereas the ancient affective action systems that produce affect bursts are very hard to study in the human species, this is not the case for the acoustic percept that an affect burst produces. The cognitive significance of vocal expression of emotion lies in the fact that the expression can be attended to and so itself becomes an input into cognitive processes (Jackendoff, 1996). When the acoustic percept produced in an affect burst is attended to, either by the producing organism itself or by another, we leave the system of affect burst behavior, and intrinsic communication, and enter the systems of intentional communicative behavior.

As a communicative process, the vocal expression of an emotional state is not the endpoint, but rather the starting point. It has been implicitly assumed in the research that others understand the expressed emotion in a natural way, maybe because they possess the same mechanisms for expressing emotion vocally, or because of the existence of universal "inference rules" (Scherer, 2003) that allow receivers to infer vocalizers' emotional states from vocal cues. However, we must keep in mind that the naturalness of an *expression* does not make its *interpretation* natural. Although a vocal expression with particular acoustic qualities might be a natural symptom of a particular affective state in all humans (and beyond), the interpretation of the expression *as* a symptom is not naturally given.[7] In order for a particular acoustic percept to be interpreted *as* an expression of happiness, the expression has to be attended to and understood. While this understanding might indeed be possible due to evolved inference systems in the case of the vocalization of raw affective states, human vocal communication of emotions clearly goes beyond that.

Imitation and the Conventionalization of Vocal Icons: Figure 13–2(b) and (c)

The vocalization of emotions in humans is not restricted to symptomatic expression. Most of the time, vocal expression

---

[7]Although fever has always been a natural expression (a symptom) of an inflammation in the organism, this *interpretation* of fever required the development of medical knowledge (Rodriguez, in press).

of emotions in humans, and possibly some other primates, also has an appeal function (Scherer, 1992). That is, humans use the voice *in order to* do something, in order to achieve a change in the state of others. Humans intentionally use their voices for communication. An understanding of the reasons for universality and diversity in vocal communication in humans therefore ultimately requires us to investigate the evolution of this communication system in its mutuality with (a) the intertwined evolution of voluntary control over vocalizations and of the phonatory apparatus (Ploog, 1992) on the one hand, and with (b) the evolution of understanding other minds on the other hand.

Crucially, in explaining possible universals as well as diversity in human vocal communication of emotions, we can no longer refer to evolved mechanisms. The reason for this is the flexibility inherent in the processes of imitation and conventionalization. This flexibility is due to the fact that any actual speech event is more complex than the properties that become semiotically interpreted by a listener (Bühler, 1934/1982). For example, the vocal expression of happiness involves communication through a variety of acoustic channels (e.g., Frick, 1985), such as pitch, rate, tension, etc. The interpretation of a vocal affect expression *as* expressing a happy state can become associated with one or several of these channels in the processes of simulation and conventionalization, coarsely represented in Figure 13–2(b) and (c). The intentional vocal communication of emotion, while initially a simulation of universal affect bursts, modifies the acoustic percept in a multitude of ways that cannot be reduced to social repressions. The iconic expression conventionally used in the vocal communication of an emotional state is constrained not only by societal rules, but also by system-internal considerations. For example, if the vocal simulations of happiness and nervousness are similar enough to be confused frequently, the conventional vocal expression of one or both of these emotions will change to make them more distinguishable.[8] This means that the motive for engaging with others through communication is itself a driving force behind the development of diversity. Such functional constraints are themselves universal, but they have the effect that overlap in the intentional vocal behavior of adult speakers across cultures will bear a complex relation to evolved affect burst systems. This positive motive for local developments of vocal communication is the reason why diversity cannot just be peeled away to reach a universal core. No known direct link leads from one to the other. Indeed, there may not exist one single path from one to the other, since propositional communication has a neural infrastructure of its own. Still there has to be some kind of interconnection between the two, perhaps in the fundamental motivational urge to communicate, which is heavily represented in limbic social-brain structures such as the anterior cingulate, which also regulate social motivation. However, it is worth considering that even lower brain functions, such as the seeking urge, driven by general purpose dopaminergic motivational systems, is a major force in promoting the desire to communicate.

---

[8]The intentional use of voice in communication does not mean that changes in the conventional vocal expression of emotion are intended. Intentional actions on the individual level lead to unintended changes in convention (Keller, 1994).

Discussion

Universality and Diversity Do Not Exclude Each Other

The major consequence that follows from the systems model we have suggested is that universality and diversity do not stand in opposition.

On the one hand, we are convinced that many affective states are, on a preconceptual level, shared by all humans. These shared affective states are surely more numerous than the modest six or so basic emotions often suggested as universal. This universality, however, does not at all diminish the fact that the expression of emotion, as soon as it involves elements of volition and creativity, might become very diverse across cultures. What is more, this diversity is not at all superficial, a package for a universal content. Rather, communication processes, including vocal communication, are a major force in the development of complex affective categories such as happiness or despair that constitute a culture's "forms of life" (Brakel, 1994). Human utterances are more than just expressions of a subjective state: they give this state a form, and thus enable its scrutiny and categorization (Humboldt, 1835/1994; Jackendoff, 1996). They become an input to cognitive and communication processes.

Conversely, diversity does not at all diminish the existence or relevance of universals. Imagine two cultures in which the conventionalization of the vocal expression of happy affective states has taken maximally diverse paths. Say, culture A has conventionalized increased pitch variation as a signal of such states, and has dramatized this acoustic prop-

erty in vocal communication. Culture B has conventionalized fast speech rate as a signal of happy states, and has dramatized this acoustic property in vocal communication. Here we have maximal diversity: the two typical expressions of happiness do not overlap in terms of their acoustic properties. Nevertheless, if presented with vocal portrayals of happiness from a member of culture B, a member of culture A might still be able to correctly identify the intended state, because she will recognize it as a *possible* simulation of happy affect burst vocalizations. This will be even more so if she is faced with a choice between, say, happiness, sadness, anger, and fear. Diversity can be absolute—this does not diminish the universal potential provided by the acoustics of affect bursts.

In order to say anything about evolved universals of affect burst vocalization, those vocalizations have to be studied in all their complexity, including neurological substrates. Hence, studying affect burst vocalization might be difficult in humans, and simpler in other animals. For instance, the topic is already being addressed in primate research (Jürgens, 2006). The study of intentional vocal portrayal of emotions, on the other hand, can address a different kind of universals. This is so because intentional vocal communication is constrained by factors that are not themselves related to the affective system.

Developing Universals

The communicative model we have presented [Figure 13-2(b) and (c)] predicts that overlap in the vocal expression of communication develops through processes of conventionalization, that is, in social contact. In this sense, universals of vocal communication of emotion are developing as networks of communication expand. These are universals that develop through histories of engagement. In this sense, diversity is ultimately not based in ethnic, geographical, or linguistic factors, but perhaps mostly in lack of mutual engagement. This is supported by research showing that cross-cultural recognition rates of vocal expression of emotions increase with the increase of telephone contact between countries (Elfenbein & Ambady, 2002). It is also consistent with the finding that within a country, minority groups are better at recognizing emotions expressed vocally by majority group members than vice versa (Elfenbein & Ambady, 2002).

Research into universality and diversity of vocal communication of emotion should take histories of engagement across groups into account.[9] For instance, the extent to which cross-cultural intercourse is resulting in imitation of emotional prosody should not be underestimated. People might consciously or unconsciously mimic the prosody of interlocutors, particularly where continuous engagement occurs, much in the manner of a "phonetic chameleon." However, this appears to be presently untested.

Units of Analysis

The basic reservation we have about much of the empirical research and its interpretation can probably be summarized thus. A communication system cannot be properly understood if the units of analysis are the individual, on the one hand, and the society, on the other. We also need to take the communicative process as the unit of analysis. Dividing individuals from society has, in the current research context, led researchers interested in universality to a fundamentally negative view of communication and sociality in general: what the public context of emotional expression does is to constrain the individual, place rules on her behavior, and force her to suppress or modify emotional expression. We have argued that this view conceals many interesting questions about universality and diversity in the vocal expression of emotions, for example, the development of universality in histories of engagement. This leads to two types of universality (Marková, 1987) in affective vocalizations: evolved universals in symptomatic systems, shared across species, and developing commonalities in iconic systems, shared within communities, which become universal as networks of communication expand.

Universals and Functionality

We might therefore reopen the question of what it means if a behavior or psychological state is universal or not. Why should vocal expressions of emotion be universal anyway? The general point that researchers interested in universality wish to claim is that vocal expressions

---

[9]The fact that it is engagement in communication rather than just exposure to communication is supported by a study showing that students of English as a second language with high proficiency in English were not better at recognizing emotions vocally expressed by a native English speaker than students with low English proficiency. The authors conclude that learning a foreign language in a classroom setting might not be sufficient to become sensitive to this channel of communication.

are universal because of phylogenetic continuity (e.g., Scherer, 1999b). This would mean that vocal expression of emotion must be, and must have been, an adaptive behavior, that is, it must be functional. Its *functionality* determines the properties of an emotional expression (Darwin, 1872). However, in the sequence model of vocal expression discussed in the second section, the local display rules also *render* vocal expression functional. A more positive view of vocal communication of emotion would suggest that the community, the culture of the speaker, is itself one of the environmental systems that influence ongoing social microevolution. In this perspective, then, there is mutuality, rather than a unidirectional influence, between the two systems discussed here: the emotional-affective action systems and the cognitive communicative systems.

Conclusions

Raw affective experiences are a gift of nature; they are not cognitively penetrable (Panksepp, 2005). However, the percepts that result from vocalization *are* penetrable for humans: they can be attended to, repeated, reflected upon, dramatized, etc. Diversity develops in communication systems because expressions of emotion involve multiple channels, including various cognitive ones, but intentional vocalization might utilize only a subsection of these. In situations of fear the voice might become tense, it might tremble, and so on. In attending to the vocalization, a listener might pick out one of the vocal qualities, and ultimately a tense voice can become associated with fear in one group, whereas in

another group a trembling voice is the more typical expression of fear. Communication systems undergo processes of conventionalization and change that are in part independent from the universal constraints of the affective system. Communication is a way of engaging the world that is distinct in principle from such evolutionarily more basic systems (Panksepp, 2005, p. 162).

The human voice comes to convey many subtle changes in emotional state —at least to somebody who has a history of engagement with the speaker. It is misleading to narrow down the universal to only a handful of emotions, in the hope that they will be the major way in which emotionality is communicated in the voice. Rather, it seems to us that there is a lot that is universal in the communication of affective states, and at the same time there is a lot that is diverse: many affective states (tiredness, playfulness, exhilaration, fear, many shades of distress, and many shades of joy) are surely felt by all people (Panksepp, 2005). However, as soon as such states are communicated, not to mention given names and thus ordered into categories, it is increasingly less fruitful to look at these vocalizations for a universal core of emotionality. Emotions become semiotically formed in communication, and emotions are easily recognizable from the voice if hearer and speaker share a history of using the same communication system. For example, it is easy to recognize contempt from the voice of a person that one knows well. However, the recognition of contempt has been very low in recognition studies (Elfenbein & Ambady, 2002).

What follows is that universality in the vocal expression of emotions can be studied in two ways. Studies of biologically entrenched action systems might be more successful with nonhuman animals and very early stages of communication development in our own species. Studies of the vocal communication of emotions in humans that have been or are becoming enculturated might more fruitfully focus on the development of universality in histories of social engagement.

Models trying to incorporate both universality and diversity have taken the form of unidirectional sequence models: An emotional state triggers a universal mechanism (a motor program for vocal expression, for example), which is then modulated according to local display rules. Fundamentally, these models use conduit-metaphors of communication (Reddy, 1979/1993), where the basic emotions are the substance that itself remains untouched, and just becomes wrapped into different cognitive-communicative packages by the local code that needs to be decoded by the listener. We have suggested an alternative model that accommodates the ambiguous results of empirical research and motivates new questions about the universality and diversity of vocal expressions of emotions.

Vocal expression of emotion is usually studied as a natural sign, with a self-evident meaning. However, the fact that we can study the acoustic properties of an auditory signal and establish acoustic regularities does not mean that the meaning of such a natural sign is self-evident. The fact that a certain percept (such as a particular pitch contour) is a natural symptom of a state does not mean that it is understood *as* a sign of this state. As long as it is not clear what the relation is between auditory perception and conscious states, the description of acoustic properties cannot be used as a consistent description of a meaning.

In sum, we have been arguing that universals of iconic vocal emotional communication develop in histories of engagement. If such a process of developing universals exists, it must necessarily build on yet other universal potentials of the brain and mind. One of these potentials is accessible in the acoustics of affect bursts. Others have to be found in consistent patterns of social cognition, which may become increasingly complex with increasingly complex manmade environments. Presumably, the universal tendencies that govern social cognition would have less variability in humans still living in natural environments, but they may vary substantially depending upon the ecological factors of those environments. Future research might attempt to address the development of universals in the intersubjective engagements that emerge in different sociocultural contexts and world environments, and the relation between such developing universals and evolved vocal action patterns.

Acknowledgments. We are grateful to Alan Costall for discussions on an earlier draft of this chapter. Jörg Zinken's research is supported by the European Union's sixth framework project "Stages in the Evolution and Development of Sign Use."

References

Albas, D. C., McCluskey, K. W., & Albas, C. A. (1976). Perception of the emotional content of speech: A comparison of two Canadian groups. *Journal of Cross-Cultural Psychology, 7*(4), 481–489.

Bachorowski, J. A., & Owren, M. J. (1995). Vocal expression of emotion: Acoustic properties of speech are associated with emotional intensity and context. *Psychological Science, 6*(4), 219–223.

Bernstein Ratner, N., & Pye, C. (1984). Higher pitch in BT is not universal: Acoustic evidence from Quiche Mayan. *Journal of Child Language, 11*(3), 515–522.

Bezooijen, R. v., Otto, S. A., & Heenan, T. A. (1983). Recognition of vocal expressions of emotion: A three-nation study to identify universal characteristics. *Journal of Cross-Cultural Psychology, 14*(4), 387–406.

Black, M. (1962). *Models and metaphors: Studies in language and philosophy.* New York: Cornell University Press.

Borod, J. C. (2000). *The neuropsychology of emotion.* New York: Oxford University Press.

Brakel, J. v. (1994). Emotions: A cross-cultural perspective on forms of life. In W. M. Wentworth & J. Ryan (Eds.), *Social perspectives on emotion* (Vol. 2, pp. 179–237). Greenwich, CT: JAI Press.

Bühler, K. (1982). *Sprachtheorie.* Stuttgart, Germany: UTB. (Original work published 1934)

Burgdorf, J., & Panksepp, J. (2006). The neurobiology of positive emotions. *Neuroscience and Biobehavioral Reviews, 30,* 173–187.

Burnham, D., Kitamura, C., & Vollmer-Conna, U. (2002). What's new, pussycat? On talking to babies and animals. *Science, 296,* 1435.

Darwin, C. (1872). *The expression of emotions in man and animal.* London: John Murray.

Elfenbein, H. A., & Ambady, N. (2002). On the universality and cultural specificity of emotion recognition: A meta-analysis. *Psychological Bulletin, 128*(2), 203–235.

Ellsworth, P. C. (1994). Sense, culture, and sensibility. In S. Kitayama & H. R. Markus (Eds.), *Emotion and culture: Empirical studies of mutual influence* (pp. 23–50). Washington, DC: APA.

Fernald, A. (1989). Intonation and communicative intent in mothers' speech to infants: Is the melody the message? *Child Development, 60,* 1497–1510.

Fernald, A., & Simon, T. (1984). Expanded intonation contours in mothers' speech to newborns. *Developmental Psychology, 20*(1), 104–113.

Fernald, A., Taeschner, T., Dunn, J., Papousek, M., de Boysson-Bardies, B., & Fukui, I. (1989). A cross-language study of prosodic modifications in mothers' and fathers' speech to preverbal infants. *Journal of Child Language, 16*(3), 477–501.

Frick, R. W. (1985). Communicating emotion: The role of prosodic features. *Psychological Bulletin, 97*(3), 412–429.

Graham, C. R., Hamblin, A. W., & Feldstein, S. (2001). Recognition of emotion in English voices by speakers of Japanese, Spanish and English. *International Review of Applied Linguistics, 39,* 19–37.

Hauser, M. D. (1996). *The evolution of communication.* Cambridge, MA: MIT Press.

Hornstein, M. (1967). Accuracy of emotional communication and interpersonal compatibility. *Journal of Personality, 35*(1), 20–30.

Humboldt, W. v. (1994). Charakter der Sprachen. In J. Trabant (Ed.), *Wilhelm von Humboldt. Ueber die Sprache: Reden vor der Akademie.* Stuttgart, Germany: UTB. (Originally published in 1835)

Jackendoff, R. (1996). How language helps us think. *Pragmatics & Cognition, 4*(1), 1–34.

Jürgens, U. (1998). Neuronal control of mammalian vocalization, with special reference to the squirrel monkey. *Naturwissenschaften, 85,* 376–388.

Jürgens, U. (2006). *Common acoustic features in the vocal expression of emotions in monkeys and man.* Unpublished manuscript.

Juslin, P. N., & Laukka, P. (2003). Communication of emotions in vocal expression and music performance: Different channels, same code? *Psychological Bulletin, 129*(5), 770–814.

Keller, R. (1994). *On language change. The invisible hand in language.* London: Routledge.

Kitamura, C., & Burnham, D. (2003). Pitch and communicative intent in mother's speech: Adjustments for age and sex in the first year. *Infancy, 4*(1), 85–110.

Kitamura, C., Thanavishuth, C., Burnham, D., & Luksaneeyanawin, S. (2002). Universality and specificity in infant-directed speech: Pitch modifications as a function of infant age and sex in a tonal and non-tonal language. *Infant Behavior and Development, 24*(4), 372–392.

Knoll, M. A., & Uther, M. (2004). "Motherese" and "Chin-ese": Evidence of acoustic changes in speech directed at infants and foreigners. *Journal of the Acoustical Society of America, 116*(4), 2522.

Knoll, M. A., Walsh, S. A., MacLeod, N. O'Neill, M. & Uther, M (2007). Good performers know their audience! Identification and characterisation of pitch contours in infant- and foreigner-directed speech. In N. MacLeod (Ed.), *Automated taxon recognition in systematics:Theory, approaches and applications* (pp. 299-310). Boca Raton, Florida: CRC Press/The Systematics Association.

Kuhl, P. (2000). Language, mind and brain: Experience alters perception. In M. E. Gazzaniga (Ed.), *The new cognitive neurosciences* (2nd ed., pp. 99–115). Cambridge, MA: MIT Press.

Kuhl, P. K. (1994). Learning and representation in speech and language. *Current Opinion in Neurobiology, 4*(6), 812–822.

Manstead, A. S. R., & Fischer, A. H. (2002). Beyond the universality-specificity dichotomy. *Cognition and Emotion, 16*(1), 1–9.

Marková, I. (1987). The concepts of the universal in the Cartesian and Hegelian frameworks. In A. Costall & A. Still (Eds.), *Cognitive psychology in question* (pp. 213–233). Brighton, UK: The Harvester Press.

Newman, J. D. (Ed.). (1988). *The physiological control of mammalian vocalizations.* New York: Plenum.

Panksepp, J. (1982). Towards a general psychobiological theory of the emotions. *Behavioral and Brain Sciences, 5*, 407–467.

Panksepp, J. (2000). The neurodynamics of emotions: An evolutionary-neurodevelopmental view. In M. D. Lewis & I. Granic (Eds.), *Emotion, self-organization, and development* (pp. 236–264). New York: Cambridge University Press.

Panksepp, J. (2003). Can anthropomorphic analyses of "separation cries" in other animals inform us about the emotional nature of social loss in humans? *Psychological Reviews, 110*, 376–388.

Panksepp, J. (2005). On the embodied neural nature of core emotional affects. *Journal of Consciousness Studies, 12*(8–10), 158–184.

Panksepp, J., & Bernatzky, G. (2002). Emotional sounds and the brain: The neuroaffective foundations of musical appreciation. *Behavioural Processes, 60*, 133–155.

Papousek, H., & Hwang, S. (1991). Tone and intonation in Mandarin babytalk to presylabic infants: Comparison with registers of adult conversation and foreign language instruction. *Applied Psycholinguistics, 12*(4), 481–504.

Ploog, D. W. (1992). The evolution of vocal communication. In H. Papoušek, U. Jürgens, & M. Papoušek (Eds.), *Nonverbal vocal communication: Comparative and developmental approaches* (pp. 6-30). Cambridge, UK: Cambridge University Press.

Reddy, M. J. (1993). The conduit metaphor: A case of frame conflict in our language about language. In A. Ortony (Ed.), *Metaphor and thought* (pp. 164–201). Cambridge, UK: Cambridge University Press. (Originally published in 1979)

Rodriguez, C. (in press). Object use, communication and signs. The triadic basis of early cognitive development. In J. Valsiner & A. Rosa (Eds.), *The Cambridge handbook of socio-cultural psychology.* Cambridge, UK: Cambridge University Press.

Saunders, B. (1995). Disinterring basic color terms: A study in the mystique of cognitivism. *History of the Human Sciences, 8*(4), 19–38.

Scherer, K. R. (1992). Vocal affect expression as symptom, symbol, and appeal. In H. Papoušek, U. Jürgens, & M. Papoušek (Eds.), *Nonverbal vocal communication: Comparative and developmental ap-*

proaches (pp. 43-60). Cambridge, UK: Cambridge University Press.

Scherer, K. R. (1999). Cross-cultural patterns. In D. Levinson, J. J. J. Ponzetti, & P. F. Jorgensen (Eds.), *Encyclopedia of human emotions* (Vol. 1, pp. 147-156). New York: Macmillan Reference.

Scherer, K. R. (1999). Universality of emotional expression. In D. Levinson, J. J. J. Ponzetti, & P. F. Jorgensen (Eds.), *Encyclopedia of human emotions* (Vol. 2, pp. 669-674). New York: Macmillan Reference.

Scherer, K. R. (2000). A cross-cultural investigation of emotion inferences from voice and speech: Implications for speech technology. *Geneva Studies in Emotion and Communication, 14*(1), 1-4.

Scherer, K. R. (2003). Vocal communication of emotion: A review of research paradigms. *Speech Communication, 40*, 227-256.

Scherer, K. R., Banse, R., & Wallbott, H. G. (2001). Emotion inferences from vocal expression correlate across languages and cultures. *Journal of Cross-Cultural Psychology, 32*(1), 76-92.

Stern, D. N., Spieker, S., Barnett, R. K., & Mac-

Kain, K. (1983). The prosody of maternal speech: Infant age and context related changes. *Journal of Child Language, 10*(1), 1-15.

Toda, S., Fogel, A., & Kawai, M. (1990). Maternal speech to three-month-old infants in the United States and Japan. *Journal of Child Language, 17*(2), 279-294.

Trainor, L. J., Austin, C. M., & Desjardins, R. N. (2000). Is infant-directed speech prosody a result of the vocal expression of emotion? *Psychological Science, 11*(3), 188-195.

Trevarthen, C. (2000). Intrinsic motives for companionship in understanding: Their origin, development, and significance for infant mental health. *Infant Mental Health Journal, 22*, 95-131.

Viscovich, N. B., Jr., Pihan, H., Peery, S., Brickman, A. M., Tabert, M., & Schmidt, M. S., Jr. (2003). Acoustical analysis of posed prosodic expressions: Effects of emotion and sex. *Perceptual and Motor Skills, 93*(1), 759-771.

Wierzbicka, A. (1991). *Cross-cultural pragmatics: The semantics of human interaction*. Berlin, Germany: Mouton.

CHAPTER 14

Voice Fundamental Frequency Changes as a Function of Foreign Languages Familiarity: An Emotional Effect?

Kati Järvinen, Anne-Maria Laukkanen, and Krzysztof Izdebski

Introduction

The ability to speak foreign languages is essential in communication among peoples and across cultures and nations, and knowledge of foreign languages is increasingly important in modern multi-cultural societies; it is especially crucial for speakers representing smaller nations or isolated language groups. The act of speaking a foreign language at all, or speaking it fluently, is a formidable task as it requires not only the acquisition of new phonologic, lexical, semantic, syntactic, and prosodic features, but also cultural know-how and acculturation in general including recognition of culturally defined emotional social patterns.

Among the parameters of language, prosodic features appear crucial to achieve accent-free production, with correct prosody being seemingly more crucial than correct articulation or lexical confidence. It is thus not surprising that bilinguals show greater lateralization in the right hemisphere for the later learned language (Evans, Workman, Mayer, & Crowley, 2003). Moreover, learning in itself is a complex process that may be stressful, and learning has been shown to be influenced by the time of the day (Maheu, Collicutt, Kornik, Moszkowski, & Lupien, 2005). Moreover, behavioral studies have demonstrated that prosody is of importance even for 3-month-old infants in native language acquisition (Homae, Watanabe, Nakano, Asakawa, & Taga, 2006).

Achievement of these skills in adulthood is often considered to be an impossible task, and foreign accent can be a hindrance to social advancement in non-immigrant societies, or when trying to define a nation based on linguistic constraints (Helly, 1995), while it actually may be an unexpected fringe benefit in a tolerant and immigrant-friendly milieu (Jones, 2004). In general, however, speaking a foreign language with improper prosody can be detrimental to comprehension and intelligibility (Sikorski, 2005) to the point that a specialized branch of speech pathology has emerged aiming at accent reduction (Malugani, 2006; Sikorski, 2005), though high intelligibility can result from a combination of acoustic-phonetic characteristics (Hazan & Markham, 2004)

One essential element of prosody is expressed by the voice fundamental frequency (F_0) and its changes. However, F_0 stability can be easily challenged, as F_0 is subject to modifications by both physiological factors, such as vocal cord conditions (Guimares & Abberton, 2005; Izdebski, 2005), and/or emotional factors including stress (Hollien, 1980; Scherer, 1981; Shipp & Izdebski, 1981; Vilkman & Manninen, 1986; Williams & Stevens, 1981) and because F_0 reactivity can be heavily weighted by psychological personality traits (Johannes, Salnitski, Gunga, & Kirsch, 2000). Also, when speakers imitate pitch contours they actively generate their own prosody, and when they do that, they are influenced by the prosodic structure of another speaker's antecedent speech (Bosshardt, Sappok,

Knipschild, & Holscher, 1997). Thus it can be speculated that a psychological load will be placed upon the speaker of a foreign language due to inadequate control of lexicon, semantics, articulation, timing, and prosody and that this load will affect F_0 levels more than by chance (Hollien, Geison, & Hicks, 1987), when speaking the less familiar language or when imitating or feigning a foreign language.

With this scenario in mind, we hypothesized that when speaking a foreign language the F_0 levels will rise above the habitual level of the native language with the level of F_0 elevation depending on the degree of familiarity or unfamiliarity (higher confidence, less stress; less confidence, more stress) with the foreign language being spoken by the speaker. Moreover, we hypothesized that a wider F_0 distance will be introduced when speaking or imitating a completely unfamiliar language, because unfamiliarity evokes stronger emotive response (Carroll & Young, 2005).

To test this hypothesis we conducted a series of studies in which speakers of one language spoke multiple foreign languages with which they were more or less familiar, were pretending to know, or were imitating. We examined the F_0 findings from these speakers producing "foreign language tasks" vis-á-vis the F_0 levels of their native language. These experiments also raised a question, whether convincing or systematic F_0 change could be expected when speakers are forced to switch to the other language, which requires adjustments in prosody, articulation, and rate, from the native tongue, and whether the degree of familiarity or unfamiliarity with a foreign language shows a systematic trend on these changes. If the acoustical correlation was found, then F_0 alteration profile would be in opposition to F_0 alteration findings noticed in normal speakers, who for example feign depression and sleepiness (Reilly, Cannizzaro, Harel, & Snyder, 2004). Moreover, the outcomes are of interest to findings from perceptual studies of native versus foreign language intonation patterns, showing that the perception of similarities and differences among intonation contours may reflect universal auditory mechanisms with outputs molded by experience with one's native language (Grabe & Karpinski, 2003), and that the precision in imitation of adult intonation patterns (at least by children) depends on pitch directionality, with falling tones depending on their position in the sentence (Snow, 1998).

Is Speaking a Foreign Language Injurious to Your Health, or to Your Vocal Folds?

Speaking a foreign language requires adopting a new phonetic-prosodic scheme for the expression of thoughts and vocally coded emotions. It may also include a more or less conscious attempt to adapt to different vocal ideals of a foreign culture. People who speak foreign languages, especially simultaneous translators or interpreters, often complain about symptoms of vocal fatigue and mental exhaustion after being on-line for more than few hours, and report increased presence of stress when exposed to a "cocktail party" effect when multiple languages are present and they understand many of the languages that are spoken simultaneously (Izdebski, 2007). Interpreters were

also shown to exhibit dysphonia, cardiovascular problems, and CNS disturbances (Khaimovich, Makarova, & Kirikova, 1995), and mounting evidence suggests that stress and distress play a role in voice disorders (Seifert & Kollbruner, 2005).

There is also both clinical and experimental evidence on the relation between vocal parameters and symptoms of vocal fatigue. In voice pedagogy and clinical practice the prolonged use of a loud, high-pitched, and hyperfunctional voice (overpressured) has been regarded as one of the potential phonotrauma mechanisms (Izdebski, 2007; Olson, Cruz,, Izdebski, & Baldwin 2004; Sodersten, Granqvist, Hammarberg, & Szabo, 2002; Vilkman & Manninen, 1986).

It seems plausible that the type of voice use largely determines the biomechanical forces related to voice production and that the forces, in turn, would cause vocal symptoms and trauma to the vocal fold tissue. Vocal fold nodules are typically formed at the anterior one third of the glottic juncture where the amplitude of vibration of the vocal fold is largest (Berry, Montequin, & Tayama, 2001). Higher impact stress (force related to the collision between the vocal folds during vibration) has been measured for higher F_0 and SPL and tighter adduction (Jiang & Titze, 1994; Reed, Doherty, & Shipp, 1992; Verdolini, Hess, Titze, Bierhals, & Gross, 1999).

Materials

The major bulk of the data reported here was based on a study conducted by the first two authors on native female speakers of Finnish language who read a text in five nonnative languages (1–3 per each subject). The second part of the reported data is based on a preliminary work by the third author ,who investigated multiple speakers speaking in multiple foreign languages of varied degrees of familiarity,[1] pretending to speak a foreign language, or imitating a foreign language.

The Finnish Experiment

Finnish or Suomi, the native language of Finland, is a language spoken by approximately 6 million people in the country of Finland and in the Baltic region. Finnish belongs to the Finno-Ugric language group, and it differs significantly from the major languages in Europe, which represent either Germanic, Latin, or Slavic based language groups.

Finnish is an agglutinative type of language, and learning Finnish is considered to be difficult, because few languages are related to Finnish, thus leaving a potential and even the European student of Finnish to learn words without reference to other European languages; this gap affects even the so-called "international words" (e.g., bank = *pankki*, computer = *tietokone*, telephone = *puhelin*, etc.).

The stress is always placed on the first syllable. Finnish words can be very long (e.g., *Saippuakivikauppias*, dealer in soapstone), yet other languages have longer words. Just for fun, let it be known that the longest word in the English language ever reported, *pneumonoultramicroscopicsilicovolcano-koniosis*, *coniosis* for short, was recognized by the National Puzzlers' League at the opening session of the organization's 103rd semi-

annual meeting held on February 23, 1935, in New York City at the Hotel New Yorker. In the Malay language the longest word is *menyetidaknyahcasdiversifika-sielektrostatikkan* (a meager compound of 46 letters), meaning "to undiversify uncharged electrostatic electricity"; in Dutch the longest word is *kindercar-navalsoptochtvoorbereidingswerkza-amheden,* a 49-letter composition, meaning "preparation activities for a children's carnival procession"; in Swedish, it is *nordöstersjökustartilleriflygspaning-ssimulatoranläggningsmaterielunder-hållsuppföljningssystemdiskussionsin-läggsförberedelsearbeten,* a monster of 130 letters meaning "preparatory work on the contribution to the discussion on the maintaining system of support of the material of the aviation survey simulator device within the northeast part of the coast artillery of the Baltic," according to the 1996 *Guinness Book of World Records.* By the way, there are short words in Swedish, such as *ö* meaning an island. In German, the longest word is *Donaudampfschiffahrtselektrizitaeten hauptbetriebswerkbauunterbeam-tengesellschaft,* a short 80-letter blurb, meaning "the club for subordinate officials of the head office management of the Danube steamboat electrical services" (name of a pre-war club in Vienna), according to *Guinness,* 1996. And although the longest word in Finnish is not the longest word in the world, the longest compound Finnish word found on a Web site listing oddities and trivia (2006) was *kaksitariffikolmivaihevaihtovirtakilo-wattituntimittari,* which means something like "dual-tariff tri-stage AC kWh

---

[1]By familiarity is meant here, the self-judgment of how comfortable each speaker was to engage in the typical chit-chat style of discourse in the given foreign language.

meter." But Finnish is plentiful in such long words; for example, consider the word *epäjärjestelmällistyttää* or *autorkaksitariffikolmivaihevaihtovirtakilowattituntimittarillaansakaan*. In Polish the long words are not so long as in Germanic languages, or in Mohawk for a matter of fact, but they do exist, either for fun (*Konsantynopolitacznykowianeczka*, meaning a female inhabitant of Constantinople) or real words like *piêædziesiêciocentówka* (a 50 cent coin), *piêædziesiêciofenigówka* (a no longer valid German 50 Pfennig coin), *piêædziesiêciocentymówka* (a pre-Euro French 50 centimes coin), *dwudziestopiêciocentówka* (a pre-Euro Dutch 25 cent coin, called in Dutch *het kwaartje*), *piêædziesiêciostotinkówka* (a Bulgarian 50 stotinki coin), *dwustupiêædziesiêcioguldenówka* (referring to a no longer existing Dutch banknote), *dziewiêædziesiêciodziewiêcioletniak,* or a 35-letter-long tongue twister meaning a "99-year-old man." To have more fun with these words, check the Internet for various Web sites on oddities, such as http://www.members.aol.com/gulfhigh2/words, or go to http://www.experts.about.com. To read more on prosody and vocal emotions of Suomi, please consult Chapter 7 in this volume).

Subjects

The subjects were 44 female native speakers of Finnish, of which 17 were teachers of foreign languages. Their mean age was 44 years (range 29–58 years of age) and their mean experience of teaching was 16 years (range 2–32 years). There were also 27 students of the University of Tampere, Finland, majoring in a foreign language. Their mean age was 23 years of age (range was 18–30 years), and their mean years of study was 3 years (range 1–6 years).

The subjects read aloud a neutral newspaper text in Finnish and in one to three foreign languages. The sample duration was approximately 1 minute for each language. The foreign languages were English (27 subjects in total), Swedish (13), German (9), French (8), and Russian (7). To eliminate the possible effect of task order, half of the subjects started with a Finnish text, the other half with a foreign language sample. The subjects were asked to mark the order of familiarity of the foreign languages in a questionnaire.

The recordings took place in two occasions. The teachers were recorded in classroom conditions by using a portable Tascam DAT recorder and a Sony ECM-MS957 microphone. The students were recorded in a well-attenuated studio with Tascam DAT recorder and Brüel & Kjær (4165) microphone. All tapes were calibrated for measurement of the sound pressure level and the distance of the microphone was 40 cm from the mouth.

Analyses

Fundamental frequency (mean, SD, and range in each sample) and voiced-voiceless ratio were analyzed using Real Speech 4.2 Program (Tiger Electronics, Seattle, Washington).

Vocal loading index was calculated as mean fundamental frequency (Hz) times duration of the voiced signal (in seconds) in the sample divided by 1000 (Rantala & Vilkman, 1999). This index indicates the number of the vocal fold vibrations in the sample and can therefore reflect the amount of loading posed on the vocal folds in speech.

Results

Mean fundamental frequency was statistically significantly higher in every foreign language compared to that in Finnish F_0. The average difference in the mean F_0 of text reading was smallest between Finnish and Swedish (4 Hz) and largest between Finnish and Russian (14 Hertz). Fundamental frequency range and standard deviation did not differ significantly between Finnish and foreign languages. Differences in SPL between the languages were statistically nonsignificant as well.

The amount of increase in mean F_0 compared to Finnish did not differ significantly between the first (and thus supposedly the most fluent) foreign language and the other, less fluent languages. The years of teaching or studying a language did not correlate with the amount of difference in the mean F_0 between Finnish and the foreign languages. English, Swedish, and German did not differ significantly from each other in the amount of difference in mean F_0 compared to Finnish, while French seemed to cause a larger increase in F_0 compared to other languages.

The voiced-voiceless ratio was slightly higher in the samples of Finnish, reflecting the different prevalence of vowels and consonants in these languages, but the difference was statistically significant only for English and German. Due to differences in voiced-voiceless ratio, the vocal loading index was significantly lower in English compared to Finnish. In other languages the difference was not statistically significant.

The Other Experiments

The other experiments were conducted on pilot bases and comprised various subsets: Polish, American English, Tagalog, and Mexican-Spanish. In the Polish part, F_0 of speech samples comprising counting or speaking spontaneously by two native male Polish speakers (mean age 46 years) was tested against multiple foreign languages spoken by these speakers.

One male participant spoke numbers in Polish against 12 different languages (American English, German, Swedish, Danish, Dutch, French, Italian, Spanish, Brazilian Portuguese, Russian, Japanese, Tagalog, and Finnish. The speech samples of Cantonese Chinese were simulated (imitated). The other male Polish speaker spoke against Swedish, Russian, German, and American English.

One of the female native Polish speakers spoke against Russian, Swedish, French, German, Italian, American English, and an Arabic dialect spoken in Morocco. The second female Polish speaker spoke against Canadian English, Russian, Spanish, and German.

Polish language (in contrast to Finnish) puts stress on the penultimate syllable, and contrary to many other languages including other Slavic languages contains more consonantal segments. To read more about the specific features of Polish please consult Chapter 5, Volume 2.

In the American English part of this pilot study, four adult native American English speakers spoke against French, Farsi, Fijian, Russian, Arabic, and Spanish and imitated Cantonese Chinese, Polish, and Swedish.

In the Tagalog part of this study a native female Tagalog speaker spoke against American English. The order of speaking foreign languages for all participants was at random, and the speakers self-judged the fluency of the nonnative language.

Results were analyzed for fundamental frequency only as opposed to the Finnish experiment, where F_0 and sound pressure level (SPL), voiced-voiceless ratio, and vocal loading index for Finnish females reading in Finnish and in one to three foreign languages were analyzed.

Results

As in the Finnish experiment, the F_0 was higher for all speakers (male and female) when the nonnative language was produced. The greatest F_0 distance was found for the least familiar or the imitated language.

For the male speakers producing familiar foreign languages the maximum F_0 difference was nearly 20 Hz, with average difference not exceeding 10 Hz. For the female the maximum difference was 30 Hz, with the average difference not exceeding 15 Hz. The F_0 distance reached 70 Hz when imitated language was produced by American English native speakers imitating Cantonese Chinese.

Discussion

The results showed that all native speakers, be it of Finnish, Polish, American English, or Tagalog and irrespectively of gender, used higher mean F_0 when speaking foreign languages as compared to their native language. The widest F_0 distance was found for the imitation condition. For the non-Finnish group a trend

of mode pitch distance between the native and "the least fluent or the completely unknown (imitation condition) language" appeared. This was interpreted as indicative of added stress factor from the idea of pitch matching to the target speaker, no matter the gender of the target speaker and the experimental speaker. In that sense, the adult speakers behaved in way youngsters behave when imitating adult prosody.

This rise in F_0 most likely can be interpreted on many grounds, but it may reflect a higher psycho-physiological activity (Orlikoff & Baken, 1988; 1989) when speaking in a foreign language, which supposedly is a more demanding and hence emotionally loading task than speaking in one's mother tongue. Elevated F_0 has also been explained as a sign of submissiveness and willingness to cooperate, as in interrogative prosody, indicating a willingness to participate in a discourse (Grabe & Karpinski, 2003).

The use of pitch and its variation are also culture and gender dependent (Lewis, 2002). It is possible that the subjects of the present study tried to some extent to adapt their voices to a certain level they imagined the native speakers of the foreign language would use. This adaptation phenomenon appears to be a useful tool in reducing the so-called foreign accent effect.

According to previous studies the average fundamental frequency in Finnish-speaking females is lower than for example in Swedish or English-speaking women (Laukkanen & Leino, 1999; Pegoraro Krook, 1988; Rantala 2000). Some subjects of the present study reported that they felt that they use a higher pitch in foreign languages but they could not explain the reason for it. Ohara has found in her studies (1992, 1999) that females speaking Japanese as a mother tongue have a lower pitch when speaking English. English-speaking females have a higher pitch when speaking Japanese as a foreign language. According to Ohara this can be caused by the fact that Japanese culture uses a clear pitch distinction to differentiate female and masculine speech. In the present study French differed significantly from the other Finnish foreign languages by causing a larger F_0 increase. Similarly, larger F_0 distances were found for the least familiar languages in the non-Finnish parts of this report, possibly relating to a feeling of elevated anxiety when speaking in a more distant language.

It would have been expected that the fundamental frequency range and standard deviation would be greater in foreign languages compared to Finnish—taking that the general impression is that Finnish uses a more restricted intonation than the foreign languages studied. In this study this was however not the case. It is possible that the subjects tried and felt they had achieved the foreign intonation in their speech merely by raising the mean fundamental frequency level. It is possible that the Finnish intonation pattern influenced their intonation also in the foreign languages and they compensated for it by having a higher fundamental frequency. Finnish people usually have problems especially with the prosodic features of foreign languages (Salo-Lee, 1995). The intonation pattern of one's mother tongue can influence the intonation of a foreign language (Grover, Jamieson, & Dobrovolsky, 1987) and according to Iivonen et al. (1987), Finnish people can raise their pitch and sound volume when trying to achieve a foreign intonation. It is also possible that

the high pitch restricted the deviation and range in F_0. If the F_0 was higher than usual, it could have made it difficult for the subjects to use variation both in frequency and in amplitude.

Higher F_0 and possibly also somewhat more hyperfunctional voice production when speaking in a foreign language obviously increase voice production-related vocal loading and can thus increase the risk of vocal fatigue symptoms. The higher fundamental frequency should raise the vocal loading index, but the only significant change in the vocal loading index was in English, where it was smaller than in Finnish. This can be due to the fact that the amount of the voiced speech naturally affects the vocal loading index, too. The vowel-consonant ratio in Finnish is 100:109, while in English it is 100:158 (Hakulinen, 1979).

A systematic study comparing languages and cultures from the point of view of vocal loading and the prevalence of voice disorders would be a difficult but interesting challenge.

References

Berry, D. A., Montequin, D., & Tayama, N. (2001). High-speed digital imaging of the medial surface of the vocal folds. *Journal of the Acoustical Society of America, 110,* 2539–2547.

Bosshardt, H. G., Sappok, C., Knipschild, M., & Holscher, C. (1997). Spontaneous imitation of fundamental frequency and speech rate by nonstutterers and stutterers. *Journal of Psycholinguistic Research, 26*(4), 425–448.

Carroll, N. C., & Young, A. W. (2005). Priming of emotion recognition. *Quarterly Jour-*

nal of Experimental Psychology A, *58*(7), 1173-1197.

Evans, J., Workman, L., Mayer, P., & Crowley, K. (2002). Differential bilingual laterality: Mythical monster found in Wales. *Brain and Language*, *83*(2), 291-299.

Grabe, E., & Karpinski, M. (2003). Universal and language specific aspects of intonation: English and Polish. *Language and Speech*, *46*(Pt. 4), 375-401.

Grabe, E., Rosner, B. S., Garcia-Albea, J. E., & Zhou, X. (2004). Perception of English intonation by English, Spanish, and Chinese listeners. *Language and Speech*, *46*(4), 375-401.

Grover, C., Jamieson, D., & Dobrovolsky, M. (1987). Intonation in English, French and German: Perception and production. *Language and Speech. 30*(3), 277-295.

Guimaraes, I., & Abberton, E. (2005). Health and voice quality in smokers: An exploratory investigation. *Logopedics, Phoniatrics, and Vocology*, *30*(3-4), 185-191.

Hakulinen, L. (1979). *Suomen kielen rakenne ja kehitys* (4th ed.). Helsinki, Finland: Otava.

Hazan V., & Markham, D. (2004). Acoustic-phonetic correlates of talker intelligibility for adults and children. *Journal of the Acoustical Society of America*, *116*(5), 3108-3118.

Helly, D. (1995). Quebecers, foreigners or citizens? The basis of the sense of belonging of immigrants to Quebec [In French]. *Revue of European Migration International*, *11*(3), 67-78.

Hollien, H. (1980). Vocal indicators of psychological stress. In F. Wright, C. Bahn, & R. W. Rieber (Eds.), Forensic Psychology and Psychiatry. *Annals of New York Academy of Sciences*, *347*, 47-72.

Hollien, H., Geison, L., & Hicks, J. W., Jr. (1987). Voice stress evaluators and lie detection. *Journal of Forensic Science*, *32*(2), 405-418.

Homae, F., Watanabe, H., Nakano, T., Asakawa, K., & Taga, G. (2006). The right hemisphere of sleeping infant perceives sentential prosody. *Neuroscience Research*, *54*(4), 276-280.

Iivonen, A., Nitti, A., Evalanen, N., Erttu, T., Ulanko, A., Eijo, R., et al. (1987). *Puheen intonaatio*. Helsinki, Finland: Gaudeamus.

Izdebski, K. (2007). Clinical voice assessment: The role & value of the Phonatory Function Studies. In A. Lalwani (Ed.), *Current diagnosis & treatment. Otolaryngology head and neck surgery* (2nd ed., pp. 416-429). New York: McGraw Hill Lange.

Jiang, J., & Titze, I. (1994). Measurement of vocal fold intraglottal stress and impact stress. *Journal of Voice*, *8*, 132-144.

Johannes, B., Salnitski, V. P., Gunga, H. C., & Kirsch, K. (2000). Voice stress monitoring in space—Possibilities and limits. *Aviation, Space, Environmental Medicine*, *71*(Suppl. 9), A58-A65.

Jones, D. (2004). The universal psychology of kinship: Evidence from language. *Trends in Cognitive Science*, *8*(5), 211-215.

Karpinski, M., & Klesta, J. (2001). The project of an intonational database for the Polish language. In (Ed.), *Prosody 2000*. Poznan, Poland: Adam Mickiewicz University.

Khaimovich, M. L., Makarova, V. N., & Kirikova, G. A. (1995). The effect of increased voice and psychophysiological loads on the health status of interpreter guides [In Russian]. *Meditsina Trudai Promyshlennaia Ekologia*, *11*, 24-26.

Laukkanen, A.-M., & Leino, T. (1999). *Ihmeellinen ihmisääni*. Tampere, Finland: Gaudeamus.

Lewis, J. A. (2002). *Social influences on female speakers' pitch*. Unpublished doctoral dissertation, University of California, Berkeley.

Maheu, F. S., Collicutt, P., Kornik, R., Moszkowski, R., & Lupien, S. J. (2005). The perfect time to be stressed: A differential modulation of human memory by stress applied in the morning or in the afternoon. *Progress in Neuropsychopharmacology, Biology and Psychiatry*, *29*(8), 1281-1218.

Mäki, E., Niemi, H.-M., Lundén, S., & Laukkanen, A.-M. (2001). F_0, SPL and vocal fatigue in a vocally loading test. In *Proceedings of the 25th World Congress of the International Association of Logopedics and Phoniatrics* [CD-ROM]. Montreal, Canada: Author.

Malugani, M. (2001). Speech pathologists build a profitable niche in accent reduction. Accessed March 3, 2006 from http://www.healthcare.monster.com/therapy/articles/accent/

McWhirter, N. D. & McWhirter, A. (1966). *The Guinness Book of Records,* [13th edition]. London: Guinness Superlatives Ltd.

Ohara, Y. (1992.) Gender-dependent pitch levels: A comparative study in Japanese and English. In K. Hall, M. Bucholtz, & B. Moonwomon (Eds.), *Locating power: Proceedings of the Second Berkeley Women and Language Conference* (Vol. 2, pp. 468-477). Berkeley, CA: Berkeley Women and Language Group.

Ohara, Y. (1999). Performing gender through voice pitch: A cross-cultural analysis of Japanese and American English. In U. Pasero & F. Braun (Eds.), *Perceiving and performing gender* (pp. 106-116). Opladen/Wiesbaden, Germany: Westdeutscher Verlagz.

Oliver, D. (2005). *Deriving pitch accent classes using automatic f_0 stylisation and unsupervised clustering techniques.* In proceedings of Second Baltic Conference on Human Language eTechnologies, April, 4-6, pp.161-166. Tallinn, Estonia.

Olson, D. E., Cruz, R. M., Izdebski, K., & Baldwin, T. (2004). Muscle tension dysphonia in patients who use computerized speech recognition systems. *Ear, Nose and Throat Journal, 83*(3), 195-198.

Orlikoff, R. B., & Baken, R. J. (1988). Fundamental frequency modulation of the human voice by the heartbeat: Preliminary results and possible mechanism. *Journal of the Acoustical Society of America, 85,* 888-893.

Orlikoff, R. B., & Baken, R. J. (1989). The effect of the heartbeat on vocal fundamental fre-quency perturbation. *Journal of Speech and Hearing Research, 32,* 576-582.

Pegoraro Krook, M. I. (1988). Speaking fundamental frequency characteristics of normal Swedish subjects obtained by glottal frequency analysis. *Folia Phoniatrica, 40,* 82-90.

Rantala, L., Vilkman, E. (1999). Relatonship between subjective voice complaints and acoustic parameters in teachers' voice. *J. Voice, 13,* 484-495.

Reed, C. G., Doherty, E. T., & Shipp, T. (1992). Direct measurement of vocal fold medial forces. *American Speech and Hearing Association Report, 34,* 131(A).

Reilly, N., Cannizzaro, M. S., Harel, B. T., & Snyder, P. J. (2004). Feigned depression and feigned sleepiness: A voice acoustical analysis. *Brain and Cognition, 55*(2), 383-386.

Salo-Lee, L. (1995). Kulttuurienvälisten viestintätaitojen oppiminen: "Prosessipuhuminen" keinona tehokkaaseen vieraskieliseen suulliseen ilmaisuun. In L. Salo-Lee (Ed.), *Kieli & Kulttuuri oppimisessa ja opettamisessa* (pp. 153-169). Jyväskylän yliopisto viestintätieteiden julkaisuja 12. Jyväskylä, Finland: Kopi-Jyvä Oy.

Scherer, K. (1981). Vocal indicators of stress. In J. K. Darby (Ed.), *Speech evaluation in psychiatry* (pp. 171-187). New York: Grune and Stratton.

Seifert, E., & Kollbrunner, J. (2005). Stress and distress in non-organic voice disorder. *Swiss Medical Weekly, 135*(27-28), 387-397.

Shipp, T., & Izdebski, K. (1981). Current evidence for the existence of laryngeal macrotremor and microtremor. *Journal of Forensic Science, 26*(3), 501-505.

Sikorski, L. D. (2005). Foreign accents: Suggested competencies for improving communicative pronunciation. *Seminars in Speech and Language, 26*(2), 126-130.

Snow, D. (1998). Children's imitations of intonation contours: Are rising tones more difficult than falling tones? *Journal of Speech, Language and Hearing Research, 41*(3), 576-587.

Sodersten, M., Granqvist, S., Hammarberg, B., & Szabo, A. (2002). Vocal behavior and vocal loading factors for preschool teachers at work studied with binaural DAT recordings. *Journal of Voice, 16*(3), 356–371.

Verdolini, K., Hess, M. M., Titze, I. R., Bierhals, W., & Gross, M. (1999). Investigation of vocal fold impact stress in human subjects. *Journal of Voice, 13*, 184–202.

Vilkman, E, & Manninen, O. (1986). Changes in prosodic features of speech due to environmental factors. *Speech Communication, 5*, 331–345.

Williams, C. E., & Stevens, K. N. (1981). Vocal correlates of emotional states. In J. K. Darby (Ed.), *Speech evaluation in psychiatry* (pp. 221–240). New York: Grune and Stratton.

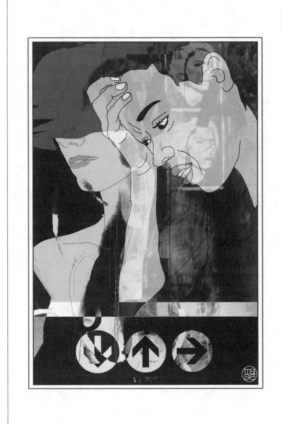

CHAPTER 15

Voice and Affect in Speech Communication

Geneviève Caelen-Haumont and
Branka Zei Pollermann

Abstract

After clarifying the semiotic status of vocal indicators of affect, we trace the role of affective components of speech communication from ancient oratory up to the present. Specific attention is given to the often neglected contribution of linguists to the study of emotional components of speech (the contribution very much present already at the turn of the 19th–20th centuries). Recent approaches to the study of both cognitive and affective components of speech prosody are also described. MELISM, a tool for automatic segmentation and coding of prosodic features of speech, is presented at the end.

The Semiotic Status of Vocal Indicators of Affect: Vocal Expression or Vocal Communication of Affect?

All observable changes in human behavior (regardless of the type of sensorial modality) can be informative of the state of the individual. However, most of such changes are not produced in order to inform other members of the species of the person's psychological or physical state. From the perceived features, the observer infers the meaning without explicit learning of the code involved. Such features are informative without having been produced to this effect. By contrast, those features that *are* produced in order to transmit information have a communicative function and are conventionalized. Wharton (2003) illustrates this distinction by comparing shivering with smiling. Shivering is a spontaneous behavior whose function is to generate heat. To an observer, shivering provides information that the individual is feeling cold. However, the function of shivering is not to signal this information. Smiling, by contrast, could be considered as intentional signaling, whose function *is* to convey information (Ekman, 1999). As Wilson and Wharton (2005) write:

> For instance, a speaker's mental or physical state may affect the prosodic properties of her utterance, enabling a hearer with the appropriate experience or background knowledge to infer whether she is drunk or sober, sick or healthy, tired or alert, hesitant or assured. As with shivering, these prosodic properties carry information about the speaker's mental or physical state, but it is not their function to do so: they are natural signs, interpreted by inference rather than decoding. (p. 1561)

In everyday speech communication, the interpretation of speech signal relies heavily on the information provided by the shared knowledge that is part of the context (concrete circumstances and culture). In the interest of the economy of communication, the spontaneously produced information found in the speaker's vocal and facial behavior is part of the shared contextual knowledge that serves as interpretative framework —the context that provides the information not contained in the verbal message itself. This information is specifically geared at guiding the hearer during the inferential phase of auditory comprehension. In this process the speaker may also use nonverbal signals intentionally in order to facilitate access to meaning, to divert the hearer from a particular interpretation or even mislead him.

Unlike in typewritten communication, in oral communication the sender of the message produces his own tool for communication. By this fact the sounds produced *on-line* necessarily carry the "signature" of their producer. The information thus provided is related to the speaker's physical conditions at the moment of speech production, as well as to his or her cognitive-affective states such as attitudes, interpersonal stances, emotions, or personality traits. Such information can be produced spontaneously or intentionally and may vary according to social context and the speaker's communicative intentions. Some vocal features can thus be interpreted as the expression (symptom) of the speaker's inner state while others will be considered as intentional communicative signals or styles (Zei-Pollermann, 2002).

Voice and Affect in Ancient Oratory

Since antiquity, the study of emotional aspects of speech has been part of philosophical, religious, literary, and artistic works. It was only later that affective speech became a subject in its own right, investigated by psychologists, linguists, neurologists, physiologists, and other scientists. Going back to Aristotle, in Book 3 of *Rhetoric*, Aristotle points out the importance of studying the subject of verbal expression and delivery, which he felt was a powerfully effective means of conducting good oratory. Aristotle writes (Russel & Winterbottom, 1972, p. 135): "This study is about the proper use of voice (loud, soft, and moderate, to express individual emotions), the proper use of accents (acute, grave and circumflex), and the rhythms appropriate to different things." While for Aristotle the whole study of rhetoric is directed towards producing belief (that is, not knowledge), for Cicero (Russel & Winterbottom, p. 250), the purpose is triple: "For the best orator is the one, who by his oratory instructs, pleases, and moves the minds of his audience. To instruct is a debt to be paid, to give pleasure a gratuity to confer, to rouse emotion a sheer necessity." At that time, and for many years to come, emotional effects of voice on the listener played a major part in oratory. Emotional effects are produced for a purpose and the delivery is one of the means.

In this context the speaker's true emotions are not the focus of attention. Only the emotional impact created on the hearer is clearly pointed out. The orator's genuine feelings are mentioned only indirectly in the context of their usefulness in making the orator appear more credible and creating the impression of naturalness for "Naturalness is convincing, artificiality the reverse. . . . One should aim at the effect attained by Theodorus' voice in comparison with other actors'; his seems to belong to the character, theirs to be imposed on it" (Russel & Winterbottom, p. 137). The instrumental use of oratory to elicit emotions in others is well described by Cicero (p. 217) in the following paragraph of his text *The Brutus:*

> The orator's audience believes his words, thinks them true, assents, approves; his speech carries conviction, . . . the crowd rejoices, grieves, laughs, cries, likes, dislikes. . . . It is angered and soothed, it hopes and fears. These effects take place according to the way in which the minds of those present are worked on by words, thoughts and delivery.

Cicero is aware that passions induced in the audience by oratory modify people's judgment so that eventually, affect dominates over truth and justice.[1] A very similar view was developed by Quitilian who adds that vocal aspects of delivery can reveal the unadmitted passions of the speaker.

It appears that Cicero's oratory excellence includes induction of two kinds of

---

[1] *De Oratore*, II. XLII. 178: Haec properans ut et apud doctos et semidoctus ipse percurro, ut aliquando ad illa maiora veniamus: nihil est enim in dicendo, Catule, maius, quam ut faveat oratori is, qui audiet, utique ipse sic moveatur, ut impetu quodam animi et perturbatione magis quam iudicio aut consilio regatur: plura enim multo homines iudicant odio aut amore aut cupiditate aut iracundia aut dolore aut laetitia aut spe aut timore aut errore aut aliqua permotione mentis quam veritate aut praescripto aut iuris norma aliqua aut iudici formula aut legibus.

emotions: esthetic or disinterested and utilitarian (Scherer, 2005). The role of utilitarian emotions (such as fear or anger) is mainly to steer the receiver's behavior presumably through empathy or identification with the speaker.

The role of disinterested emotions would be to provide esthetic experience or disinterested pleasure (Kant, 2001) resulting either from intrinsic qualities of sensorial experience (visual or auditory) or from the pleasure of intellectual discovery of the truth. For Cicero the delivery skills do not only include the voice, they also include the orators' facial expressions and body movements, which "signify in what sense everything they say is to be understood" (Russel & Winterbottom, p. 242). This statement from Cicero clarifies the role of nonverbal aspects of communication, which is to guide the interpretation of the words by providing the psychological context (in terms of knowledge and affect). It is nevertheless important to keep in mind that in ancient oratory the main focus was on use of language and of the argument, while the delivery played a role of providing the right emotional context for winning an argument. Voice and feelings continued to be inherently related to each other in the centuries to come. St. Augustine considered the human voice as capable of stimulating the soul and producing physical pleasure as the voice is considered to contain the whole range of the feelings of one's soul: "*tutta la scala dei sentimenti della nostra anima.*" (St Augustino, 397/1969). Following St. Augustine, the medieval scholastic tradition considered the speaker's voice as emanating from the soul and the rhetoric figures as superfluous because the preacher's strong emotion (*grandis affectus*) provided all the force to his discourse.

It is interesting to note that in medical writings on vocal disturbances, the voice was also regarded as a reflection of thought activities in general and thought disturbances in particular (Paparela, 1556).

Rhetoric's reputation suffered during the Age of Enlightenment, when it was condemned as meaningless bombast or unwelcome ornamentation—the view in agreement with the Enlightenment Movement that advocated rationality as a means to establish an authoritative system of ethics, esthetics, and knowledge.

In conclusion to this very sketchy presentation of the link between voice and emotion in ancient oratory, we must point out that voice was considered to have an emotion eliciting effect only in conjunction with the words and other nonverbal expressions.

The Study of Affect in Everyday Speech Communication: The Contribution of Linguists

Notwithstanding Darwin's (1872) impetus on research of emotional expression, the study of vocal indicators of affective states remains mainly in the domain of linguistics and literature. For example, Bourdon (1892) surfaces as the first one to engage in empirical study and theoretical modeling of the effects of emotions on speech communication. His work describes in quite some detail the effects of emotions and emotional tendencies on vocal intensity, pitch height, timing of speech, pauses, intonation contours, and accentuation. He defined the term *ten-*

dencies as a person's stable patterns of emotional reactions including behaviors; it is close to the concept of temperament.

At the beginning of the 20th century, as it is well known, Ferdinand de Saussure's teaching brings a decisive contribution to the constitution of linguistics as an independent science. The linguists' debate focalizes on the relation between the subjective, ever-changing aspects of speech vs. the stable and conventionalized aspects of language. Charles Bally (1905) studied the affective components of speech on both semantic and prosodic levels, and laid the foundations for the stylistics of ordinary spoken language. In the wake of Bally's stylistics, Troubetzkoy (1939)—an active member of the Prague linguistic circle—proposes a term *phonostylistics* for a science whose aim would be to study two domains of speech: (a) expression, as a symptom of the speaker's state and (b) appeal, as a set of conventionalized vocal features fulfilling specific social functions. His proposal is based on Buhler's (1934) *organon* model of the semiotics of speech communication. Troubetzkoy concedes that it is not always easy to separate the spontaneously expressed features related to the speaker's psychophysiological state from those used intentionally for purposes of communication—like for example the use of an accent characteristic of a social class.

The study of phonostylistics continued in the works of Spitzer (1961) as well as Dámaso and Bousoño (1951), who classified speech styles according to the types of affect expressed.

Among the first empirical studies were those of Seashore (1927), Fairbanks and Pronovost (1939), as well as Fairbanks and Hoaglin (1941). The subsequent works of Williams and Stevens (1972), Bolinger (1945; 1946; 1965; 1972), and Crystal (1975) were fundamental. Their aim was to establish a repertory of acoustic features related to various emotional states. Fónagy (1971) makes a considerable contribution to the study of affect in speech. He suggests a model of *double coding* where speech communication involves two successive coding procedures: (a) linguistic coding by which an idea is transformed into a speech signal composed of a sequence of phonemes (e.g., "It's very kind of you") and (b) paralinguistic coding, which adds emotional components to the phonemic sequence (e.g., the feeling of hate or contempt). Fónagy's rich work on the prosody of emotions also includes experimental comparative studies of emotional prosody and music (Fónagy & Magdics, 1963).

Within the framework of phonostylistics and by analogy to the concept of a phoneme, Pierre Leon (1970; 1971; 1976) coined the term *phonostyleme*, defined as a bundle of distinctive features relevant for the vocal differentiation of emotions. These features were mean F_0, F_0 range, intonation contour, tempo, and vocal intensity. None of the features was considered to be able to characterize an emotion in an independent manner. Faure (1970; 1973), Fónagy (1973), I. Fónagy, Bérard, and J. Fónagy (1982), Fónagy and Sap (1997), and Fónagy (1982a, 1982b) contributed substantially to research on the acoustic patterns of emotions.

A frequent problem in social sciences is lack of consensus on the labeling of key concepts related to the object of the study. Drawing on the works of Crystal and Quirk (1964) as well as that of Laver (1968), Roach (2000) proposed a rather comprehensive prosodic and paralinguistic labeling, comprising 36 labels. The prosodic coding presents four characteristics related to F_0 height and range, four for intensity, and eight for tempo. In addition, the paralinguistic code includes nine labels for voice quality, five for speech fluency, and three for expressions such as laughing, crying, and tremulous voice.

In the past 20 years many studies have tried to determine the acoustic patterns of emotions (Zei and Archinard, 2001). Prosodic features listed by the various authors overlap considerably. Table 15–1, elaborated by Murray and Arnott (1993, Table 1, pp. 1106), describes the main prosodic features in the English language for five basic emotions. These features seem to be applicable to many other languages.

Other numerous works were undertaken within the broader framework of linguistic or semantic studies. Notable research was done for Spanish and American English by Bolinger (1945; 1946; 1965; 1972), for British English by Crystal (1975), and for French by Faure (1970; 1973), Fónagy and Bérard (1973), I. Fónagy, Bérard, and J. Fónagy (1982), as well as Fónagy and Sap (1997).

These studies were characterized by a search of acoustic profiles based on the quantification of F_0, intensity, timing, and pace parameters related to the speakers' emotional states and attitudes.

For example Fónagy and Bérard (1973) and Fónagy et al. (1982) studied melodic

Table 15–1. Summary of human vocal emotion effects. The effects described are those most commonly associated with the emotions indicated, and are relative to neutral speech.

	Anger	Happiness	Sadness	Fear	Disgust
Speech rate	slightly faster	faster or slower	slightly slower	much faster	very much slower
Pitch average	very much higher	much higher	slightly lower	very much higher	very much lower
Pitch range	much wider	much wider	slightly narrower	much wider	slightly wider
Intensity	higher	higher	lower	normal	lower
Voice quality	breathy, chest tone	breathy, blaring	resonant	irregular voicing	grumbled, chest tone
Pitch changes	abrupt, on stressed syllables	smooth, upward inflections	downward inflections	normal	wide, downward terminal inflections
Articulation	tense	normal	slurring	precise	normal

Note. From "Toward the Simulation of Emotion in Synthetic Speech: A Review of the Literature on Human Vocal Emotion," by L. R. Murray and J. L. Arnott, 1993, *Journal of the Acoustical Society of America, 93*(2), pp. 1097–1108. Copyright 1993 by American Institute of Physics. Reprinted with permission from L. R. Murray and J. L. Arnott.

clichés of Parisian French related to different speaking styles. Fónagy (1982a; 1982b) specialized in studying various speaking styles such as storytelling, reading the daily news, and expressing attitudes and emotions.

Bolinger studied prosodic systems in various languages as of 1945. His position about an inherently paralinguistic emotive role of intonation is well illustrated in the following statement: " . . . while intonation may well play a grammatical role, it does so by virtue of its emotive power; intonation is supportive where grammar is concerned, but it is not definitional: there is no intonation that is the property of any one grammatical category" (Bolinger, 1986, p. 13). Similar findings were reported by Faure (1970; 1973) and Caelen-Haumont (1978/1981). Bolinger (1986) showed that accent or intonational prominence simultaneously signals the speaker's interest that a given word has for him (*interest accent*) and his emotional involvement such as earnestness (*power accent*). The latter type of accents obeys the principle of climax that explains why a final accent tends to be a strong one and why we so often encounter right-shifted accents, for example, "At Putnam dodge in Burlingàme" (Bolinger, 1986, p. 14). Conversely, if the speaker wants to tone down his utterance to reduce its power, he may move the word accent leftward: "It's bigger than Ténnessee" rather than "It's bigger than Tennessée." Bolinger also convincingly demonstrated his view that "melody expresses other forms of arousal, especially those of sustained feeling, and its opposite, rest" (p. 15). For him, it is much more important to apprehend the fundamentally emotive and metaphorical character of intonation denoting meanings, such as pacification, prompting,

reprimanding, irony, deep concern, than to "pursue it down the byways of syntax and morphology" (p. 20).

The above-mentioned meanings of intonation are conceptually close to Scherer's set of design features of affective states (Scherer, 2004) such as moods, interpersonal stances, or personality traits. They also correspond to what Caelen-Haumont and Bel (2000) termed *ordinary emotion* states related to beliefs, values, and subjective feelings.

Empirical findings related to prosodic cues of emotions and attitudes are found in the work of Léon (1970), who presented evidence that high register and wide F_0 range were associated with joy, self-consciousness, and lightness, while a low register with a narrow F_0 range were associated with sadness, confidence, and graveness. The contour type was not considered to be discriminating by itself, whereas vocal intensity was proportional to the strength of the expressed feeling.

Much of the research done in this field was characterized by association of F_0 parameters to different phrase modalities. O'Connor and Arnold (1973), for instance, found that "wh-questions" realized with a *high drop* were perceived as *vivid, businesslike, not unfriendly, lively,* or *interested*. For Halliday (1994), wh-questions with a rising tone characterize a continuity and are tentative, whereas yes-no questions with a falling tone are peremptory. He also found that declarative sentences with a high rise contour could be perceived as "challenging, aggressive, defensive, or indignant."

Scherer and colleagues' "configuration" model (Scherer, Ladd, & Silverman, 1984) also explored the relationship between the intonation contour and the type of sentence. The authors found that the reversal of standard English patterns (i.e., final pitch lowering for wh-questions, and final pitch rising for yes-no questions) produced negative connotations. As Wichmann (2002) pointed out, deviations from conventional tonal realizations may generate negative attitudes. In general, one notices that deviations from vocal stereotypes can often be perceived as vocal markers of affect. Wichmann also studied the influence of social context on affective prosody. She found that in private conversations among friends, the sentences ending with *please* have a final pitch rise, while final pitch fall is used in public situations demonstrating a display of social power or status. Wichmann concludes that the meaning thus depends to some extent on the power relationship between the speaker and hearer. These results are congruent with Ohala's *frequency code* (1983), which relates dominance to low-pitched and submissiveness to high-pitched voices.

Drawing on Ohala's frequency code, Piot (2001) investigated the prosodic expression of two cognitive parameters in French: *ignorance* and *desire to know*. He investigated whether the degree of pitch rise was related to the degree of *ignorance* and/or a *desire to know*. Using speech synthesis (by varying F_0 parameters, intensity, speech rate), he showed that (a) F_0 peak value was positively correlated with the degree of ignorance and the desire *to know or to inform*, (b) increased rate of delivery was related to the desire to know, but not to the desire to inform, (c) sentence final level of intensity was positively correlated with both cognitive parameters only in assertions, but not in questions. The experiment also revealed the importance of vocal range and the final pitch contour in the perception of attitudes, as well as the role of the tonal height in signaling novelty.

In the wake of Scherer's models of covariance and configuration, Ladd and colleagues (Ladd, Silverman, Tolkmitt, Bergman, & Scherer, 1985) undertook three experiments where subjects were to assess the emotion carried by statements in which the pitch range, the sentence contour type, and the voice quality were systematically changed. The results showed that pitch range and voice quality had the strongest influence on the subject's inference of the speaker's arousal and on the inference of cognition-related attitudes at the same time. The contour type alone was not significantly related to the classification of attitudes, but rather the classification of emotions. An important conclusion was drawn from these experiments, namely, that the three prosodic cues, pitch range, contour type, and voice quality, all function independently of each other.

Kehrein (2002) studied the relation between vocal parameters and emotional dimensions of valence, arousal, dominance, and unexpectedness. The latter dimension is known to be related to an increase in F_0 maximum (Caelen-Haumont, 1991, to be published). Based on intersubjective attribution of categorical emotional and attitudinal meanings, Kehrein measured the acoustic features of utterances whose speakers were judged as *excited/agitated, uncertain, eager or angry, calm/relaxed, content, delighted, uncertain/perplexed, apologetic, resigned, frustrated, and disappointed*. His findings confirm a *compositional approach to emotional meaning* because individual acoustic parameters contribute to the constitution of a variety of perceived emotions and attitudes.

As the attribution of emotional meaning is dependent upon the verbal elements and the context of the interaction, Kehrein concludes that assessment of vocal expression of emotions can only be done in context.

We support the above conclusion in that the vocal aspects of emotions should be considered within the whole interactive context including the language, the concrete material context, and the speaker's nonverbal displays. As communication is a multichannel process, the contribution of each channel is a function of simultaneous presence of all the others.

Melism as Expression of the Speaker's Subjective Emotional Space

Prosody appears to be a particularly suitable means of expressing the subjective dimension of speech communication. Subjectively tinted prosody is a precious source of contextual information that helps disambiguate the interpretation of meaning.

As pointed out by Caelen-Haumont and Bel (2000), in the prosody of French language, the syntactic and pragmatic functions of intonation usually acquire normative strength leaving little space for the speaker's expression of his or her individuality. Nevertheless, the speaker's prosodic *decision latitude* can be exercised locally on the level of word prosody, mainly in lexical but also in grammatical words. Caelen-Haumont termed such prosodic marking as *melisms.* The notion of melism has been borrowed from the domain of singing and refers to pitch

excursions (melodic movements) spread over the duration of the word, such that the number of notes perceived is higher than the number of syllables in the word. Melisms can coincide with syntactic and/or syntagmatic structure of the intonation, just as they can diverge significantly from the canonical intonation contour. The divergence is either local—on a single word or a syntagmatic unit—or it can spread over several units. Melisms are considered to be a prosodic reflection of the subject's basic affective states and attitudes such as doubts, beliefs, or value-invested thoughts as well as emotions. Such basic underlying affective states are conceptually close to Russel's *core affect* (Russel, 2003), where various shades of emotions are conceptualized as departures from a neutral point on two bipolar (valence-arousal) axes of his dimensional model of emotions. When projected into the prosodic space, Russel's arousal dimension appears to have an acoustic counterpart in the so-called *effort code* (Chen, Gussenhoven, & Rietveld, 2002) whereby the effort expended on speech production is proportional to the span of pitch excursions (de Jong 1995), the steepness of their rising or falling slopes (Caelen-Haumont, 1991, to be published; Caelen-Haumont & Bel, 2000), and the magnitude of intensity peaks. The effort code thus appears to reflect the speaker's personal involvement, which in turn is prosodically manifested in melisms realized on the lexical items relevant to the speaker's interaction with the hearer. Melisms can temporarily disturb the cohesion between intonation and the linguistic structure, but the underlying syntactic organization can allow the speaker to take this liberty and mark the utterance by his personal touch.

MELISM—An Automatic Method of Segmentation and Melodic Coding of Speech

To allow accurate descriptions of melodic salience, an automatic analysis tool, MELISM, was developed by Caelen-Haumont and Auran (2004; 2005). MELISM procedure is based on Praat software (Boersma & Weenink, 1996) and allows automatic detection of melisms, their segmentation into *tonal syllables*, and their positioning on a nine-level scale based on a stylized F_0 curve generated by MOMEL[2] (Hirst & Espesser, 1993). The tonal syllables are mono- or bitonal sequences obtained at the points of change of melodic slopes. MELISM requires (a) a preliminary segmentation

of the signal into linguistic units considered as relevant (e.g., single words or prosodic words), and (b) a stylization of the F_0 contour by determining target points with MOMEL algorithm.

Table 15–2 illustrates the nine-level scale based on Delattre's four-level model (Delattre, 1966) and obtained by dividing the space between each of the four levels into three segments. The nine-level scale is expressed by the following symbols: a = Acute; s = Supra; h = High; s = Elevated; c = Central; b = Bottom; I = Infra; g = Grave. The more acute ones (A, S or H) are involved in the definition of melisms.

To illustrate the MELISM procedure, two spontaneous speech samples are presented here, one expressing the emotion of joy and the other two attitudes.

Table 15–2. Matrix of tonal sequences describing the melodic configurations of words

	Melisms								
Tone	Acute a	Supra s	High h	Elevated e	Middle m	Central c	Bottom b	Infra i	Grave g
a	aa	as	ah	ae	am	ac	ab	ai	ag
s	sa	ss	sh	se	sm	sc	sb	si	sg
h	ha	hs	hh	he	hm	hc	hb	hi	hg
e	ea	es	eh	ee	em	ec	eb	ei	eg
m	ma	ms	mh	me	mm	mc	mb	mi	mg
c	ca	cs	ch	ce	cm	cc	cb	ci	cg
b	ba	bs	bh	be	bm	bc	bb	bi	bg
i	ia	is	ih	ie	im	ic	ib	ii	ig
g	ga	gs	gh	ge	gm	gc	gb	gi	gg

[2]MOMEL (Hirst & Espesser, 1993) allows stylization of fundamental frequency contours as a combination of their macromelodic and a micromelodic components. This is assumed to correspond to the global pitch contour of the utterance, which is continuous and independent of the nature of the constituent phonemes. It corresponds approximately to what we produce if we hum an utterance instead of speaking it.

Figure 15-1 presents the analysis of a spontaneous speech sample evoking a joyful childhood memory: *"Cela m'a marquée, petite (rires) je me rappelle le grenier (rires) / It struck me when I was little (laugh), I remember the attic (laugh)."* One notices that the F_0 contour evolves in the upper part of the speaker's register relative to her mean F_0 (170 Hz), with tonal peaks reaching high values: a, s, and h.

Figure 15-2 displays the analysis of an utterance expressing controlled irritation and irony: *"Non, c'est des matières sur l'étude de l'agronomie (pause), comme c'est intéressant . . . / No, they're courses in agronomy study (pause), how interesting . . . "* The highlighted part of the utterance expresses *"controlled irritation."* The latter is related to the fact that she was obliged to study agronomy despite her wish to pursue economic studies. One observes a sequence of F_0 rises—each marking a lexical word. Levels extend from *b* to *h*, mostly between *b* and *c*. The segment after the pause expresses *irony*. It is characterized by narrower F_0 range: between *b* and *m*, with an initial plateau at level *b*, which gives it a rather flat contour that is in contrast with the semantic content of the utterance *"how interesting."*

We believe that prosody is characterized by the interaction of two contradictory forces: one related to the grammaticalization of prosodic contours congruent with linguistic structures, and the other related to local deviations expressing the speaker's personal affective state. This *freedom* is linked to the potency dimension of affectivity (see Zei Pollermann & Izdebski, Chapter 3). Indeed, it is in the act of speaking that the subject can assert his or her personal *numerical identity* as opposed to a *collective iden-*

tity related to his or her belonging to a group of language users.

That everyday speech carries information about the speaker's cognitive-affective state is well known and has been adequately documented in the works of linguists and psychologists for well over a century. Some of the earliest influential readings in this field were those of Steel, 1775; Bourdon, 1892; Bréal, 1897; Bally, 1905; Marty, 1908; Sapir, 1927; Seashore, 1927; Buhler, 1934. Most of these authors—just as ancient Greek and Roman orators—pointed out the joint action of nonlinguistic and linguistic aspects of speech in speech communication. They had a global view of a coordinated action of verbal and nonverbal channels of communication, including facial and body movements. Such parallel coding is inherent to the speech act, and can serve to regulate interpersonal relationships on the level of the interaction partners' emotions, their mutual status and role, and the felt success of their communicative efforts.

In this chapter we have tried to highlight the historic continuity of the role assigned to vocal affect in speech communication. We could thus say that the study of vocally communicated affect started within a global framework of interaction between verbal and nonverbal aspects of communication. In ancient rhetoric, the semantic components of speech were interpreted in relation to the emotional messages carried by the human voice. With the introduction of experimentally more rigorous methods often referred to as the *standard content paradigms* (Davitz, 1964), much of research on the communication of affect was stripped off the semantic component of speech, in spite of evidence that

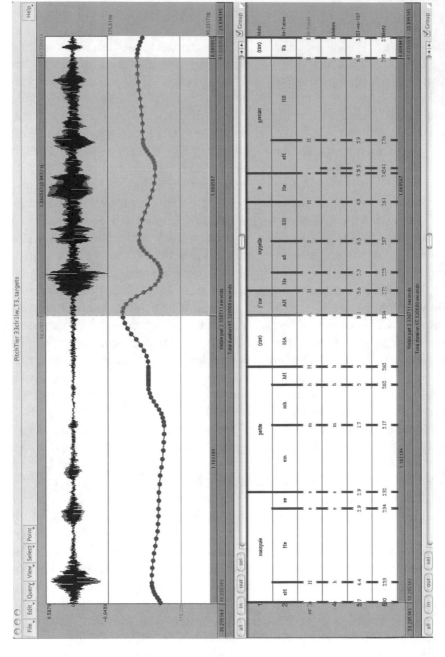

Figure 15–1. From top to bottom: Wave form of the sound; pitch contour generated with MOMEL (Hirst & Espesser, 1993); pitch contour with mean F_0 marked by a straight horizontal line; Tier1: text of utterance; Tier 2: melodic tunes of linguistic units; Tier 3: melodic tones—tonal targets of F_0 in semitones; Tier 4: alphabetic coding of melisms; Tier 5: F_0 in semitones relative to the subject's mean F_0 of 170 Hz; Tier 6: F_0 in Hertz.

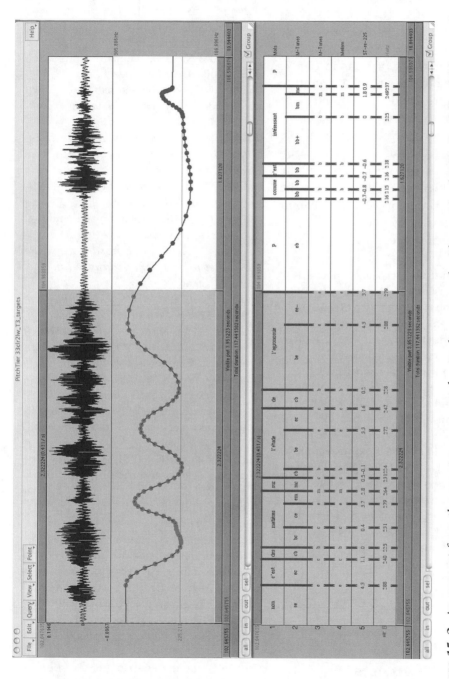

Figure 15–2. An excerpt from the spontaneous speech sample expressed with restrained irritation followed by irony: "Non, c'est des matières sur l'étude de l'agronomie (pause), comme c'est intéressant . . . No, they're courses on agronomy (pause) how interesting . . ." From top to bottom: Wave form of the sound; pitch contour with mean F_0 marked by a straight horizontal line; Tier1: text of utterance; Tier 2: melodic tunes of linguistic units; Tier 3: melodic tones—tonal targets of F_0 in semitones; Tier 4: alphabetic coding of melisms; Tier 5: F_0 in semitones relative to the subject's mean F_0 of 225 Hz; Tier 6: F_0 in Hertz.

linguistic and nonverbal cues can contribute in an additive fashion to listeners' judgments of affect (Ladd et al., 1985; Scherer & Oshinsky, 1977). More recent research on attitudes (Wichmann, 2002) as well as the work of Kehrein (2002) illustrate the necessity of integrating verbal elements and social context of interaction into the research paradigms. Caelen's study of melisms is an example of how the attribution of affective meaning depends on both the context and the semantic content of the utterance. In the concluding paragraph of their chapter on vocal expression of emotion, Scherer and colleagues wrote:

> Apart from studying vocal communication process as a whole, it may also be time to drop the assumption of separate linguistic and nonlinguistic channels, together with the hermeutic separation of the respective research traditions. As we have shown, there is much evidence that a large part of emotion signaling in voice and speech is dually coded, in both linguistic and nonlinguistic features. Thus a rapprochement between researchers interested in expression and those interested in language, is highly desirable, as is a more intensive interaction between researchers studying vocal and facial expression, two research areas that have had little contact so far, even though they have a common origin in the underlying emotion, and are often interpreted as a Gestalt by a perceiver (Scherer, Johnstone, & Klasmeyer, 2003, pp. 451–452).

References

Bally, C. (1905). *Précis de stylistique: Esquisse d'une méthode fondée sur l'étude du français moderne.* Geneva, Switzerland: A. Eggimann.

Boersma, P., & Weenink, D. J. M. (1996). *Praat, a system for doing phonetics by computer.* Amsterdam: Institute of Phonetic Sciences of the University of Amsterdam.

Bolinger, D. (1945). Spanish intonation, Review of Tomás Navarro, Manual de entonación española. *American Speech, 20,* 128–130.

Bolinger, D. (1946). The intonation of quoted questions. *Quarterly Journal of Speech, 32,* 197–202.

Bolinger, D. (1965). *Forms of English: Accent, morpheme, order.* Cambridge, MA: Harvard University Press.

Bolinger, D. (1972). *Intonation.* Harmondsworth, UK: Penguin Books.

Bolinger, D. (1986). Intonation and emotion. *Quaderni di Semantica, 7,* 13–21.

Bourdon, B. (1892). *L'expression des émotions et des tendances dans le langage.* Paris: Alcan.

Bréal, M. (1897). *Essai de sémantique (science des significations).* Paris: Fayard.

Bühler, K. (1934). *Sprachtheorie. Die Darstellungsfunktion der Sprache* (2nd ed.). Stuttgart, Germany: Gustav Fischer.

Caelen-Haumont, G. (1978). *Structures prosodiques de la phrase énonciative simple et étendue.* Unpublished doctoral dissertation. Université de Toulouse-le-Mirail, Toulouse, France.

Caelen-Haumont, G. (1981) *Structures prosodiques de la phrase énonciative simple et étendue.* Doctoral dissertation, Hamburger Phonetische Beitrage, band 34. hamburg Buske.

Caelen-Haumont, G. (1991). Stratégies des locuteurs en réponse à des consignes de lecture d'un texte: Analyse des interactions entre modèles syntaxiques, sémantiques, pragmatique et paramètres prosodiques. Unpublished doctoral dissertation, Université de Provence, Aixen-Provence, France.

Caelen-Haumont, G. (à paraître). *Prosodie et sens: une approche expérimentale.* Doctoral dissertation (doctorat d'état). L'Harmattan-Marges Linguistiques.

Caelen-Haumont, G., & Auran, C. (2004). The phonology of melodic prominence: The structure of melisms. In B. Bel & I. Marlien

(Eds.), *Proceedings of Speech Prosody 2004*. Nara, Japan, 143-146. France: Université de Provence.

Caelen-Haumont, G., & Auran, C. (2005). Manuel d'utilisation de la procédure MOMEL-MELISM sous Praat, 1-57. Retrieved 2005 from http://www.lpl.univ-aix.fr/~lpldev/MELISM/

Caelen-Haumont, G., & Bel, B. (2000). Le caractère spontané dans la parole et le chant improvisés: De la structure intonative au mélisme. *Revue Parole, 15-16*, 251-302.

Chen, A., Gussenhoven, C., & Rietveld, A. (2002). Language-specific uses of the Effort code. In B. Bel & I. Marlien (Eds.), *Proceedings of the Speech Prosody 2002 Conference* (pp. 215-218). France: Université de Provence, Aix-en-Provence

Crystal, D. (1975). *The English tone of voice*. London: Edward Arnold.

Crystal, D., & Quirk, R. (1964). *Systems of prosodic and paralinguistic features in English*. The Hague: Mouton and Co.

Dámaso, A., & Bousoño, C. (1951). Seis calas en la expresión literaria española, Madrid, Spain: Gredos.

Darwin, C. (1965). *The expression of the emotions in man and animals*. Chicago: University of Chicago Press. (Originally published 1872)

Davitz, J. R. (1964). Auditory correlates of vocal expressions of emotional meanings. In J. R. Davitz (Ed.), *The communication of emotional meaning* (pp. 101-112). New York: McGraw-Hill.

de Jong, K. J. (1995). The supraglottal articulation of prominence in English: Linguistic stress as localized hyperarticulation. *Journal of the Acoustical Society of America, 97*, 491-504.

Delattre, P. (1966). Les dix intonations de base du français. *French Review, 40*, 1-14.

Ekman, P. (1999). Emotional and conversational nonverbal signals. In L. Messing & R. Campbell (Eds.), *Gesture, speech and sign* (pp. 45-57). Oxford, UK: University Press.

Fairbanks, G., & Hoaglin, L. W. (1941). An experimental study of the duration characteristics of the voice during the expres-sion of emotion. *Speech Monographs, 8*, 85-90.

Fairbanks, G., & Pronovost, W. (1939). *Speech Monographs, 6*, 87-104.

Faure, G. (1970). Contribution à l'étude du statut phonologique des structures prosodématiques. *Studia Phonetica, 3*, 93-107.

Faure, G. (1973). Tendances et perspectives de la recherche intonologique. *Travaux de l'Institut de Phonétique d'Aix-en-Provence*, 5-29.

Fónagy, I. (1971). Double coding in speech. *Semiotica, 3*, 189-222.

Fónagy, I. (1982). Variations et normes prosodiques. *Folia Linguistica, XVI, 1-4*, 17-38.

Fónagy, I. (1982). *Vive voix. Essais de psycho-phonétique*. Paris: Payot.

Fónagy, I., & Bérard, E. (1973). Questions totales et implicatives. *Studia Phonetica, 8*, 53-98.

Fónagy, I., Bérard, E., & Fónagy, J. (1982). Les clichés mélodiques. *Folia Linguistica, 161*(4), 153-185.

Fónagy, I., & Magdics, K. (1963). Emotional patterns in intonation and music. *Zeitschrift fur Phonetik 16*, 293-326.

Fónagy, I., & Sap, J. (1997). Traits prosodiques distinctifs de certaines attitudes intellectuelles et émotives. *Actes des 8e Journées d'Études sur la Parole*, 237-246. France: Université de Provence, Aix-en-Provence.

Halliday, M. A. K. (1994). *An introduction to functional grammar* (2nd ed.). London: Edward Arnold.

Hirst, D., & Espesser, R. (1993). Automatic labelling of fundamental frequency using a quadratic spline function. *Travaux de l'Institut de Phonétique d'Aix, 15*, 71-85. France: Université de Provence, Aix-en Provence.

Kant, E. (2001). *Critique de la raison pure*. Paris: Garnier Flammarion.

Kehrein, R. (2002). The prosody of authentic emotions. In B. Bel & I. Marlien (Eds.), *Proceedings of the Speech Prosody 2002 Conference* (pp. 423-426). France: Université de Provence, Aix-en-Provence,

Ladd, D. R., Silverman, K. E. A., Tolkmitt, F., Bergman, G., & Scherer, K. R. (1985). Evidence for the independent function of intonation contour type, voice quality, and F_0 range in signalling speaker effect. *Journal of the Acoustical Society of America, 78*, 435-444.

Laver, J. (1968). Voice quality and indexical information. *British Journal of Disorders of Communication, 3*, 43-54.

Léon, P. R. (1970). Systématique des fonctions expressives de l'intonation, Analyse des faits prosodiques. *Studia Phonetica, 3*, 56-71.

Léon, P. R. (1971). Essais de Phonostylistique. *Studia Phonetica, 4.*

Léon, P. R. (1976). De l'analyse psychologique à la catégorisation auditive et acoustique des émotions dans la parole. *Journal de Psychologie, 3-4*, 305-324.

Marty, A. (1908). *Untersuchungen zur Grundlegung der allegemeinen Grammatik und Sprachphilosophie* (Vol. 1). Niemeyer, Austria: Halle.

Murray, L. R., & Arnott, J. L. (1993). Toward the simulation of emotion in synthetic speech: A review of the literature on human vocal emotion. *Journal of the Acoustical Society of America, 93*(2), 1097-1108.

O'Connor, J. D., & Arnold, G. (1973). *Intonation of colloquial English.* London: Longman.

Ohala, J. J. (1983). Cross-language use of pitch: An ethological view. *Phonetica, 40*, 1-18.

Piaget, J. (1970). *Epistémologie génétique.* Paris: PUF.

Piot, O. (2001). Ignorance, empathie et motivation: Une évaluation de leurs expressions dans la prosodie du français. In V. Auberge, A. Lacheret-Dujour & H. Loevenbruck (Eds.). *Actes des Journées Prosodie,* 139-143. France: Grenoble.

Roach, P. (2000). Techniques for the phonetic description of emotional speech. *Proceedings of the ISCA Workshop on Speech and Emotion,* Belfast. Proceedings on line. Retrieved from http://www.qbc.ac.uk/en/isca /proceedings

Russel, J. A. (2003). Core affect and the psychological construction of emotion. *Psychological Review, 110*(1), 145-172.

Russel & Winterbottom (Eds.) (1972). Ancient literary criticism. Oxford, UK: Clarendon Press.

St. Augustino (1969). Le confessioni, Libro X. In C. Carena (trans.),. Rome, Italy: Città Nuova.

Sapir, E. (1927). Speech as a personality trait. *American Journal of Sociology, 32*, 892-905.

Scherer, K. R. (1984). On the nature and function of emotion: A component process approach. In K. Scherer & P. Ekman (Eds.), *Handbook of methods in nonverbal behavior research* (pp. 293-318). Hillsdale, NJ: Erlbaum.

Scherer K. R. (2004). Which emotions can be induced by music? What are the underlying mechanisms? And how can we measure them? *Journal of New Music Research, 33*,(3), 239-251.

Scherer, K. R. (2005). Unconscious processes in emotion: The bulk of the iceberg. In P. Niedenthal, L. Feldman-Barrett, & P. Winkielman (Eds.), *The unconscious in emotion* (pp. 312-334). New York: Guilford.

Scherer, K. R., Johnstone, T., & Klasmeyer, G. (2003). Vocal expression of emotion. In R. J. Davidson, K. R. Scherer, & H. Goldsmith (Eds.), *Handbook of the affective sciences* (pp. 433-456). New York: Oxford University Press.

Scherer, K. R., Ladd, D. R., & Silverman, K. E. A. (1984). Vocal cues to speaker affect: Testing two models. *Journal of the Acoustical Society of America, 76*(5), 1346-1356.

Scherer, K. R., & Oshinsky, J. S. (1977). Cue utilization in emotion attribution from auditory stimuli. *Motivation and Emotion, 1*, 331-346.

Seashore, C. E. (1927). Phonophotography in the measurement of the expression of emotion in music and speech. *Scientific Monthly, 24*, 463-471.

Sebastiani, (1562). *Medicorvum doctrinam, Biblioteca medica storica della Ducale Università Coruzzi.* No 493.

Spitzer, L. (1961). *Stilstudien. Erster Teil: Sprachstile/Zweiter Teil: Stilsprachen* (Vols. 1–2). Munich, Germany: Max Hueber Verlag.

Steele, J. (1974). *An essay towards establishing the melody and measure of speech to be expressed and perpetuated by peculiar symbols.* (Also listed as *Prosodia Rationalis.*) Microfiche reproduction published by London: Scolar Press. (Originally published 1775)

Troubetzkoy, N. S. (1939). *Grundzüge der Phonologie: TCLP* (Vol. VII). Prague, Czech Republic: Travaux du Cercle Linguistique de Prague.

Wharton, T. (2003). Interjections, language and the 'showing-saying' continuum. *Pragmatics and Cognition 11*, 39–91.

Wichmann, A. (2002). Attitudinal intonation and the inferential process. In B. Bel & I. Marlien (Eds.), *Proceedings of the Speech Prosody 2002 Conference* (pp. 11–16). Aix-en-Provence, France: Université de Provence, Aix-en-Provence.

Williams, C. E., & Stevens, K. N. (1972). Emotions and speech: Some acoustical correlates. *Journal of the Acoustical Society of America, 52*(4/2), 1238–1250.

Wilson, D., & Wharton, T. (2006). Relevance and prosody. *Journal of Pragmatics, 38*(10), 1559–1579.

Zei, B., & Archinard, M. (2001). Acoustic patterns of emotions. In E. Keller, G. Bailly, A. Monagham, J. Terken, & M. Huckvale (Eds.), *Improvements in speech synthesis* (pp. 237–245). Chichester, UK: Wiley.

Zei-Pollermann, B. (2002). A place for prosody in a unified model of cognition and emotion. In B. Bel & I. Marlien (Eds.), *Proceedings of the Speech Prosody 2002 Conference* (pp. 17–22). Aix-en-Provence, France: Université de Provence, Aix-en-Provence.

Index